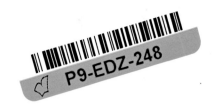
P9-EDZ-248

Household Homeopathy

A Safe and Effective Approach to Wellness for the Whole Family

Vinton McCabe

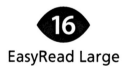

16

EasyRead Large

RHYW

Copyright Page from the Original Book

The information contained in this book is based upon the research and personal and professional experiences of the author. It is not intended as a substitute for consulting with your physician or other healthcare provider. Any attempt to diagnose and treat an illness should be done under the direction of a healthcare professional.

The publisher does not advocate the use of any particular healthcare protocol but believes the information in this book should be available to the public. The publisher and author are not responsible for any adverse effects or consequences resulting from the use of the suggestions, preparations, or procedures discussed in this book. Should the reader have any questions concerning the appropriateness of any procedures or preparation mentioned, the author and the publisher strongly suggest consulting a professional healthcare advisor.

Basic Health Publications, Inc.
8200 Boulevard East
North Bergen, NJ 07047
1-201-868-8336

Library of Congress Cataloging-in-Publication Data

McCabe, Vinton.
    Household homeopathy : a safe and effective approach to wellness for the whole family / by Vinton McCabe.
        p. cm.
    Includes bibliographical references and index.
    ISBN 1-59120-070-9 (alk. paper)
    1. Homeopathy. 2. Self-care, Health. I. Title.

    RX73.M378   2004
    615.5'32—dc22

                                                2004020643

Editor: Karen Anspach
Typesetting/Book design: Gary A. Rosenberg
Cover design: Mike Stromberg

Printed in the United States of America

10   9   8   7   6   5   4   3   2   1

TABLE OF CONTENTS

We believe that the expressions of disease are uniform, and always have the same meaning, and that the actions of remedies are something definite and uniform— 'that like causes always produce like effects.' If we properly study our cases, so as to determine a definite condition of disease, and know the direct actions of remedies in such conditions, we will have a certain and rational practice of medicine.

—JOHN SCUDDER, *SPECIFIC DIAGNOSIS*

AUTHOR'S NOTE

On Patients and Practitioners

For the purposes of the study of homeopathy, and for simplicity's sake, I have decided to refer to all those who are in need of homeopathic treatment as "patients." I do not use this term to imply the traditional doctor/patient relationship as it exists in Western medicine.

Further, for the purposes of this book, I use the term "practitioner" as a general purpose term for all those who make use of over-the-counter homeopathic remedies for self-treatment, and to assist their loved ones and pets in times of need.

When referring to those who have medical degrees that allow them to make use of homeopathic treatments as part of their therapeutic processes, I use the term "medical professional."

Finally, please be aware that since this book's focus is on the acute cases the reader may encounter in household situations, I have opted, again for simplicity's sake, to make use of the masculine pronoun "he" in these pages for all patients, whether male or female. I do this because, while homeopathic remedies may be somewhat gender linked in their constitutional use, these same remedies are gender neutral when they are used in the treatment of those with acute ailments. (The terms "acute" and "constitutional" are explained later in this book.)

PREFACE

Who Is John Scudder?

So, just who is John Scudder, anyway? Or, more correctly, who was he, as he has been dead for a good long time now.

The same question may be asked about Samuel Hahnemann, although more readers are likely to have some sort of an answer for that name. But what about Stuart Close? Or Margery Blackie? Or John Clarke? Or James Tyler Kent?

For these names, and for hundreds of others, the answer is the same: they have each contributed a concept, or, in some cases, many different concepts, that combined together have created modern homeopathy. They are the forefathers and mothers of a healing practice considered to be just over two hundred years old, that shot from obscurity to being a household name in the past handful of years. Certainly homeopathic remedies like Arnica, once considered arcane, have become common in American medicine chests.

While most readers may instantly recognize Samuel Hahnemann as the "Father of Homeopathy," they must also realize that no one person could have created a practice so complex and based on such a wide range of principles and philosophies, as homeopathy. Indeed, a study of the history of homeopathy reveals that many of the ideas that would one day be termed *homeopathic* were practiced by Hippocrates himself in ancient Greece, and by the wildman-healer Paracelsus, whose methods and origins of practice have largely been lost to the ages. It seems that the drumbeat of homeopathy has always been a part of medicine. Homeopathic concepts have been practiced by herbalists and healers in the Western world from a time that predates written history. Homeopathic concepts are also present in Eastern medicine, as we can see in the practice of acupuncture, which works in a manner closely related to homeopathy. The Eastern concept of treating the patient as a whole being rather than a collection of symptoms, organs, chemicals, and the like reinforces the parallels between Asian medicine and homeopathy.

But more on this later, and more on Chinese medicine in Chapter Four. Here I am discussing this book, *Household Homeopathy,* and why I decided to put it together. After fifteen years of teaching classes in homeopathy to medical practitioners and lay persons, and after fifteen years of tackling the role of president for the Connecticut Homeopathic Association (a role that always seems to involve begging for money or services from someone so that the not-for-profit educational group could continue to function), I decided that it was time to step aside and let others take on the tasks of teaching, organizing, fund-raising, and class production.

I also decided to try to go out with a bang.

I put together a class called Household Homeopathy. With it, I tried to do something new—I decided to treat acute homeopathy just as seriously as practitioners treat constitutional treatments. Acute treatments are those whose goal is to restore "status quo"—to restore the patient to the level of health they had before the onset of illness. Constitutional treatments are those that seek to permanently improve the overall or given state of the patient's health; they are both curative and preventative.

Most classes in acute homeopathy are taught for the sake of homemakers who want to know what to do when their child gets a cold or falls down on the playground. And laudable as that goal is, these classes are usually as limited in content as they are in attendees' expectations.

I decided to try to create the most in-depth and fully rounded class in acute homeopathy possible. It would be a year in the teaching, and each month's lecture would build upon what had come before and lead into what would follow next. The idea is that acute prescribing is, in actuality, not easier than constitutional prescribing: it is simply different.

It is my belief that the acute prescriber has to know more about the materia medica (the sources, nature, properties, and preparation) of homeopathic remedies—and has to have more working knowledge of homeopathy in general—than do constitutional prescribers.

How many times have we gone to a degreed professional homeopath and had our case taken, only to have the homeopath say that he will call in a day or two with his prescription? Such a thing cannot happen in acute homeopathy because there often is no time in an acute case for deep reflection. The practitioner must be ready with a remedy in mind and an action to be taken.

And I often have been given a remedy by a constitutional practitioner only to have it changed a month later when it failed to work. The acute practitioner, again, needs to get it right the first time. He does not have the grace period of trying one remedy, and then another.

So, you see, those lay persons who learn their remedies cold, and who can recognize the symptoms that require them when they see them walking around in human or animal form, often know more about homeopathy than the practitioners who have come to depend upon computer programs and libraries of materia medicas as the source of their treatment strategies.

I first heard of John Scudder and his work as an eclectic physician during the Civil War era about the same time that I was forming this class in my mind. I began to develop my class a little differently after I read that, when selecting his remedies, he ignored all subjective symptoms and used only the objective symptoms of a case for speed and simplicity's sake.

Scudder, you see, had reminded me of things that I had heard early on in my study of homeopathy. I once attended a class in Nyack, New York, taught by S.K. Bannerjea, who comes from a long line of homeopaths in his native India. Bannerjea, I remember, would laugh when he talked about the way American homeopaths tend to sit and take a long interview and case history for every case, no matter the ailment or its history. He said that there would be a riot if the homeopath tried to spend an hour or more with each new patient in India, with the long lines of patients standing and waiting outside the door.

No, he said, in India it was very different. There, the homeopath looked at his patient, studied him, and asked only a few questions as needed. He then treated the patient with the remedy suggested by his own experience and objective observation of the patient. In fact, Bannerjea told us, the practice of homeopathy in India was heavily based in the senses of the practitioner. The practitioner was taught to use all his senses (except for, one hopes, taste) in his evaluation of his patient.

Bannerjea told us that, as his final exam, he was told to sit down at a table and look at the window in front of him. A light came on behind the window and he saw a large baby. The baby was held up for him to see.

"What do you give this baby?" he was asked.

He looked at the child. It was a large baby—doughy, fleshy. It seemed to have a large head and to be having trouble holding its head upright. The head rolled backward and forward, and from side to side.

Based on this information, Bannerjea said, "Calcarea Carbonica."

He passed.

So perhaps it was something in my early training, and my need to find something deeper and truer, that combined into "Objective Homeopathy," my final class.

And certainly Scudder and his methodology had come along just at the right time.

This book is based on the notes I used in teaching that class. It is intended to be a companion to the other books I have written, but it is also meant to carry those works a step forward, as it offers a shorthand version of acute case taking—one based in the ideas of the American homeopath John Scudder, and my Indian teacher S.K. Bannerjea. Acute case taking is the process of matching the symptoms of a self-limiting ailment with the actions of a homeopathic remedy ("artificial" symptoms versus "natural" symptoms). The closer the match, the better the remedy will perform.

Since I have written rather exhaustively on acute homeopathy in the past, I will try to minimize duplicating information, while still making this book one that stands on its own. You can pick up this text and find a good deal of useful information in it without previously having read a work about homeopathy.

Part One of this book will introduce the concepts that, together, make up the practice of homeopathy. We will spend a good deal of time considering symptoms and learning the difference between subjective and objective symptoms, as well as examining the other ways in which a given patient's symptoms can be grouped and considered in determining homeopathic treatment.

We will take a closer look at John Scudder, his work and his times, and the ideas that he has contributed to homeopathy. In the same way, we will take a brief look at Chinese medicine and the ways in which homeopaths can improve their practice by studying it. Then we will look at homeopathic case taking, at remedy selection, and at case management—all for acute treatments only.

There is something somewhat new in Part Two. I call it an "Objective Materia Medica." This lists the fifty-two remedies that I consider to be the most important for the home homeopathic kit, and stresses the objective symptoms when each is indicated. In other words, it lists the remedies and tells you, remedy by remedy, what you are likely to see and to otherwise sense when you come across the patient needing that remedy.

Part Three turns that presentation around, and gives the reader an understanding of what remedies are likely to be suggested by certain specific ailments and conditions.

And the Appendices give you lists—lists of homeopathic organizations, websites, and pharmacies; lists of historic homeopaths and their contributions; and a list of the books that I think are essential for every homeopathic home. In addition, there is a section called The Wisdom of John Scudder, in which I give extended quotations from Scudder's books to give the reader a chance to share the writings of a master homeopath.

All together, I hope that this text leaves you as satisfied and informed as the students who took my final class. I hope that you learn to respect the power of homeopathy, and through it, your own ability to improve your life and the lives of those you love.

INTRODUCTION

Homeopathy in Your Household

You may already have experience with homeopathy when you begin this book. You may have visited a professional homeopath, or tried taking remedies on your own. Or, you may have no experience at all with this topic, other than having heard the word "homeopathy." You may never have attended a class or read a book on this subject. Whatever your previous background and reason, you want to learn something about homeopathy, and that's great. But let me tell you this right up front: it will take time, energy, and commitment.

The allopath, the doctor who practices conventional Western medicine, often only has to learn about a few favorite medicines. This is particularly true of traditional medical specialists, who see the same handful of conditions over and over again. Homeopathy, in contrast, is the full expression of holistic medicine, and it views people as whole beings in body, mind, and spirit. In the holistic perspective all symptoms are both interconnected and interrelated, and there can be no specialists.

Homeopathy is a nonspecific form of medicine. It demands that we search out the "totality of symptoms" in all cases before we can give a remedy. We must assemble a portrait of the patient as a whole, and give each symptom the full weight and respect it deserves, before we undertake any sort of treatment.

Yet, in another way, homeopathy is the *most* specific form of medicine, in that each remedy is selected specifically for an individual person, who is suffering from a set of symptoms known as a disease. Therefore, there is no homeopathic remedy for the condition of backache. There is, instead, a long list of remedies that may be useful in treating the patient with backache among his symptoms. It is up to the practitioner to decide upon the remedy in that list that best matches the patient's backache, as well as the rest of his symptoms.

Those of you who want to learn homeopathy will first have to come to grips with its basic concepts and "peculiarities," and then take it upon yourselves to read as much as you can and seek out classes on the subject. As you progress, you will likely want to link up with a study group at some point—a circle of peers with whom you can share your successes and failures.

To understand homeopathy, you will need to study many things. The first and most important is the pharmacy of homeopathic remedies and their actions. These remedies can be found alphabetically listed in books called *materia medicas.* Although these have been authored by many different practitioners, each serves the same purpose—to give insight into the full range of actions that each remedy offers. A good materia medica is essential in the study of homeopathic remedies and their uses.

You will also have to study the repertory, which is the homeopathic handbook of symptoms and the remedies that treat them. Each repertory is unique, so you will have to become familiar with the principles by which they are all used, and then really understand the one you choose to use and make your own.

Also, you will have to understand what Hahnemann calls "the nature of disease," which involves both the study of homeopathic philosophy and what an allopath would call pathology. Finally, a class in physiology at your nearest junior college certainly wouldn't hurt.

You see, there's a lot to learn. And that is where commitment comes in.

I feel that it is very important that you determine your own personal level of commitment and goals for personal mastery of the subject at the beginning of your studies. Those of you who want to learn a few remedies that might be of help to yourself and your loved ones will certainly find that information here, as will those of you who want to build a home kit of the homeopathic remedies that are most often associated with household emergencies.

But those of you who wish to master acute homeopathy—to be able to look at a case and determine what remedy will work to bring about healing—will have your work cut out for you. You will have to use this book only as a starting point. To complete your education, you will have to seek out a homeopathic study group, or form one if none exists in your area. You will have to find classes in both the philosophy and practice of homeopathy. And you will have to learn to separate the wheat from the chaff in those classes and groups, and from this book and others. You will soon come to learn that, unlike the practitioners of allopathic medicine, no two homeopaths seem to agree on just what homeopathy is, and how it is practiced.

THE GOAL OF THIS BOOK

This book can only give you my ideas as to how homeopathic remedies can best be used for day-to-day acute situations in the home. This book is as down-to-earth and practical as I can make it, to bring the rules of homeopathic practice into the everyday world. That's why I named it a "household book." In the pages that follow, I will do my best to describe the methods by which our most common homeopathic remedies can be used most safely and effectively. And, just as important, I will explore how they may most easily be used.

The goal of this book is to provide the reader with the knowledge of how homeopathy is practiced in the acute sphere, and how to select the remedies, handle them, and use them wisely. While I do not intend that anyone begin to practice medicine without a license, it is my goal that you learn how we all can promote healing in our own lives and in the lives of our loved ones and how we can make a healing impact in our own homes.

THE GOAL OF MEDICAL TREATMENT

Before we can begin a study of acute homeopathy, we have to expand our thinking and consider the goal of medical treatment. By this I mean *any* medical treatment, whether homeopathic or allopathic, because both forms of medicine have the same treatment goal, even though they differ in their concept of how that goal can be reached.

The goal of any medical treatment is to bring about some sort of change within the life of a human being. It is, of course, hoped and expected that the change will be for the better, and that the person will be better after the treatment than he was before. It is certainly not the goal of treatment that the patient remain unchanged.

But ask yourself if in your own experience that goal of improvement has always been met once you took that goal from the sphere of philosophy into the real world. Have you always been better off for having had a medical treatment? Have you ever been worse off for having had a medical treatment? Have you ever undergone treatment—perhaps long and painful treatment—only to find yourself in the same condition after treatment that you were in before?

Given the fact that you are considering the option of homeopathic treatment, the answer to at least one of those questions is likely to point to a less than successful experience with medicine in general, and specifically with allopathic medicine. One of the reasons people come to homeopathy is because other forms of medicine have failed them.

Homeopathy shares the general goal that those receiving treatment should experience a positive change in their lives. But I can promise you that if it is used correctly, homeopathy can never have a negative impact. The patient will either experience a good deal of positive change, or nothing whatsoever will happen. This is one of the most powerful benefits of homeopathic treatments: if the remedies are used appropriately, the worse case scenario for a failed treatment will be no change in the patient's condition. The patient's condition will not worsen, and some new condition will not be created as a result of the treatment.

We work with the idea of effecting a change in our lives whenever we study any form of medicine or seek out any specific treatment. In doing so, we are trying to find out how change can occur, and what part medicine plays in the concept of positive change in our lives.

The Goal of Allopathic Treatment

We are all experts in allopathic medicine in the United States. We learn about it before we are even born. We experience prenatal care and prenatal education in the medicine that is the norm for our society.

Think about the goals of allopathic medicine.

The first, without a doubt, is the ending of pain. The majority of our allopathic practice is geared to putting some form of medication between the patient and his or her pain. Consider something as simple as a headache. When you take a Tylenol, does that medicine have anything to do with actually ending your headache or preventing the next one? No, it doesn't; it simply blocks your body's ability to sense the pain that it is experiencing. Allopathic medicine, in large part, still relies on the body's ability to heal itself, and uses medication as a means of making the patient more comfortable while the healing takes place. In other words, the major goal of allopathic medicine is the ending or blocking of pain.

The second goal of allopathic medicine is eradication of disease. For the allopath, disease is thought of as a third party, as if the office contained the patient, the doctor and the disease. Disease is seen as an invasive and attacking entity, and the patient as the innocent victim. Therefore, allopathic medicine seeks to track down and to destroy diseases as the government does terrorists. The allopathic medical model is very similar to the military model—we have wars on specific diseases, war on AIDS, and war on cancer; it is as if, were we able to truly wipe out these specific diseases, no other diseases could ever rise up and cause harm. As if a successful war on cancer would act as a warning to all the other viruses and bacteria to just mind their own business, and we will leave them alone in the rain forest, or wherever else they choose to hide.

Finally, there is the allopathic viewpoint of symptoms. Symptoms are seen as bad things that should be removed. They are signs of invasion and aspects of disease that cause pain and shorten lives. The idea here is that, if you, as a patient, are experiencing five different aspects of pain associated with a specific disease, then we, as allopathic doctors, will remove these five things and leave the rest of you alone. You can be considered healthy because you no longer have those five things.

This is the allopathic mindset: disease is an outside force, an entity unto itself, which attacks the innocent victim. Symptoms—the aches and pains of disease—are bad things that need to be removed as quickly as possible by whatever means possible. And, underneath it all, healing is still a natural mechanism, but one that needs the assistance of medication to control pain while healing takes place.

The Goal of Homeopathic Treatment

In his major work, *The Organon of Medicine,* Samuel Hahnemann, the German physician who formulated the homeopathic method, writes that each patient is entitled to a cure that is "rapid, gentle and permanent."

All three things at once—that's the hard part. Proper homeopathic treatment should yield quick results. You should begin to feel better anywhere from a few hours to a few days into treatment. The treatment should be gentle. The remedy should lead to such a gentle change that usually the patient has to be asked whether or not he still has his symptoms before he realizes that, indeed, they have lifted. And the change is to be permanent. Since homeopathic treatment draws forth the symptoms and permits nothing to be suppressed or held within the body, mind, or spirit, once the symptoms are gone, they are gone forever.

Allopathic medicine, on the other hand, tends to believe that achieving any two out of these three goals is fine, and in fact, excellent. Many allopathic treatments are quick and permanent (think of the result of any operation) but not gentle, or quick and gentle (think of the result of many allopathic drugs) but not permanent, or gentle and permanent (think of herbal treatments) but certainly not quick.

But what is the deeper goal underneath the idea of the rapid, gentle, and permanent cure? The goal of homeopathic treatment is to end illness by working with its cause, and not just with its symptoms. For the homeopath, disease cannot be seen as an invasion of outside forces, but as an expression of self. It is part of us. It comes from within rather than from the outside. The illness is our own unique reaction to a catalyst, which may be a virus, a bacteria or another form of stress. That is why, for the homeopathic practitioner, no two illnesses suggest the same treatment. Since each illness is a unique being's reaction to stimulus, the medicine required will be unique as well.

And if illness is our reaction to a catalyst, then our symptoms are a sign of the reactive nature of our being. Something has happened on some level of being—physical, mental or spiritual—which has caused us to react in a manner that has left us susceptible to disease. And as a result, disease has taken root. From the homeopathic approach, if we simply attempt to pull that disease out by its roots, we will weaken the overall system. Homeopathy attacks the problem holistically instead, and seeks to strengthen the whole being, the whole system. As the being becomes stronger, it is able to throw off the illness in a rapid, gentle, and permanent manner. That is the goal of homeopathy.

Considering Homeopathic Treatments

While it is certainly possible to do a great deal of good through the understanding and use of only a few homeopathic remedies—Arnica, for instance, can be very useful in the household and will, even if it is the only remedy learned and used, effect a good many cures—even those interested in learning only the most basic and simplified level of homeopathy must have some basic understanding of the philosophy that underlies and informs homeopathic treatments.

You will quickly begin to understand that the homeopathic viewpoint towards disease and its cure is very different from the allopathic, and its treatment methodology is very different from the allopath's mode of treatment. In the same way, the homeopath sees the patient in a very different manner than the allopath does.

In the first chapter of this book, we will look more closely at homeopathy itself, and at the principles by which it is appropriately practiced.

Levels of Homeopathic Treatment

While all homeopathic treatments work from the same basic philosophy, the depth of homeopathic treatments differs according to the goals of the specific treatment, and according to both the practitioner's and the patient's definition of the concept of "the totality of the symptoms."

It may be said that there are three distinct levels of homeopathic treatment, each with its own specific intent, and each with a different definition of success.

The first level of treatment is the *acute.* This treatment speaks to a specific ailment or situation that is said to be "self-limiting." In other words, it may be an illness like a cold or flu that will, in time, conclude on its own. No treatment of any sort may be required—indeed, in many acute situations like colds, many types of medical treatment may be totally ineffective.

This is not to say that acute situations are never dangerous or life threatening. Most mechanical injuries, from playground falls to car accidents, no matter how serious, may be said to be acute in nature. The flu outbreak of the early part of the twentieth century was an acute epidemic, and those cases of influenza were acute in nature, but killed many millions worldwide. Even today, flu kills thousands of people annually.

It is the goal of the acute treatment that separates it from the other levels of treatment. The acute treatment assumes that the patient was in a state of relative good health before the onset of the acute distress, whether it is mechanical or infectious in nature. The goal of this level of treatment, therefore, is the preservation of the earlier status quo. The practitioner seeks to return the patient to that same level of health he enjoyed before the onset of the acute situation.

This means that, for the acute prescriber, the term "totality of symptoms" refers to all those symptoms that arose with the onset of the acute situation. If a patient, for instance, has become very thirsty for cold water since the onset of a cold a few days earlier, that is an important symptom for the acute case. If that patient has been thirsty for cold water for a period of months or years, then it is of no importance to the acute case, except as a reference point for what would be considered the norm for the patient when in a state of normal good health.

The acute prescriber, therefore, considers what has changed in the patient's life in the past few days since the onset of ill health, and considers these aspects as well, to find a remedy that best addresses every factor to restore the patient to a state of normal good health.

It should also be noted that in the selection of a remedy the acute treatment should not attempt to include any other sets of symptoms that could be considered a chronic condition of any sort. It is very likely that the patient with high blood pressure before his cold will still have high blood pressure at the successful conclusion of his acute treatment, if the correct remedy is selected.

The second level of homeopathic treatment is the *constitutional.* This is a deeper level of treatment. The constitutional treatment seeks to bring about a healing of the immediate situation and improve the patient's overall general health. It also is likely to be used for the patient with a chronic condition that has been in place for a number of months or years.

There may be no easy way in which a base point of "normal good health" can be found for this level of treatment. The patient may have been sick for quite some time, and his life may have been defined and structured around the illness for so long that it is difficult for him to remember how he felt before the onset of illness. The practitioner may have to explore the patient's whole lifetime to get a feel for that patient's condition and an idea of what remedy or remedies may be helpful in his treatment.

What can be more clearly understood is the concept of "totality of symptoms" as it relates to the constitutional treatment. Here the concept of totality does refer to all the symptoms, good, bad, or indifferent, that the patient experiences. It is also important that the practitioner get a feel for how those symptoms have evolved over time, and how the symptoms may combine or alternate with each other. The modalities of the symptoms—what makes them feel better or worse—are of particular importance in the constitutional case.

The goal of the constitutional treatment is not only to improve the patient's overall health, particularly where the chronic conditions are involved, but also to make the patient less likely to become ill in the future once treatment is concluded. Thus, the constitutional treatment seeks to fundamentally improve the patient's health and nature. The constitutional treatment should not be undertaken by anyone who has not mastered all the skills necessary for this level of homeopathic care.

The third level of treatment is called *miasmic.* It relates to the term "miasm" as used by Samuel Hahnemann. The term itself means "blot" or "taint." In using it, Hahnemann spoke of what we might now call a genetic predisposition to a specific illness or to a group of illnesses. Ailments like heart disease, drug or alcohol abuse, or even some forms of cancer, may be said to be miasmic in nature, especially when they occur in more than one member of a family.

In taking the case for a miasmic treatment, it is very helpful for the practitioner to include in his "totality of symptoms" not only the patient's own long-term and recent symptoms, but also those common to the patient's family. The practitioner may wish to know what ailments the patient's parents and grandparents suffered, as well as the causes of their deaths. In doing so, the practitioner seeks to uncover which of several specific miasms are active in the patient's system, and which may lie latent.

This is the deepest level of homeopathic treatment, one that may be said to be of a transformational nature. The goal of this level of treatment seeks no less than to bring the patient into a state of total freedom, in which his life is in no way defined by illness of any sort. It should be noted that miasmic treatment is the most complex type of homeopathic treatment, and it should only be undertaken by a master homeopath. Like the constitutional treatment, it should not be undertaken by anyone who has not mastered all the skills necessary.

While it may be somewhat ironic, it is worth noting that the number of different remedies, and the doses and potencies used at each level of treatment, work with reverse logic depending upon the depth and range of treatment.

The acute treatment will likely use more different remedies and potencies and a higher number of doses than the constitutional treatment, which in turn will often include more remedies and potencies than the miasmic treatment. The acute treatment will often call for two or three remedies given in rapid succession (never, however, with more than one remedy given at the same time) to restore the status, while the constitutional treatment may call for a single remedy given somewhat continuously for an extended length of time. And the deepest level of treatment, the miasmic, may actually be resolved by a single dose of a single remedy, or by successive doses of that same remedy.

So although it is important to know the goals and practices common to each of the three levels of treatment, it should also be understood that the widest gulf in treatment methodology separates the acute from the constitutional and miasmic. The skills needed for a practitioner to successfully conclude an acute treatment are often different from those needed in a chronic or miasmic case.

Considering the Acute Homeopathic Treatment

Finally, let us consider the task of selecting and using homeopathic remedies in acute situations. This is, I think, the most misunderstood aspect of homeopathic care.

For the more than twenty-five years in which I have been actively studying homeopathy, attending classes, clinics, and conferences, it has always been stated that, while the overall practice of homeopathy is best suited to medical professionals, it is all right if lay people want to practice acute homeopathy.

Since we all have the legal right to self-medicate—as long as the medications used are legal and available over the counter, if not prescribed for us by a physician—it is certainly understandable that the leaders of homeopathic community had to recognize the right of the lay person to select and use remedies for themselves and their loved ones. But more than two decades of hearing that acute homeopathy belongs to lay persons while constitutional prescribing and miasmic care are the domain of the professional have created the false assumption that the practice of acute homeopathy is simpler than is the practice of constitutional care. In my experience, this is simply not the case. In fact, I often have seen constitutional cases that seemed almost elegantly simple and acute cases of extreme complexity.

The simple truth is that acute and constitutional treatments are different (I include miasmic as a subset of constitutional treatment in this context), but one does not, by its nature, require any less skill, knowledge, or dedication than the other to do correctly. They simply require a different set of muscles.

Think about allopathic medicine for a moment. Our society does not think less of the acute caregiver than of the doctor who treats chronic cases, or specializes in specific ailments. In fact, we tend to love the acute caregiver. The top rated television show of the last decade, *ER,* celebrated the skills of those who must make quick life and death decisions under intense acute circumstances.

But when we get into the homeopathic arena, these same decisions are largely put in the hands of the wife and mother, who stores her kit under her bed. (This is not to say that these decisions are not in safe hands, however. Some of the finest homeopaths I have ever known have been lay practitioners—many of whom I would want at my bedside should I ever need emergency care.)

This thinking seems a little odd to me.

After all, when we are dealing with a chronic condition like an allergy or digestive trouble, especially one that has been in place for a number of years and is not inherently life threatening, the homeopath is in the happy position of being able to research the case and take all the time he needs before even giving the first remedy. And should that remedy fail to work as expected, he again has all the additional time he needs to find a second, or even a third remedy, until he find one that will finally move the case along toward healing, even if it is not totally curative.

The acute prescriber has no such time available, and very few second chances with remedies. The acute prescriber has to correctly assess the case the first time, and discern which symptoms should be considered to be a part of the "totality" to be included in the sphere of treatment.

Further, he has to know his materia medica so well that he can recognize the remedies "on the fly." He has to know a Pulsatilla when he sees one, and be able to tell the difference between that Pulsatilla and the Natrum Mur that he might otherwise confuse it with.

Also, the acute prescriber cannot give multiple remedies in the short space of time available without making the case untreatable by confusing it with their various actions. Usually, the acute prescriber gets only two chances: the remedy of first choice, and a follow-up. If he blows these selections he has lost the opportunity to cure the case.

Above all things, the homeopath wants to avoid the pitfalls of polypharmacy—giving more than one remedy at a time. Hahnemann railed against this method of treating a patient in both acute and constitutional treatment, and in both homeopathic and allopathic treatments. Every medicine affects the patient. If they are selected well they create a number of artificial symptoms that lead the patient toward healing, but when too many remedies are used in too short a period of time, the artificial symptoms confuse the case. Ultimately neither the patient nor the prescriber can know what is natural to the disease state, and what was artificially grafted onto it.

The acute prescriber has to know the remedies and how to use them. He has to be skilled at the selection of appropriate potencies and the correct number of doses. And the greatest difference between acute and constitutional prescribing skills is that the acute prescriber must remain in the moment with the patient. Anyone who has ever visited a professional homeopath's office, only to watch him flipping through book after book (or typing into the homeopathic software on his computer), while supposedly taking a case, already knows this. The acute prescriber must learn to take a case in minutes, ask as few questions as possible, and assess the case largely on the basis of the observable and tangible symptoms, which are known as *objective symptoms.*

This concept brings us to the heart of this book. Learning to quickly and accurately assess an acute situation and appropriately use homeopathic remedies to restore health is a powerful goal for any homeopath, whether professional or lay. My years of experience have taught me that this can best and most easily be accomplished almost completely through the use of the objective symptoms. The acute prescriber must learn to use all of his senses in case taking and not simply rely on a verbal interview as so many do, especially those who dedicate themselves to constitutional care.

The purpose of this book, therefore, is to give those who want to increase their skills with homeopathy "on the fly" some tools to help them achieve their goals.

The first part of the book is called "Objective Diagnosis," a title used as a tribute to John Scudder, an American homeopath who practiced approximately 150 years ago and wrote a book of the same name.

You will find some basic information about homeopathy in the first chapter of this section. You may find this information especially helpful if you are new to homeopathic medicine.

The second chapter concerns itself with Scudder and his methods of diagnosis. It contains a brief history of his work and methods, as well as an overview of how he developed all five of his senses to make himself a better diagnostician.

The third chapter looks at the world of traditional Chinese medicine, and the time-tested methods by which Eastern physicians use the same objective symptoms in diagnosing their cases.

The fourth chapter puts all of the previous information together, blending these techniques into a plan of action for case taking. Samuel Hahnemann gives us the structure for homeopathic case taking in his book *The Organon of Medicine.* Given time, training, and education, that structure can help you master the art of acute prescribing.

Finally, the fifth chapter gives you information on managing the acute case, including what notes to make and how to keep them, how to learn from your successes, and, especially, from your failures. It also describes the care and storage of homeopathic remedies.

The second part of the book contains what I like to call an "Objective Materia Medica." While other materia medicas tend to stress the persona of the remedies, this one focuses on the physical aspects of the case and on outward demonstration of the emotions of the patient. A few charts compare and contrast the remedies to help clarify your understanding of them.

This part is followed by a section that discusses the most common household health emergencies and the remedies most frequently used to treat them.

Please note that this book is not an exhaustive text. Rather, it is one that I hope will demystify homeopathy, and give readers a basic understanding of the most common remedies and their uses.

This book will show readers that concentrating on the objective aspects of any acute case is the fastest and simplest method to assess the case and form a plan of action, and how to most safely and effectively use the remedies selected for the healing process.

PART ONE

Objective Diagnosis

The question—How do you feel? Elicits a loose, wandering description of the patient's sensations, and is only important in that it suggests special questions and examinations. The question—Where do you feel it? Is pertinent, and will elicit valuable information of local disease.

—JOHN SCUDDER, *SPECIFIC DIAGNOSIS*

1

What Is Homeopathy?

As a specific form of medical treatment, homeopathy dates back just over 200 years, to the work of the German physician Samuel Hahnemann, who practiced in the late 1700s. Hahnemann was applying principles of healing that dated back to Hippocrates, for use in his own medical practice. Hahnemann took two Greek words, *homios* and *allos* and combined them with the Greek suffix *pathos* to coin the terms *homeopathy* and *allopathy* in 1896, after years of clinical tests. He used these terms to define what he saw to be two distinct schools of medical treatment. The term "homeopathy" literally means "similar suffering," in that "pathos" means "suffering" and "homios" may be translated as "similar." In the same way, "allos" translates as "different," making allopathic medicine "different suffering." Both terms were coined by Hahnemann, but refer back to an older medical philosophy.

As a general concept homeopathy dates back to some two thousand years before Hahnemann. Hippocrates, and others who practiced medicine with him on the Isle of Cos, taught that medical philosophy fundamentally consisted of three aspects: how any given practitioner identified the symptoms of discomfort associated with disease; what that practitioner thought might be the originating factor or factors of that disease state; and how he worked with his patient in restoring that patient to health. Hippocrates said that there were only two forms of medicine, and that those two forms were like two streams placed side by side that flowed in opposite directions.

In coining the words homeopathy and allopathy, Hahnemann gave names to those two distinct rivers of healing. Hahnemann wrote that the allopathic doctor was taught to see the symptoms of disease as a bad thing, as a sign of an invasion of the patient's system from outside, and as a form of attack that must be fought against to restore the patient to health. The allopath therefore works to eliminate the symptoms associated with a specific disease state. If they cannot be effectively removed, the alternative is to suppress them and restore the patient to a state of "quasi-health." Although the ailment lingers, the patient does not experience the full discomfort associated with the disease state.

The allopath in his philosophy and practice of medicine, therefore, works from a disease diagnosis, in which a given set of symptoms are clustered together under a specific title or disease name. When a specific disease is identified in any patient, the diagnosis then implies a map to cure. Specific symptoms require specific medicines.

The word allopathy literally refers to the concept of "different suffering," which refers to the fact that the medicines allopaths use in treatment are capable of creating a set of *symptoms* in the patient that are counter to those identified as a natural part of the disease state. Therefore, the person with nasal discharge from seasonal allergies is given antihistamine to counter the natural symptoms and stop the discharge. The allopathic treatment of disease always works in this manner—a medicine is given that acts in opposition to the natural set of symptoms. Whatever flows is dried, and whatever is dry, flows.

As we will see, allopathic treatment methods are in direct conflict with homeopathic treatment. The two forms of medicine have opposite views both in philosophy, regarding the nature of symptoms, and in practice, where the two use very different forms of medicine in very different ways.

But there is perhaps a more fundamental difference between the two forms of treatment, one that has to do with the nature of the patient, as well as the nature of disease.

HOMEOPATHY AS "DIVERGENT MEDICINE"

It may help the reader understand the concepts of "divergence" or "convergence" as medical philosophies if I acknowledge that I spent seven years of my life as a vision therapist, after first spending five years as a patient of vision therapy. It was from this work, and my ensuing perspective on the concept of vision that my thoughts on "divergent" and "convergent" medicines came about.

It is the job of the vision therapist to take the optometrist's diagnosis of vision disorder and turn that diagnosis into a set of vision exercises that best harmonize (improve) that patient's vision.

As a vision therapist, you quickly learn that in the United States today, the most common vision ailment involves over convergence. In other words, the problem most patients have is that their eyes turn inward—a problem commonly called cross-eyed. The cause of this is the amount of detail work performed by the average person. Students spend their days reading from books, employees spend the day in front of the computer screen, and their eyes turn inward to see the small print. After years this creates stress, which is expressed as headaches, shoulder pain and the like, as well as the over convergence.

So, from my viewpoint as a vision therapist, allopathic medicine (the dominant form of medicine in the Western world) can be said to be a form of "convergent medicine." It requires that the practitioner converge upon, or narrow down, his view of his patient to a set of very specific details—the patient's symptoms—while largely ignoring the patient as a whole being. This is detailed medicine—eyes turned inward medicine. Consider how the practice of allopathy has been broken down into the practice of many, many different specialties. In the area of vision alone there are specialists working with the cornea, and others working with the retina, to name just two. But specialists are something you never find in homeopathic medicine.

In the same way that a vision therapist would consider allopathy to be "convergent," the same therapist would consider homeopathy to be "divergent medicine," because the homeopathic practitioner must place the details of a patient's discomfort within the context of his whole being to find an effective treatment. This practitioner can be compared to a vision therapy patient with divergent eyes, in that his eyes turn outward. The divergent patient has a good deal of trouble dealing with details, because turning his eyes inward at all creates a good deal of both psychological and physical discomfort. The divergent personality type is a person for whom the "big picture" is most important, and for whom details are a pain. In the same way, the homeopath will put the details aside or assemble them into a whole picture before choosing a treatment path, even if he studies the details of a case for a long period of time. What is important is the case as a whole, and the matching of that whole with the portrait of a remedy's whole sphere of activity.

To summarize the difference in the perspective of the allopath and the homeopath, we could say that should an allopath and a homeopath stand together and look at one of Seurat's most famous paintings, the allopath would see myriad colored spots, while the homeopath would see *Sunday in the Park.*

This same divergent attitude holds not only for the patient, but also for the homeopath's remedies and his approach to them. The specific details that usually are associated with the disease diagnosis are often put aside in favor of what the homeopath calls his "drug diagnosis." With the "drug diagnosis," a specific remedy is selected because it is most suited to the patient *in toto* —body, mind, and spirit—even if it is not the remedy that would be considered the leading contender for a case of migraine, eyestrain, or flu. In fact, most homeopaths will name their cases by the remedy diagnosis rather than by the disease diagnosis, and say a real Natrum Mur case, instead of a case of seasonal rhinitis.

It is, therefore, important to remember that there is no such thing as a homeopathic specialist. No homeopath ever looks at just one organ or one system in the body in order to treat the whole. Also, the remedies themselves cannot be limited in their scope. There is no such thing as a cold remedy or backache remedy; there is simply the matching of the remedy in its action with the patient and his disease in its full range of symptoms. For simplicity, homeopathic texts (especially those on acute treatments) tend to group Arnica, Rhus Tox, and the like as if their actions were limited solely to first aid, but we should always be aware that remedies have a wide range of actions, all of which are equally important.

Remember, in homeopathic medicine it all comes down to the totality of the patient—total body, total mind, and total spirit.

Perhaps British homeopath Margery Blackie expressed it best when she titled her book *The Patient, Not the Cure.* In doing so, she reminds us that unlike the allopath, the homeopath is not treating disease, but is instead treating the patient who finds himself diseased. The fact that she gives her book the subtitle "The Challenge of Homeopathy" points out just how hard it is to be an effective homeopath.

Symptoms and the Homeopath

For the homeopath, the symptoms associated with any given disease are not seen as invaders from outside, but as part of the patient's own system or self that have been made active and visible. They are the equal and opposite reaction that the body has to the action created by the presence of a disease germ. The symptoms are not created by the germ itself, as is commonly believed, but by the body's attempts to eliminate the germ and to bring itself back into healthy balance. Thus, the virus does not cause the runny nose; the nose runs because the body is trying its best to wash the virus out of the system.

Because of this, the homeopath seeks to honor the symptoms and study them as the master plan by which the body is seeking health. The homeopath works *with* the symptoms, encouraging them, to assist the body's movement toward health.

Therefore, the homeopath seeks to bring the symptoms forward, and, ultimately, out of the patient's body by strengthening the patient as a whole being. This is accomplished by stoking the patient's life energy, which is called *Chi* in traditional Chinese medicine and *Vital Force* in homeopathic medicine.

Referring back to the fact that the term "homeopathy" translates as "similar suffering," it is important to keep in mind that a homeopath selects a remedy by matching the symptoms the patient is experiencing and the homeopath's knowledge of the symptoms associated with the given disease, with the artificial symptoms the remedy is known to create. In constitutional homeopathy, those symptoms would include those being experienced by the patient at the given moment, along with those that he has experienced in the past.

In acute treatments, matching the symptoms of the natural disease with those created by the impact of the remedy is a fairly simple thing if the patient was considered to be in a healthy state before the onset of the acute illness. The patient may have had allergies and insomnia, but for the sake of the acute treatment, he is considered to have been in a healthy state before the onset of the flu symptoms.

It is the goal and power of the acute treatment only to restore the patient to the state of health he enjoyed or suffered before the onset of the acute treatment. Therefore, our allergic insomniac will still have insomnia and allergies after the flu has left him.

Because the acute treatment only restores the status quo as it was before the onset of the acute condition, the matching of the condition and the remedy become fairly simple. We are zeroing in on only a few defined aspects of the patient: those things that became distorted with the onset of disease, such as a patient who was never particularly thirsty but suddenly craves large amounts of cold water, or a patient who was always rather warm and usually slept with the window open, but now wants things closed up tight and wraps himself in blankets. And the patient who has always been filled with humor, but now is suddenly in the blackest of moods.

These symptoms, aspects of the patient's overall being that have suddenly changed with the disease, along with the more commonly considered symptoms—mucus, red and sore throats and the like—are the indicators that will lead us to the remedy that treats them.

That's why so much of this book studies the natural symptoms and the remedies they suggest, in addition to the remedies and the symptoms they can artificially create. Homeopathic treatment is impossible without the knowledge of at least our most commonly used remedies, and without a basic knowledge of disease and the symptoms that can be associated with any given acute condition.

Homeopathy, Equal and Opposite

A few paragraphs back, I referred to a patient's symptoms as being "the equal and opposite reaction" that his body is having to the initial action created by the presence of a disease germ. I must now again consider the idea of equal and opposite, because it is just about the most important thing I can tell you about homeopathy. In fact, it explains the very heart of homeopathy, and why, in the end, it is a cleaner and more effective form of treatment than allopathic medicine.

In my classes in homeopathy, I used to tell new students that they already knew everything they needed to know about homeopathy, in that they had studied it in the seventh or eighth grade.

Then I asked them to fill in the blank. "For every action," I would say, "there is—blank." And the class would answer, "An equal and opposite reaction." "Exactly," I would say, "I told you that you all knew everything you needed to know about it."

And I was right. We all know the scientific principle that for every action there is an equal and opposite reaction. We apply it to physics, to astronomy, and to math, but we don't apply it to medicine. We ought to. It explains so very much.

Let's say that Paul is a very tired little man. He cannot sleep. Night after night, he cannot sleep. Such insomnia. He turns to an allopath for help, and is given a sleeping pill. The first night that he takes it he sleeps like a baby. It is like a month in the country. The second night, everything is fine. But, by the tenth night, the pill is not working so well anymore. Paul finds that he is restless again and cannot sleep. He finds that he needs two pills in order to sleep, and then three, and then more. Ultimately, he finds that allopathic sleeping medicine keeps him awake.

Paul finally crawls into a homeopath's office. Here he is given Coffea, a remedy created from coffee. At first, Paul feels a little buzzed by the medicine, a little worked up, but then he falls asleep and continues to sleep well ever after.

Why? Because the homeopath worked with the state that Paul was already in when selecting his remedy. And because the nature of the remedy matched the natural disease state very well, in the symptoms it was capable of creating.

Look at it this way: because the allopathic medicine worked in opposition with the natural disease state, and because our universe dictates that for every action there is an equal and opposite reaction, Paul was bounced around like a Ping Pong ball allopathically. He was, by his diseased nature, sleepless. He was then given a medicine that created an artificial sleep state. His own system was at first surprised by the medicine and had no defense against it. This was the initial honeymoon state, during which the medicine seemed to be working so well. But as the medicine was continued nightly, Paul's system began to create an equal and opposite reaction to the medicine's action, and sleeplessness began to set in again. If Paul continued to take the medicine, more and more would be needed to overwhelm Paul's system and allow for sleep. Ultimately, the allopathic treatment for Paul's sleeplessness would completely rob him of sleep, while leaving him dependent upon his sleep medicine.

Now look at the homeopathic treatment. Paul was given a remedy that, in a healthy person, would create the very sleeplessness from which Paul suffered. Paul felt an increased restlessness as the remedy had its initial impact, but he fell asleep once his system reacted against the action of the medicine. And the problem was solved, because this sleep state was the natural reaction his body had to the homeopathic medicine and was not artificially created. Paul should need no more medicine of any sort in order to sleep.

Homeopathic medicine works so well and so quickly because it works with the universal principle that for every action there is an equal and opposite reaction. In fact, homeopathic treatment depends upon the equal and opposite reaction that your system will have to the medicine's action to bring about healing. You see, it is not the medicine that heals. The medicine merely acts a catalyst. It is your system that heals itself. The homeopath creates a situation in which cure is possible, by giving the remedy that is most similar in its action to the natural disease state and encouraging the body to work in an equal and opposite reaction to the action of the remedy. That's what makes homeopathy such an elegant form of medicine, and such a safe one as well. That, and the method by which homeopathic remedies are both created and tested, a method created and refined by Hahnemann himself.

THE CREATION OF HOMEOPATHIC REMEDIES

Samuel Hahnemann was a pioneer in the creation of new medicines, in that he tested his remedies only on healthy humans. He felt that, should he test his medicine on those who were sick, he would only be testing its impact on that specific disease state in that particular patient. Instead, he tested his remedies on a large group of healthy persons, and he was able to create a complete portrait of that remedy and its wide range of impact by studying and carefully analyzing the impact of each medicine on each individual.

It should be noted that, unlike allopathic medicine, which considers each medicine to have a primary action or use and a number of other actions that are termed "side effects," homeopathic medicine makes no such distinction, but, instead gathers information on the full range of effects of each medicine. These are all considered when matching that medicine to the patient whose case incorporates multiple facets of that remedy's "sphere of action."

The role of the homeopathic physician in the selection of a remedy, therefore, is matching the patient's full range of symptoms to the remedy that would create these same symptoms in a healthy person. The remedy that creates the symptoms of the illness in a healthy person will eliminate the same symptoms in the person who has the illness.

Thus, homeopathy, as a "divergent medicine," places far more emphasis on the totality of a patient's symptoms and the total sphere of a remedy's action than it does on the naming of diseases and the development of a strategy in combating any specific disease.

Each patient is viewed as a whole and unique being, so the medicine that is required, no matter what that patient's condition, may follow no set pattern of treatment. Because homeopathy contains no classifications that identify specific medicines as being "pain medication" or "heart medication," each treatment must focus completely on each individual patient and his own unique needs. In other words, there is no map to follow in homeopathy.

It should be noted, before we move more specifically into the practice of homeopathy, that, based upon what has been written above, all forms of medicine fall within the realm of being either allopathic or homeopathic. Whether the school is Eastern or Western, or ancient or modern, this division has determined its viewpoint of and treatment of symptoms. Chinese medicine, for instance, contains both types of medicine within its traditions: herbal treatments, which are allopathic by nature, and acupuncture, which is homeopathic both in philosophy and healing action.

In establishing a system of treatments that functioned within the tenants of his homeopathic philosophy, Hahnemann brought together several diverse principles that combine to form the practice of homeopathy. As the American homeopath James Tyler Kent expresses it, these treatments have to be "homeopathic" in two ways—in the way the medicines are created, and in the ways they are used.

It took Hahnemann years to develop the process for creating homeopathic medicines that he ultimately distilled into two component parts: dilution and succussion.

Given that Hahnemann had only the medical pharmacy of his time to work with, which included such toxic substances as arsenic, it should come as no surprise that his first priority was to find a way to avoid killing his patients with the medicines at his disposal. He did this by simply diluting these substances. Through years of testing, he set up two scales of *dilution* to dissolve the substances from which the medicine is created; the *decimal scale* (to the tenth part) and the *centesimal* (to the hundredth part). He ultimately created what today is called the "microdose" through multiple levels of dilution—a level of dilution at which not one molecule of the original substance remains. In doing so, Hahnemann created a medicine that had no possible physical toxicity. Ironically, the medicine seemed to become more powerful the more it was diluted. Hahnemann was unable to conclude why this might be, but modern homeopaths believe that while the original energy signature of the substance remains after the multiple levels of dilution, its physical nature falls away. Homeopathic medicine can therefore be seen as a means by which the energy, or Vital Force, of another substance is utilized to balance the patient's own blocked or unbalanced life force.

The second aspect in the creation of a homeopathic remedy, *succussion,* simply involves shaking, or blending, the remedy in liquid form at each level of dilution. Hahnemann found that the succussion of the remedy made the remedy more potent than it was if simply diluted. Thus he instituted a process, called potentization, by which any natural substance could be shaped into a homeopathic medicine.

The Three Laws of Cure

Hahnemann set forth "Three Laws of Cure" in determining how a medicine may be used in order to safely cure the sick. These are the principles by which homeopathic remedies are most correctly used. To understand the importance of these laws, remember Kent's statement that homeopathic remedies are homeopathic in their action only if they have been both created and used properly. It is possible for the homeopath to take the most perfectly created remedy and ruin its curative action by using it a manner that is not in harmony with these three laws. In this situation the impact of the remedy would be allopathic. It is vital, therefore, that you understand both the creation and usage of a remedy before you handle it: that you both understand and abide by the Three Laws of Cure.

The first law, the *Law of Similars,* is perhaps the heart of homeopathy. It refers to the idea that for every action there is and equal and opposite reaction. It is simply states that "like cures like." To remember this law, think back to the literal meaning of the word homeopathy itself, and to the fact that the homeopath will use the remedy that is most *similar* in action to the situation at hand to bring about a cure. It is for this reason that homeopathic remedies are not classified by the diseases they treat, but by the type of person who needs them.

The second of these laws, the *Law of Simplex,* states that only one remedy at a time should be used in the treatment of any patient for any disease. Hahnemann's reasoning in the creation of this law was that only one remedy is needed to improve a patient suffering from a number of symptoms because each remedy is capable of creating a panoply of changes in the human system. Since each remedy could and would create a number of symptoms, you only had to match the appropriate remedy to the patient to achieve cure.

Further, Hahnemann believed that because each medicine creates a number of changes in the human system, it is actually dangerous to use more than one remedy at a time. The practice of polypharmacy would artificially create a wide range of symptoms in the patient's system, making it all but impossible to know what medicine had created what change. Although the process of dilution ensured that none of the medicines would have a toxic impact, the use of more than one at a time could hopelessly confuse the case and make it all but impossible to track the healing process. Hahnemann, in fact, deplored polypharmacy in all forms of medicine, and begged both homeopathic and allopathic practitioners to avoid using more than one medicine at a time. All medicines, whether allopathic or homeopathic, create a wide range of artificial symptoms in the human system.

The final law, the *Law of Minimum,* has two parts. The first part states that homeopathic remedies should be given in the lowest effective potency, and the second states that the reme-dies should always be given in the fewest number of effective doses in order to achieve a cure.

The homeopath must know the remedies themselves and how they act in various poten-cies since homeopathic potency is determined by the degree of dilution, and potencies become more powerful with each level of dilution. He must be able to determine the strength of the patient's Vital Force, and the degree to which that vitality has been impaired by the force of the disease. Just as the homeopath must be able to match the remedy to the patient, he must also be able to match the potency of the remedy to the patient's innate vitality.

Finally, the homeopath must give the reme-dy only when and how it is needed, as more cases are worsened by giving too much medicine than by giving too little. The home-opath judges the case by the patient's Vital Force, and how this life energy is improved by the use of the remedy. This is a careful process, because even the case in which the patient's symptoms are not immediately improved may be said to be on the right track if the patient shows general improvement in energy and clarity. An improvement to the symptoms spe-cific to the case follows this initial general improvement. According to the law of Minimum, no further doses of any remedy should be given once that improvement begins, unless the patient experiences a setback. And those cases should be carefully considered before the potency of the medicine is increased or a different remedy is used.

Remember, it is a goal of homeopathy that the patient stop taking any and all medicine as soon as possible, especially in the acute case. Unlike the allopathic realm, in which medicines are given for a lifetime, homeopathic remedies are given only until improvement begins, and then are repeated only if absolutely required. The wise homeopath knows that more cases are ruined by giving too much medicine than by not giving enough.

When it is used in this classical method, as set forth by Samuel Hahnemann, homeopathy presents a safe and effective method of treatment for many types of patients suffering from a wide range of symptoms.

2

What Is "Objective" Homeopathy?

In the two hundred years since Samuel Hahnemann first coined the term homeopathy, its practice has taken on many forms. Some practitioners choose to ignore the Law of Simplex, and give medicines made up of many different homeopathic remedies. Others give remedies only in low doses, and still others give treatments only in high potencies. The manner in which they select the needed remedy remains more or less the same, however. It all has to do with symptoms, no matter how they use the homeopathic remedies in treating their cases.

For the homeopath, symptoms are signs that the patient's immune system is not working to some level or other, and that the patient's system is trying to heal itself of disease. The symptoms are not the direct result of the presence of a disease state, but the attempt of the body to bring itself into balance. Therefore, the coughs, sneezing, and runny nose that we associate with a cold are not caused directly by the cold virus, but by the body of the infected person as it tries to flush that virus from its system.

Perhaps the most common symptom that illustrates this is a fever. When the body moves into a fever state, it is trying to raise the temperature of the internal body climate to one in which the germs present cannot survive, in an attempt to kill off the invaders without harming the body itself. Therefore, when we work to lower a nonlife threatening fever, we are working against body's own attempt to get well.

With this understood, let's go a bit deeper and think about symptoms themselves for a moment. What are symptoms? When I ask that in class, I mostly get a list of aches and pains. Symptoms are headaches, sore throats, swollen and itchy eyes, runny noses—things that tell you that you are sick.

But this is a rather narrow definition of the word symptom.

First of all, are symptoms limited to just physical complaints? Can they be emotional as well? In other words, can an acute illness have as much impact upon your mood as it does on your body? Think about it. Have you had illnesses in the past during which you just seemed to be in the worst mood all the time? During which you complained and argued so much with everyone that no one wanted to take care of you? Have you ever had an illness during which you were afraid all the time, perhaps afraid of dying from that illness? Or an illness during which you actually were kind of having fun—having such a good time watching movies on television, playing cards, and reading magazines that it almost seemed more like a vacation than an illness?

All of these are, for the homeopath, legitimate emotional responses to illness, and all are symptoms as much as any ache or pain. Symptoms can take place on any or all planes of being—body, mind, or spirit.

Things that seem completely benign to the patient can also be symptoms to the homeopath. If we have a patient who was never thirsty until he got sick, and is now drinking a great deal of water, that's a symptom. If a previously thirsty person stops drinking, that is a symptom. If a patient was once warm and is now freezing cold and needs to be covered up, or if he now craves cold air, and so on.

So, in its broadest possible working definition, a symptom is any change that is a result of illness. Anything that changes about a person after he or she becomes ill may be considered a symptom by the homeopath, and used in determining the selection of a remedy.

This principle by which we define and identify symptoms has largely to do with the genius of Samuel Hahnemann. First, it comes from his decision to test his new remedies only on healthy human beings—creatures capable of understanding the impact that the medicine was having on their system. And, second, it comes from the manner in which he tested those remedies on those healthy people.

Hahnemann gave each of his test patients a diary as well as a dose of the medicine. Patients wrote down everything they could sense that the medicine was doing in their system and all the changes it seemed capable of making, whether for apparent good or bad. Hahnemann compared the notes in the diaries when the tests were completed. Symptoms that were created in all the patients who took the remedy were considered to be the most important. Hahnemann also gathered information about the other symptoms, those that were not experienced by all of the patients. These are the symptoms the allopath gathers together and calls side effects, and acts as if they are best ignored.

It was of vital import to Hahnemann that he understand the entire sphere of activity caused by each of his remedies. He wanted a solid understanding the many ways that each remedy was a catalyst to change in the human system before he put his remedies to use with sick patients. To do this properly there could be no false division between effects and side effects, because each was a part of that remedy's sphere of action and might at some time be of vital import in the selection of a remedy for some patient.

Remember that, for the homeopath, "like cures like."

This means that, in selecting a remedy, the homeopath wants as broad an understanding as possible of the patient's symptoms as they appear naturally in his disease state, and he wants to compare these disease symptoms with the symptoms artificially created by the remedy. He also wants to compare both sets of symptoms as broadly as possible, and consider symptoms in body, mind, and spirit. The remedy with the artificial action that most completely matches the disease's natural action will be the most curative. Like cures like.

Hahnemann referred to his remedies as "artificial diseases" to illustrate the fact that his remedies created artificial symptoms that could balance out and remove natural disease symptoms. He meant that his remedies could create as many different symptoms, on as many different levels of being, as could viruses and bacteria. But these artificial states could be intentionally created by giving the proper dosage of a specific remedy to a healthy subject, because the remedies had been created using methods tested again and again.

Hahnemann believed, and homeopathic treatment has proven over the course of time, that you will allow a patient to heal himself if he is suffering from a group of symptoms that can be called a disease, and you give him a remedy that creates those same symptoms in a healthy person. The one proviso is that the artificial disease must be slightly more potent than the natural one in place. This is why homeopathic remedies come in so many potencies—so the practitioner can choose one just slightly more potent than the natural disease. When the remedy is administered, the patient's immune system will rise up against the medicine as if it were a new disease in the system. In doing so, the body heals itself of the natural disease and when the remedy's impact fades, the patient is left in good health.

So, it's all about the symptoms: what they are, and how they can best be removed.

SYMPTOMS: SUBJECTIVE AND OBJECTIVE

Because homeopaths consider their patients' symptoms to be of the utmost importance, they have spent the last two hundred years largely in developing methods for grouping symptoms so they can be better understood and treated. We will look at most of these different methods in later chapters, but we need to review the most basic aspects of symptoms at this point:

At their most basic level, symptoms are considered to be either *subjective* or *objective* in nature.

Subjective symptoms are those that are largely hidden and unknowable to anyone but the patient. They are the symptoms that the patient feels and knows about, but we do not. They are the patient's own sensations of illness.

Subjective symptoms are those by which each individual's experience of illness may be gathered, but they are just that—an *individual* experience of illness. The degree to which such symptoms are helpful is largely limited by the patient's self-awareness, as well as by his ability to express himself.

So here is the most valuable source of information—the first hand account of the patient himself. But it is also a source that is limited by the patient's character. Some patients may tend toward the dramatic in the telling of their ills, and make the disease into something much greater than it is, while others may greatly underplay their true aches and pains. Still others may simply not be paying enough attention to their own body to be of any great help when it comes to relating their actual symptoms, especially when they are asked when a symptom began, and how it has shifted in the course of the illness.

Uncovering subjective symptoms involves an interview between the patient and the practitioner. During this interview the skilled practitioner creates an atmosphere of trust and honor between the patient and himself. The interview can yield a great deal of helpful information, if it is done correctly, and if the patient is, over time, taught just what information is most important in the selection of a homeopathic remedy. The interview process can be almost useless, however, if the interview is bungled or if the patient is noncommunicative for any reason.

The other subset of symptoms are the *objective* symptoms. These symptoms are visible to and comprehended by the practitioner without any explanation from the patient. They are quantifiable, like laboratory findings.

Therefore, when a patient says, "I feel much less dizzy when I lie down," we have a subjective symptom that the patient must provide. But, when we look at a patient's throat and it is red, shiny, and swollen, we have the objective signs of a sore throat. For the knowledgeable homeopath, these objective symptoms specifically indicate a sore throat requiring the remedy Apis.

Case Taking in the United States

In the United States, we are used to thinking of homeopathic case taking as a very long and verbal process. Many homeopaths spend hours interviewing their patients, gathering information to assist them in selecting a remedy, and then spend many more hours processing the information before making a diagnosis. Historically and geographically, this is not and has not always been the case. The majority of practitioners across the planet today take their cases with an emphasis on the nonverbal indications of symptoms rather than the verbal. And historically, many of the world's best homeopaths stressed the use of objective symptoms in the process of diagnosis.

Homeopathic case taking seems to have evolved as a verbal process in the United States, however. Our practitioners are taught to structure much of their case taking on the basis of the homeopathic interview, even though all good homeopaths certainly physically examine their patient as well. Much of what is written on the subject of homeopathy—for practitioners and the lay public alike—stresses this method of verbal case taking, and emphasizes the use of subjective symptoms in diagnosis over the objective case taking. In this book, however, we will look at the nonverbal approach.

So, the question must be posed: can a case taking, a diagnosis, and a pattern of treatment be effectively based primarily on the objective symptoms, those which can be witnessed by the practitioner? For the answer, we have to go back a few years and across the face of the planet to ancient China.

For five thousand years, practitioners of traditional Chinese medicine (TCM) have made use of the specific information contained on a patient's tongue, his pulse (Chinese practitioners recognize several pulses) and his countenance for deciding the sort of condition the patient is in, and how best to restore that patient to health. (See the next chapter for more information on TCM and how its methods of diagnosis can give the homeopath a pattern for diagnosis.)

It was, in fact, my own experience with a skilled practitioner of TCM that gave me the idea for this approach to acute homeopathic practice.

Last time I was on my acupuncturist's table, with the acupuncturist looking down at my tongue while she took my pulse, I suddenly wondered why these same sources of information could not be used in the selection of a homeopathic remedy, especially in an acute case.

I have been working with this method since that time, and have found, again and again, that you can find the correct remedy if you can read the patient's countenance (a wonderful if somewhat antiquated word, which, for our purposes should be considered the whole face, including the expression and emotional impact) and learn to garner information from their objective status. This method of remedy selection can be greatly informed and enhanced by a study of traditional Chinese medicine. In the next chapter, I offer some ideas as to how the Chinese method can be translated into homeopathic practice.

From the moment it first occurred to me that one could base a good deal of the practice of homeopathy—especially acute homeopathy—from objective symptoms, I became very excited. It seemed that the use of objective symptoms are a safer and surer method of acute prescribing, because it is based on all that can be witnessed of the patient by his practitioner's senses. This method of prescribing actually forced the practitioner to stay "in the moment" with, and pay full attention to, his patient. This seemed superior to the method I was familiar with, in which the practitioner asks question after question of his patient, but spends his time only half listening to the answers. Instead, the practitioner is taking notes and flipping through the pages of this or that homeopathic reference book.

For a while, I managed to fool myself into thinking that I had invented the notion of basing acute prescriptions on objective diagnostic symptoms. I have since learned that I certainly was not the first to think in this way.

The Concept of "Specific" Diagnosis

John M. Scudder (1829–1894) left his mark on homeopathy during the period of the Civil War in the United States. A well-named method of treatment called *eclectic* medicine was on the rise in this country at that time. As the term implies, eclectic physicians like John Scudder would gather different forms of medical philosophy and practice together to treat their patients. Everything was considered, from homeopathic to herbal and allopathic treatment. Eclecticism was the foundation from which naturopathic medicine would arise a century later.

Scudder was an eclectic physician and a noted teacher. He was interested in Hahnemann's writings and in his theory of medicine. As an eclectic physician, Scudder was known to incorporate many different philosophies into his practice, so it surprised no one when he began to incorporate homeopathy into his practice as well. He became known for blending homeopathy and allopathy, and for using both poisonous and chemical medicines, after having diluted them to the level of a 3x homeopathic remedy. (3x refers to a remedy that has gone through three distinct stages of dilution, through which it has been transformed or potentized to take it into the form of a homeopathic remedy.) Scudder felt he could make use of allopathic drugs in such a manner that they could cause no harm. He also based the use of these medicines upon homeopathic principles to further enhance their safety.

His method certainly does not represent "classical homeopathy" in any form. Indeed, it can only be called a very sloppy practice of homeopathy at best. But I mention Scudder for his genius as a diagnostician rather than for his skill with remedies.

From all reports, Scudder was very interested in homeopathy and quickly adapted much of Hahnemann's method. But, as an eclectic physician, Scudder's particular bent was that the medicine at hand should yield to his use of it: he should never have to change his methods of practice to incorporate a particular new medicine. Because of this practice, Scudder knew early in his study of homeopathy that he would have a few problems with the underpinnings of homeopathic practice.

What Scudder had the most trouble with was the materia medica, the homeopathic resource volume that lists each remedy and details the entire sphere of action for each entry. He read Hahnemann's materia medica, as well as those written after Hahnemann's death, and he felt that they were almost useless because they were too large and all-encompassing. He would look at a listing, for instance, for Sulphur, and see that it was useful for those with diarrhea and well as for those with constipation along with many, many more pages of symptoms impacted by that remedy. He finally would just slam the book shut, saying that if you took the book at its word, all the remedies would cure anything and everything.

In the end, Scudder studied his materia medica and its companion volume, the repertory, which lists specific symptoms and the remedies that treat them in a format similar to a dictionary—but he studied them in a particular manner.

Scudder felt that he had learned the practice of medicine in a particular way, and that it had served him well before homeopathy and would continue to serve him well after homeopathy. He said he could only understand disease by the symptoms he could recognize. He therefore based his homeopathic prescription on pulse, tongue, and countenance, and a very few selected symptoms, which he said gave indications of what was wrong with the patient's life. He then matched the wrongs to the specific medicine that suited that particular pattern.

In other words, he gathered some specific information from the homeopathic texts and simply ignored the rest. In doing so, he followed the role of the eclectic and adapted homeopathy to his method, rather than adapting his method to homeopathy. And, along the way, he streamlined the process of homeopathic diagnosis.

He developed a new way of working with homeopathic remedies through this practice. The system was called "specific diagnosis" and "specific medication," in that he all but threw out the full range of homeopathic diagnosis, and based his diagnosis solely on the specific objective symptoms of the case.

In the late 1800s, Scudder wrote two books that put forth his philosophy of treatment. The first, published in 1874, was called *Specific*

Diagnosis, and it contained much of the methodology he had developed for forming a drug diagnosis based solely on objective symptoms. The second, written in 1890, was called *Specific Medication.* This volume was as close to a materia medica as Scudder was likely to get, as it listed the medicines he commonly used, the formulas for their dilution where necessary, and the diseases treated by each medicine.

Note that, in his use of the word *specific,* Scudder implied a meaning somewhat different from the one you or I might give. For Scudder the word specific linked a unique remedy to a single ailment. Unlike a homeopath, who would never think that the diagnosis of a specific disease implied the need for a specific medicine, Scudder in his practice of allopathic homeopathy thought that the idea of the specifics as a great boon to medicine.

In fact, Scudder injected eclectic medicine in general with a new jolt of energy with his new concepts. What had once been a dying medical practice has now become part of the instruction in several medical schools in the United States, thanks to Scudder's teaching.

Others, most especially Frederick Humphreys, M.D., jumped on the bandwagon. Humphreys, for his part, felt that the idea of specifics—that a homeopathic remedy or remedies could be linked to a specific disease diagnosis—had great implications, not only for medical professionals, but also for lay persons. After all, thought Humphreys, didn't this just simplify the whole process of homeopathic treatment, which in its traditional form seemed so difficult and required so much study?

Humphreys published *Humphrey's Mentor,* a home guide to the use of specific homeopathic remedies in 1898, which contained a listing of diseases and their symptoms. At the end of the description of each disease were the Humphreys' Specifics, which could be used to treat a case of the disease. These Humphreys' Specifics were the first combination remedies, as each contained several remedies. The idea was that one of them would surely work for the patient, making for a much simpler practice of homeopathy, or at least quasi-homeopathy. The patient just wrote to the address in the back of the book to order their specifics.

The reaction of the homeopathic community would have been easy to prognosticate—outrage, pure and simple. Humphreys, like Scudder before him, was seen as half a homeopath at best, a besmircher of homeopathy at worst. Despite this, the public had a great deal of interest in both Scudder's methods and Humphreys' combinations. Like today, lay people who lacked education in pure homeopathy saw the combination remedies as a simple solution. The fact that the combinations broke Hahnemann's Law of Simplex did not trouble them. Humphreys' Specifics were very popular.

This is not to say that Scudder's methods were accepted within the homeopathic community. In fact, Scudder's methods were quite controversial in his day, and his legacy remains controversial with homeopaths who disdain anything other that the Hahnemannian form of homeopathic practice.

But what amazed Scudder's critics in both the homeopathic and eclectic schools was how often his prescriptions were correct. Even those in both camps who disagreed with Scudder's odd blend of the homeopathic with the allopathic could not help but see that his methods of diagnosis were leading him in the right direction.

Over the years, Scudder self-published several books about his practice, including those mentioned earlier, and his methods were adopted by many eclectic physicians, for whom homeopathic remedies became a regular part of their practice. For this reason, Scudder may be considered the physician who helped to shape modern naturopathic medicine, in that he put homeopathic remedies into the hands of the eclectics.

Scudder, Homeopathy, and Specific Diagnosis

Scudder published the first of his two books based specifically on his practice of medicine in 1874. He called it *Specific Diagnosis,* and in it he gives the foundation and framework for his method of diagnosis. I wanted to include Scudder's opinions on the topics of symptoms, disease, health, and other topics of import to our discussion, so some rather lengthy passages from *Specific Diagnosis* follow because his book was self-published, and is now scarce and long out of print. (His other major work, *Specific Medication,* was written from the point of view of the eclectic physician and not the homeopath, so it is of lesser import to our discussion and is not dealt with in these pages.) Be warned that the writing style makes Scudder's work a bit of a tough go, but it is well worth the effort.

On the topic of symptoms, Scudder writes in *Specific Diagnosis:*

Disease has certain expressions, which we call symptoms, as health has certain expressions. We find that the manifestations of life in health are very uniform, and consistent, and one can hardly mistake their meaning. So in disease, the expression of morbid life is uniform, and constant, and does not vary in different individuals, as many have supposed. If we determine in any given case the expression of diseased life, we will find it the same in all cases.

It has been claimed, and tacitly admitted that symptoms of disease were so changeable and inconstant, that they could not be depended upon with any certainty. This was certainly true to those who made their diagnosis according to the received nosology (the classification of diseases), and then prescribed at the name. For as very diverse pathological conditions would be grouped under each name, the symptoms would of course vary, and the treatment would show the element of uncertainty in so marked a manner that idiosyncrasy would be constantly called in to explain the trouble.

We propose studying the expressions or symptoms of disease with reference to the administration of remedies. It is a matter of interest to know the exact character of a lesion, but it is much more important to know the exact relationship of drug action to disease expression, and how the one will oppose the other, and restore health. If I can point out an expression of disease which will almost invariably be met by one drug, and health restored, I have made one step in a rational practice of medicine.

I have no hesitation in affirming that if we have once determined such relationship, we have determined it in all diseases alike, in all persons, and for all time to come. If, with this symptom or group of symptoms, my Aconite, Nux or Podophyllum cures to-day, it will cure tomorrow, next year, and so long as medicine is practiced. If it cures Tom, it will be equally applicable in the same condition to his father, mother, wife or mother-in-law.

"Do you mean to say," asks the reader, "that the present system of nosology is useless?" Yes, so far as curing the sick is concerned, that is just what I mean to say. Not only useless, but worthless—a curse to the physician and patient—preventing one from learning the healing art, and the other from getting well. But you ask, "how would you make out the certificate for the under-taker?" That's just what we wish to avoid, we don't care about furnishing subjects, and would very much rather people should die of old age, and then we would write it in English—"old age."

The first lesson in pathology we want to learn is that disease is wrong life. The first lesson in diagnosis is, that this wrong finds a distinct and uniform expression in the outward manifestations of life, cognizable by our senses. The first lesson in therapeutics is, that all remedies are uniform in their action; the conditions being the same, the action is always the same. We learn to know the healthy man—know him by exercising all our senses upon him. We want to know how he feels, how he looks, how he smells, how he tastes, and what kinds of sound he makes. Then we want to learn the diseased man in the same way, and compare him with our healthy standard—certain expressions of life meaning health, and certain other expressions meaning disease. Then we study the action of the drugs upon the sick, and when we find them exerting an influence opposed to disease and in favor of health, we want to know the relation between the drug and the disease—between disease expression and drug action.

I do not say that we should not study drug action in health—indeed, I think it a very important study. You may, on your own person, study a wholly unknown drug, and determine its proximate medical action. How? Easy enough. You will feel where it acts; that points out the local action of the drug, and as a matter of common sense, you would use it in disease of that part, and not a part on which it had no action. You will feel how it works—stimulant, depressing, altering the enervation, circulation, nutrition and function.

The Goals of Homeopathic Treatment

More than once now I have said that the use of objective symptoms alone is usually enough for appropriate treatment in the acute context, which is the first level of treatment. This leaves us with the implication that the constitutional and miasmic treatment levels require something more or different in the gathering of symptoms before selecting treatment. This is certainly true. Each level of treatment has a different goal, and each requires different amounts of symptom gathering.

The goal of acute treatment is a relatively simple one: restore the patient to the status quo of health enjoyed before the onset of the acute illness—so the symptom gathering is also relatively simple. Since constitutional treatments work on a deeper level, a greater and deeper amount of information is required to select the appropriate remedy. The transforming power of miasmic treatment requires even deeper and more skilled symptom gathering and consideration. This book addresses acute considerations alone, so it is appropriate that we primarily consider objective symptoms, and use subjective symptoms as backup information.

We must be careful not enter into the world of specific treatments, which is something Scudder considers more or less correct, when we read his words, and especially when we put them to use.

Accept the wisdom from his text that we must treat the whole of the being and consider the whole of the patient's symptoms when we treat homeopathically. If we become too bogged down in the details of the symptoms, especially those compiled from a subjective interview, and never put them together into a whole picture, we will only be able to select a treatment for the details and not for the whole being. At some point it is vital to the selection of remedies that the homeopath sit back and see the patient as a whole. How did he or she look? How did he dress? How did he speak? How did he act? These are just as important—indeed, often more important—than the specific details of his or her symptoms.

Add information from the objective symptoms—how his pulse felt, how her tongue looked, the color and type of his nasal discharge—to the consideration of the whole patient, and you will likely have a basis for homeopathic treatment in the acute context.

Scudder and Hahnemann, Disease, and Health

Scudder invites us to consider a new standard of consideration both for health and for disease because he weds the skills of the eclectic physician and the homeopath. In doing so, he attempts to simplify what we know as classical homeopathy.

But Hahnemann is the true revolutionary in his approach to disease and its cure. As the father of homeopathy, he was the first to observe that the clue to the cure of a disease is in the nature of the disease state itself: that like must always cure like. Perhaps more important, he was the first to take this simple observation (which had, in fact, been made before, by Hippocrates himself) and turn the philosophy into a workable practice, based on the observation of the patient and his symptoms.

Scudder insists that we must learn to observe the state of health just as we do the disease state, and that we must consider the health state to be fairly consistent from person to person in the same way that the disease state is consistent. That freedom of movement, clarity of thought, and other such characteristics are all important aspects of health. That it is the grouping of symptoms that determine the naming of and consideration of the disease, even though each individual will experience a disease state in his or her own way. In fact, the naming of any disease state is actually only the gathering together of the specific combination of symptoms that make up the disease. You may have a cold with a sore throat in which the symptoms are worse on the left side of your body, and I may have worse symptoms on the right, but both of these variations are still consistent with the nature of the disease called the common cold.

In the same way, each of us has a unique blend of symptoms that make up our state of good health. Sleep patterns, sex drives, clarity and speed of thought and speech, and so on may vary, but all remain within the sphere that may be defined as "good health."

In learning to work with homeopathic remedies in acute health crises in the home, it is important to take the time, in advance, to identify what each potential patient's state of good health looks like, as well as his characteristics in that healthy state. Every mother knows when her child is healthy and when he is not, what her child's energy level is like when he is healthy, what foods he likes and does not like, when he tends to get sleepy at night, his patterns of thirst, and what his moods and emotional states tend to be. She can very quickly spot when there is a variation in any aspect of this health pattern.

It is important, therefore, to take notes and pay attention to just how that child's healthy state may be defined. A case should be taken while the child is healthy, and these records should be kept so that any stranger would be able to identify any changes in this normal state by reading them, and use this information in a health crisis to properly select a homeopathic remedy that could set things right.

The beginning of the acute homeopathic treatment lies in the normal state of good health for any given person. It is the specific symptoms that represent any deviation from this healthy state, especially if they can be objectively observed, that determine the nature, and perhaps the name, of the disease state. This "totality of symptoms" should be gathered for the acute case and used in the selection of the remedy. Remember, the goal of the acute treatment is to maintain the patient's status quo, and return him to the normal state of good health enjoyed before the onset of the symptoms associated with the disease.

If acute treatments can be considered in this way they can be fairly simple, especially if one can keep in mind Scudder's comment that if a particular remedy cures a specific set of symptoms today, then it will cure them for all time. This is a strong argument for the study of the materia medica and the homeopathic remedies themselves, in addition to the simple fact that no one should ever use a remedy with which he is totally unfamiliar. For instance, Arnica, may be the only remedy with which you are truly familiar—the only one you can honestly say you understand in terms of its action in the human system and the situations for which it is most commonly used. If it is the only remedy that you can identify, based on objective symptoms and without having to ask a patient sitting before you a single question, then that is the only remedy you should use. This is not to say that you should give Arnica to all of your patients, but that you can only truly be trusted to treat Arnica patients. You will only able to help when Arnica is and must be the remedy of choice, which may sound insignificant. But Arnica, like any other remedy, is a powerful healing tool when it is used correctly. You may do a great deal of good with that one remedy. So use only that remedy and use it well, and when you learn a second remedy, add it to your kit only when you truly understand both its objective and subjective symptoms. Then it will be totally safe to use, and will greatly benefit those who receive it in treatment.

This is the best way you can learn to use the remedies in your home kit. Start with the one remedy, Arnica, and add others as you study their full use. In a very short time you will have a home kit of about fifty core remedies, and will be skilled in their safe and appropriate use.

The Education of the Senses

In another section of *Specific Diagnosis,* Scudder gives his insights into how the homeopathic practitioner must make use of all his senses when approaching a patient during case taking. He wrote:

We have already seen that the education necessary to make a good physician, is not from books, or the memory—both good in their place, but insufficient. The education that gives the best results, and makes the successful practitioner, is of the senses, and of the brain to receive impressions, and make deductions.

We have called attention to the proper study of anatomy, by which one may *know* the structure of the human body of himself; and the right study of physiology, by which one may *know* the various activities of this mechanism. To make these attainments requires study—not midnight oil burned in reading books, but the continuous exercise of our senses upon the human body, living or dead...

If the senses, then, are the instruments by which we obtain knowledge, it will at once be patent to the reader that their development and goodness will be the measure of our ability and our attainments. Hence the man of educated and acute senses will be far superior to and have every advantage over the man who has not been thus trained and developed.

Most persons seem to think that the human senses are natural, not acquired—that they are born to us, and not the result of education. That is a very great mistake, and a grave error to the physician. Man is born with an organism that, so to speak, has germinal capacities for use, and its future development is by normal use. The child at birth has perfect hands and arms, every bone, muscle, blood vessel and nerve being there; but they are yet wholly useless. Its feet and legs have all the parts of the adult, but it can not walk, or even wag its toes under the influence of will. Its eyes are perfect, yet the images formed upon the retina are wholly without meaning, and might quite as well be a blank.

The child slowly learns to use its hands, and months pass before it can hold an object, and a still further time before it can move the object, and a still further time before it can move the object in obedience to the will. We see it day by day learning to see, slowly taught by its surroundings. And the adaptation of the nether limbs to walking is the persistent work of the first twelve or sixteen months. Compare the child of these attainments of one year with the child of two years, and you see a wonderful difference, the education has been continually going on during the period, and with continued use in the right directions comes increased development. At the third year, there is further improvement; and thus, as we go on to the fifth, the tenth, the twentieth year, we observe a continued education of the senses, and a better development of them...

Many who would admit that the human senses are acquired, think of them as being acquired very much as the man increases in stature and weight, and something essentially belonging to this period of growth.

They conclude that the senses grow with the body, and attain maturity when it has reached the full size and stature of a man; and now a man, having his full capacity, will find neither increase nor diminution so long as he may live. They measure a man in all his parts in this way; his every function in now developed for life. A greater mistake we could not make.

The law of development is always in operation in the human body, as it is throughout the animal and vegetable world. *As any organ or part is rightly used, it grows in capacity.* Not only in infancy, in childhood, up to adult years, but each and every year of a man's life to old age. It is more marked, of course, when the reproductive powers are active, but it is always a law of life. The man between thirty and forty years, will find that he still has the germs of a large capacity, which needs but the right use for development. He may grow legs, arms, body, chest, lungs, brain, the sense of touch, of taste, of smell, of hearing, of sight, if he will; all that is necessary is that he should rightly use that he has...

Man has five senses—of touch, of sight, of hearing, of smell, or taste—all of which are useful in this study, and all require training. The physician of unskilled touch, sight, hearing, smell, taste, can never be successful...

Note that the italics above are mine. Having introduced the law of development, Scudder now gives more detail into the education of the senses:

How May We Cultivate the Senses?—This is the really important question, though the answer has been partly given in the above study. We cultivate the senses by continuously using them, and their education is the work of months and years. We can always find objects to exercise them upon, the training school is all about us, and we have only to make intelligent use of the facilities at our command. It is well, however, to have an intelligent plan and follow it up assiduously, recollecting that "time, patience and perseverance will accomplish all things."

The senses are intimately associated with the brain, and their education implies a mental training as well. Whilst we develop the organ of sense by use, we develop the brain upon which the impression is made, and the higher brain which takes cognizance of, and analyzes the sensations. The development is thus a double one, and both are essentials in correct diagnosis. A plan presupposes thought, the act of the rational mind, as well as orderly activity.

The Touch—The tactile sense has its highest development in the hands, and it is in this locality, especially, that we purpose cultivating it...

A plan of use? It suggests itself at once—we will exercise our touch upon every object we come in contact with. Here are objects large and small, long and short, rough and smooth, of varied form, with special inequalities of surface, of varied consistence, and we purpose feeling them until we can recognize them as well in the dark as in the light...

Sight—The sense of sight is one of the most important in diagnosis, and it, like others, requires education, both as to the eye which receives and the brain upon which impressions are made. The eye receives impressions of color, and by education learns to detect the form, size, distance, and many of the physical properties of objects.

Color being one of the prominent characteristics of health and disease, the ability to accurately distinguish colors must be a great to the physician. The uneducated eye receives the impress of color very much as it does light and shade, attaching about the same meaning to it, but when trained by use, it readily detects slight variations...

The practical education of the eye to color is completed upon the human body. We find distinct varieties of color in health—of skin, of mucous membranes, of parts where the circulation is superficial, showing arterial blood, of veins, of the eye, the nails, the hair. We want to learn to know the healthy man by his color, and we may know him by this...

Hearing—Physicians do not seem to have realized the importance of the ear in diagnosis. It is true that we have a system of physical diagnosis for diseases of the chest, which the student is advised to learn; but, unfortunately, the advice is not supplemented by the lesson we are trying to teach—that these organs must be educated. The student applies his untrained ear, and hears nothing, or is unable to distinguish variation in sound, and becoming disgusted, gives physical diagnosis over to the expert or the specialist. Even if he persists in trying to learn, he finds that he can not hear the sounds described in the books, (simply because there are no sounds produced), and is thus discouraged.

All nature is vocal with sound, and the sounds are the expressions of life ... All nature is vocal with sound, but to the uneducated ear it might quite as well be still, for it expresses naught to him. Train the ear, and educate the brain, and we have a "concourse of sweet sounds," taking the entire range of life, expressing all its feelings, its hopes, its fears, its griefs, its cares, its pleasures, its pains. It recognizes the love song of the bird, the tone of wedded bliss, the gush of parental affection, the cry for assistance, the shriller cry of assault, the song of victory, the wail of defeat, and the moan of death...

In auscultation (which is the act of listening, either by ear or by mechanical means, specifically as a means of diagnosis), the first lesson is in learning to hear. It requires close and continued study to hear the respiratory murmur distinctly, and this study must be continued if we expect to recognize the variations of this and the sounds produced in the bronchial tubes. Skill in physical diagnosis does not come by nature; it is the result of study, and the education of the ear and brain. No man can expect to succeed in it unless he is willing to give months to it, first to educate the ear to the hearing and analysis of sound, and next to the hearing and analysis of the sounds heard in the chest.

Smell—Of still less importance is the sense of smell, and yet it has its place in diagnosis. A good nose is a good thing, and the sense of olfaction should not only be a safeguard to the individual, warning him of noxious influences, but should be a source of pleasure as well. To some extent this sense is instinctive, especially as it warns against irritant substances, and leads to their avoidance. But it is one that may be educated to a very high degree...

We want a good nose for the purposes of diagnosis, and we especially want a good nose that it may look after the hygienic surroundings of our patients. There is an abundance of bad smells about the sick room, some peculiar to the condition of disease, and some the result of want of cleanliness and ventilation. We want to know them, and to do so we require an educated nose.

What is an educated nose? It is so trained by use that it transmits sensations to the brain, which has also been trained by use to receive and analyze them. In other words, it is the association of the brain and nose in the work. This sense is educated in the same manner as the others...

Taste—Whilst the sense of taste is a good thing, and should be well cared for, we do not propose to make much use of it in medicine. It is well, however, to use it upon the food prepared for the sick, because we find a great many wrongs here.

It can be concluded from Scudder's writings that he demands that the homeopath open all his senses to the patient in front of him. He must also set aside all judgments, all considerations of lifestyle and character—and certainly, he must set aside any snap judgments as to what remedy will act curatively for the patient—and just witness all the information that his senses can bring him.

Too often, homeopaths are quick to decide what disease they are dealing with or what remedy will be needed, and close their minds and senses to the person in front of them. This is one of the great mistakes in case taking. Some homeopaths, especially beginners, will be more concerned with making sure that they ask all the right questions associated with their case taking than they are with paying attention to their patient. I promise you that more will be discovered during case taking by saying little and paying attention to what the patient says and does, and how he looks and smells, then will ever be learned by looking through books or making remedy lists while the patient speaks.

It is much more important that the practitioner is the patient's witness, noting and recording the patient's mood, behavior and objective symptoms through the strength of the practitioner's own senses.

This concept of educating our senses is perhaps where Scudder is most similar to the practitioner of traditional Chinese medicine. We will explore TCM, and how its practitioners stress the use of all of their senses as the tools by which they learn about their patients, diagnose illnesses, and consider treatments in the pages that follow.

For more quotations from Scudder's text, turn to Appendix Three in this book.

3

Case Taking in Traditional Chinese Medicine: A Pattern to Follow

In the homeopathic philosophy, we call good health—that perfect balance in all levels of body, mind, and spirit—*homeostasis.* To achieve this balanced state in the practice of traditional Chinese medicine (TCM), physicians seek to balance yin and yang—energetic opposites that together form a complete circle and a complete balance. To the Chinese physician, the yin represents the female qualities: the moon to the yang's male sun.

When this philosophy is translated into medical treatment, the quality of yin represents "internal" ailments that are not caused by sources outside the body. The yin illness comes from within, is chronic, and often is seemingly causeless. These illnesses tend to be functional in nature rather than pathological. In homeopathic jargon we refer to these illnesses as *psoric* in nature. They belong to the body of illnesses (and the miasm called *psora)* that are more often the result of lifestyle rather than contagion, and are often passed down to us as a part of our genetic legacy. Illnesses such as low blood sugar or arthritis may be considered yin ailments.

The yang illness is one which seems to attack from without, and is referred to as an "external" illness in TCM. Any acute illness is always considered to be a manifestation of yang in Chinese medicine, and will therefore require a yang response. This concept supports the idea that the acute homeopathic treatment is always more "active" than the constitutional treatment. The acute homeopathic treatment is a yang response in a yang situation. It always involves more remedies given more often and in more varied potencies than will a constitutional treatment corresponding with a chronic disease and yin treatment.

TCM provides an excellent context in which to consider constitutional and acute homeopathic treatment, as well as a guide to follow when determining our diagnosis and our pattern of treatment.

THE PRINCIPLES OF YIN AND YANG IN DIAGNOSIS

No matter the medical discipline, the process of diagnosis is always one of seeking information: seeking clues, if you will.

In traditional Chinese medicine, balance is the key to good health—balance between heat and cold, between excess and deficiency, and between yin and yang.

Among the earliest surviving Chinese medical texts, now many thousands of years old, is the *Classic of Medicine,* said to have been written by a mythical healer called the Yellow Emperor. According to this text, the principle of yin and yang underlies everything in the universe. It is the source both of life and of death. The male force, yang, may at times stand for creation and at other times for destruction. The female force, yin, stands for conservation. Yang leads to disintegration. Yin gives shape to things. Balance between these two forces is therefore required for health and wholeness.

The Yellow Emperor writes, "If Yang is overly powerful, then Yin may be too weak. If Yin is particularly strong, then Yang is apt to be defective. If the male force is overwhelming, then there will be excessive heat. If the female force is overwhelming, then there will be excessive cold. Exposure to repeated and severe heat will induce chills. Cold injures the body while heat injures the spirit. When the spirit is hurt, severe pain will ensue. When the body is hurt, there will be swelling. Thus, when severe pain occurs first and swelling develops later, one may infer that a disharmony in the spirit has done harm to the body. Likewise, when swelling appears first and severe pain in felt later on, on can say that a dysfunction in the body has injured the spirit..."

The text tells us that yang symptoms are linked to a boisterous and coarse person. It further tells us that when yang dominates, the body is not only hot, but also that the pores are closed and the patient begins to pant. As symptoms mount, the patient will have a mouth that is dry and sore. He becomes feverish, his stomach begins to feel tight, he becomes constipated, but he will not perspire. When yang is stronger, the patient is able to endure winter but not summer.

On the other hand, when yin is stronger, the patient will be cold, covered in cold perspiration and will tremble with chills. The colder he gets, the more rebellious his spirit becomes, and the less food he will be able to digest. When yin is stronger, the patient is able to endure summer but not winter.

Therefore, the patient must have yin and yang in balance if he is to be able to endure the changes of seasons, as well as all the changes that life periodically brings. Each must take its place of dominance and each must flow into a passive role as required.

The Yellow Emperor concludes, "By observing myself I learn about others, and their diseases become apparent to me. By observing the external symptoms, I gather knowledge about the internal diseases. One should watch for things out of the ordinary. One should observe minute and trifling things and treat them as if they were big and important. When they are treated the danger they pose will be dissipated. Experts in examining patients judge their general appearance; they feel their pulse and determine whether Yin or Yang predominates. With a disease of Yin, Yang predominates. When one is filled with vigor and strength, Yin and Yang are in perfect harmony."

Therefore, as we approach the process of diagnosis for any given case in TCM, we do so with an underlying understanding of the principle of yin and yang and use this principle as the basis for our diagnostic process.

The Four Examinations

We have to travel back to the fourth century in order to understand the concept of the "four examinations." At that time, a Chinese doctor named Pien Cueh first taught his method of evaluating his patients and the nature of their ailments. It is a technique that uses all of the practitioner's senses, like the best homeopathic evaluations.

Also, like homeopathic evaluations, the four examinations of TCM come out of a desire to treat the patient on a more fundamental level than just treating his disease.

Practitioners of TCM usually make a disease diagnosis, but like modern homeopaths, they seek to base their treatment on something more. In the same way that the selection of the homeopathic remedy is based upon the "totality of symptoms," the principle of pattern discrimination, called "bian zheng lun zhi," requires that the practitioner of TCM look deeper, beyond the disease, and understand the patterns and ebb and flow of the illness.

This is the information the TCM practitioner seeks through the process of the four examinations, which take place in the following way:

The First Examination: *"Looking."* Just as in homeopathy, the case taking in TCM begins, not with the first question, but when the practitioner first sees the patient. The physician inspects his patient from the moment of first sight, taking in all details that he can, but paying attention to the patient's movements, posture, clothing, and, especially, face. As part of this examination, the practitioner must pay close attention to the patient's tongue. The tongue is called "the gateway to the interior of the body."

The tongue provides important information, because it is the only visible part of the digestive tract. In TCM, it is said that the tongue reveals the patient's internal "climate." Knowledge of the tongue can lead to an understanding of specific ailments to which the patient is prone.

According to traditional Chinese medicine, the healthy tongue is pinkish-red, and is neither too dry nor too moist. It fits perfectly and moves freely about the mouth, and seems neither too large nor too small. This healthy tongue will likely have a thin, translucent white coating.

In terms of diagnosis, three elements of the tongue's nature must be studied and noted: the shape, the body of the tongue, and the coating. Any abnormality (any change from the state of perfect health noted above) in the tongue's texture, shapes and color helps guide the practitioner toward treatment.

Any abnormality in the tongue itself is also important, because the various areas of the tongue relate to other parts of the body. The tip of the tongue relates to the heart. Therefore, a discoloration of the tip may suggest a problem with the patient's heart. The area behind the tip, covering about the first third of the tongue, relates to the lungs. The center of the tongue relates to the spleen and pancreas, and especially to the stomach. A tongue that has a thick white coating in the center, therefore, usually means that the patient has a disordered stomach. The sides of the tongue relate to the liver and gall bladder, and the back or root of the tongue relates to the kidneys.

A more detailed study of the nature of the tongue in both TCM and homeopathy follows. For now, let us continue to consider the aspects of diagnosis.

The Second Examination: *"Listening and Smelling."* This aspect relates well to traditional homeopathic case taking, in which questions are asked and answered to establish not only the situation at hand, but also the general medical history of the patient. It may take place before the actual case taking, or may be a part of it. The practitioner must pay attention to the sound of the patient, including the pitch of his voice and his manner of speech, as much as to the actual words he is saying.

We go into detail on the actual verbal case taking both in terms of homeopathy and of TCM later, but I cannot stress enough now that the smelling part comes right up there with the listening in TCM. Therefore the physician can never afford to sit back and *passively* listen. He must always pay attention to the nonverbal as well as the verbal information his patient offers. This is why case taking by telephone is so very difficult, and taking a case over a computer is all but impossible.

The practitioner must be able to know how that patient smells, and what ailments and remedies are suggested by that smell. Just as any mother knows that her child is ill by his smell alone, it is said that the Chinese physician can diagnose medical problems before any word is uttered.

In this aspect of examination, it is vital that the practitioner pay attention to the manner in which the patient gives his information, because this manner itself will be suggestive of a path to follow in treatment. The sounds of a patient's voice, breathing, and/or cough are also important. A loud voice, for instance, often indicates excess yang, as will a sudden, violent cough.

In the same way, a patient with a quiet and weak voice is indicating deficiency. Note, however, that if the patient has lost his voice altogether this may indicate either deficiency or excess—more information is required to make a diagnosis.

In TCM, the patient who whines or speaks in a singsong manner is thought to have a disordered stomach, or to have problems in the spleen or pancreas. The patient who weeps may have issues in his large intestine or in the lungs. The patient who groans may be indicating kidney ailments or discomfort within his urinary system. The patient who shouts or speaks aggressively may have liver or gall bladder issues. And the patient who laughs inappropriately may have ailments related to the heart or the small intestine.

The Third Examination: *"Asking."* This is the actual verbal case taking, which follows a pattern in Chinese medicine that is almost identical to the homeopathic model. The patient is asked not only about his aches and pains, but also about his life, his whole being, and the modalities of the case. As in homeopathy, it is important that the questions not be leading, but, instead, simply give a platform upon which the patient may expound.

For the practitioner of TCM, perhaps the most important question has to do with how the patient responds to the external world and to his immediate environment. This certainly is a key question in homeopathic case taking as well, especially in the acute situation.

Among the basic questions asked are:
- What type of pain, if any, the patient is experiencing or recently experienced
- If the patient has suffered from either dizziness or headaches
- The patient's reaction to heat and to cold
- How much the patient perspires and when, and on what specific parts of the body
- The patient's appetite, what he craves and what he dislikes
- The patient's thirst patterns, what he craves, when he craves it, the temperature of the liquid he craves, and so on
- The patient's bowel and bladder function
- The patient's sleep patterns
- The patient's sex drive, sexual function; it may also be important to ask about the patient's reproductive history

Along with these questions, the patient will be asked to give his physician a general medical history, and a record of his physical activity, or lack thereof.

The patient may also be asked about his emotional history, the depth of the emotions he feels, and the patterns in which he feels them, because the patient's emotions are as important in TCM as they are in homeopathy.

The Fourth Examination: *"Touching."* At this point the practitioner must actually touch the patient. As in Western medicine, the practitioner of TCM uses *palpation,* or the touching of specific points on the abdomen and limbs of the patient. This aspect of the examination also usually involves touching the part of the body affected by the illness—the glands under the jaw, for example, for those with colds or flu—to get an idea of the exact site of the pain and the ways in which the illness has affected the body.

The most important part of this aspect of case taking is the taking of the pulse. For the practitioner of TCM, this is perhaps the most important diagnostic tool. It certainly is the aspect of case taking that takes the greatest amount of experience to master.

The pulse reading is most often taken from the radial artery near the wrist, although it may be taken from any pulse point on the body. Just as the tongue is considered a visible signpost of the internal climate of the body, the pulse offers a way to read the internal climate of his patient through the sense of touch. The pulse reveals three aspects of the patient's being: his energy, his blood circulation, and the condition of the different organ systems in the body.

The pulse is also evaluated on three levels—the superficial, the middle, and the deep level. The normal pulse is the middle-level pulse. That pulse rate is usually four or five beats per complete inhalation/exhalation of breath.

The most common descriptions of the pulse in TCM are: floating, slippery, choppy, wiry, tight, thin, empty, full, slow, and rapid.

The pulse is broken down into four categories of information: rate, rhythm, shape, and force. Of these, the rate is most commonly used as a diagnostic tool, as it is in Western medicine. A fast pulse usually suggests the presence of an infection and/or fever. It may also indicate pain. The rhythm relates to the regularity of the pulse beat, and is also considered in Western medicine.

The shape of the pulse, however, is unique to TCM. It is somewhat difficult to explain, in that it refers to the nature of the pulse itself, and whether it is hard or soft, and wide or narrow. While the shape of the patient's pulse is highly important to diagnosis in TCM, this aspect of a case does not translate into homeopathic practice. This is mostly due to the fact that the shape of the pulse has never been considered by homeopathic researchers, so no body of information is available about it.

Finally, there is the force of the pulse, which is an indicator of the patient's Vital Force. For instance, you should be able to feel the pulse while just lightly touching the skin in a normal healthy person. If the pulse punches out at you, it indicates there is too much yang. If it is hidden and hard to find, there is too much yin.

All told, there are twenty-eight different categories of pulse in TCM. Although homeopathic investigations do not use an equivalent level of detail for recording the information taken by pulse reading at this point, it is still an important aspect of homeopathic diagnosis because the manner and speed of the pulse will suggest specific remedies to the practitioner. Take a look at the chart on pulse diagnostics for more specific information.

The diagnostic tool of Touching also yields important information about the patient's unique response to being touched. Many practitioners of TCM touch key acupuncture points on the patient's body to test their response. Reflexology points on the patent's feet may also be used for the same purpose.

The four stages of case taking in traditional Chinese medicine—Looking, Listening, Asking, and Touching—not only parallel homeopathic case taking, but also enhance the homeopathic process, particularly in acute cases. I particularly encourage those who are new to homeopathic case taking to try to develop their use of each of these steps. Practice on those near and dear to you.

Try to see what information you can obtain about a person just by looking at them, listening to them, and touching them. Then fill in the rest with what you can learn verbally.

We must become better practitioners by relying less on the patient as the ultimate source of information and more our own eyes, ears, and hands, when we gather information concerning disease and formulate a plan for health.

Comparing and Contrasting: Diagnostic Tools in Homeopathy and Traditional Chinese Medicine

The TCM practitioner uses the four examinations to gather information for pattern discrimination, the method used to identify the overall pattern of illness in a patient. The pattern is identified through three unique groups of information obtained from the four examinations. The first set of information is based on the patient's specific symptoms, as described by the patient and witnessed by the practitioner during the examination. The second is based on the information obtained by reading the patient's tongue. The third is based on the information revealed by the patient's pulse. The practitioner safely and comfortably makes his diagnosis only by comparing these three independent sets of information.

Diagnosis in TCM is, therefore, a balance between objective and subjective case taking, weighted toward the objective. Tongue and pulse readings are totally objective, and symptom gathering is both objective and subjective, so the case taking methodology in traditional Chinese medicine mirrors the concept of Objective Homeopathy almost perfectly.

Let us consider the use of the tongue and pulse readings in TCM on a deeper level, and look at the ways this information can be put to use in homeopathic diagnosis to understand this better.

How information may be gathered concerning the patient's symptoms, and how this information can be processed and put to use in creating a diagnosis and formulating a treatment will be the topic of the next two chapters.

The Tongue as a Diagnostic Tool in TCM

The use of tongue diagnosis in traditional Chinese medicine is said to date back to the Shang dynasty, which began in 1600B.C. More and more information concerning tongue diagnosis has been added to the canon of TCM since that time, and it has become one of the most important of TCM's diagnostic tools.

In TCM, the tongue is considered to be an exterior part of the body and the only visible part of the digestive tract. It is therefore uniquely positioned to give specific information about the health of the body and the strength of the immune system.

In fact, some practitioners of TCM may go so far as to say that the tongue represents a microcosm of the entire body, and if it is interpreted correctly, all the information needed to treat the patient appropriately and correctly is located in and on the body and coating of the tongue.

A practitioner will examine the general and local shape of the tongue and the color of the tongue's body and coat. When you think of a healthy tongue, picture a kitten's tongue in your mind. A healthy tongue is pink, moist but not too wet, and has a thin white coat on it.

The tongue's body is the fleshy mass of the organ itself. It has color, texture, and shape, which must be considered separately from the color and texture of the coating on top of the tongue. The physician examining the patient's tongue looks first at the tongue's body, color, size, and shape. He also checks any coating of the tongue and any abnormalities. Finally, he checks the moistness or dryness of the tongue, and of any coating of the tongue.

Tongue body color. The color of the tongue's body is an important consideration in diagnosis, and can provide a great deal of information regarding the health of the patient. Tongue colors are categorized as follows:

• *Pale Tongue*

A pale tongue may range from one that is completely white to one that is only slightly paler than the healthy "kitten" pink. A pale tongue is also likely to be a very moist tongue, and is often plumper than usual. The pale tongue may also be "indented," in that it is swollen enough to show the indentations of the teeth running along its side.

A pale tongue indicates a deficiency of yang. It also indicates a lowered metabolism, low blood pressure, anemia, and poor circulation. Some practitioners of TCM believe that a pale tongue indicates a long, slow recovery from illness.

- *Red Tongue*

A red tongue indicates an excess of heat or of yang in the body. It always indicates a pathological condition: some condition has raised the basal metabolism and changed the tongue's color to red.

A bright red tongue is an indication of fever.

A bright red tongue that is very dry is an important indication of acute dehydration.

In general, a red tongue is likely to be an indication of inflammation in the body. It will be found linked to cases of upper respiratory infection, pneumonia, and fever.

- *Purple Tongue*

The so-called purple tongue may actually be bluish, purplish, or reddish-purple in color. Whatever the color mixture, it is known as the "cyanic tongue." It is an indicator of sluggish Chi, which in homeopathy is called "Vital Force."

The bluish tongue is especially indicative of sluggish blood flow. It may be a sign of long-term heart or circulatory disease. It may also indicate high blood pressure.

The purple tongue may be a strong indicator of alcoholism. It may be an indicator of liver disease.

No matter the specific diseases indicated, the cyanic tongue is always a sign of a sluggish life force. It is also a sign of long-term illness.

Note that the cyanic tongue may not always be entirely purple or blue. Some tongues may have only some parts that have become purple, usually the tip and sides, while the rest of the tongue is still pink. This tongue should still be considered cyanic.

Tongue coating. A tongue's coating may be described as "moss" or "fur." The coating is created when small amounts of impurities arise from the digestive tract. When the stomach and spleen are acting in balance, the coating will have a uniform density, with a slightly thicker area in the center of the tongue. A thick coating, in general, indicates excess. A thin coating, in times of illness, indicates deficiency. Note that the thick coating is usually attributed to good health. The color of the tongue's coating is also important:

• *White Coating*

A white coating is the color most commonly seen. Unless this coating is very thick or fuzzy, it is a sign that the patient is more or less in good health, and that there is nothing signifi-cantly wrong with the patient.

• *Yellow Coating*

A yellow coating is the next in terms of level of health or illness. The coating may be anywhere from pale yellow to nearly a shade of brown. This is a sign that the patient is becoming more ill and can indicate anything from fever to, most commonly, digestive disorder.

• *Gray to Black Coating*

A gray to black coating indicates that the patient is suffering either from a long-lasting illness or from one that is quite serious. Note that drug addiction and the use of antibiotics can also lead to a black coating of the tongue.

Other tongue characteristics. The size of the tongue also indicates deficiency or excess. A small tongue relates to deficiency, while a swollen tongue indicates excess.

Remember, the healthy tongue is ruddy, it moves quickly and easily around the mouth, and it is constantly moist. The more aspects of a healthy tongue a patient's tongue displays, the better his overall health. Therefore, a tongue that is moist and supple and moves easily even though it has a gray or black coating still indicates a fairly strong and healthy patient. On the other hand, a shrunken and dry tongue that is sluggish in its movement and causing slurred speech indicates poor health, even if it has only a very thin white coating.

Abnormalities may also yield important information. For instance, cracks in the tongue are very common. They usually run from front to back in the center of the tongue. Shallow cracks are usually considered to be a fairly benign symptom, if they are a symptom at all. Other cracks include the long or short horizontal, which run from side to side; the transverse, which run along the tongue's sides; the irregular, which resemble little islands on the tongue; and vertical cracks, which are usually very deep and run from the center of the tongue to the tip.

The child who is born with a cracked tongue may be considered by some to have a weakened constitution.

Those who are born with what are called "hills and valleys" on the tongue are said to have a "geographic tongue." This is also known as a "mapped tongue," because the tongue has a maplike appearance. This characteristic is created by atrophy of the tongue's papillae, and the lack of formation of some papillae, in well-defined areas. Some mapped tongues may peel in several areas at once, which is called "denuded tongue."

While many Chinese practitioners believe that this abnormality is benign, some TCM practitioners believe that it also indicates a congenital weakness in the patient's constitution.

Another noted abnormality is the "indented tongue." This is also known as a "scalloped tongue," and it refers to a swollen tongue that has indentations of the teeth running along the sides of the tongue. In TCM the indented tongue is a sign of many different conditions, such as high blood pressure. In homeopathy, it is a powerful indicator of a handful of remedies, including Mercurius.

Diagnostic Indicators in Homeopathic Medicine: The Tongue

If we can adapt the methods of TCM and apply them to homeopathy, then we can learn to read the patient's tongue for clues to the nature of his disease and the remedies that might lead to cure, and we will have a powerful tool for healing.

While homeopathic research has not yet turned its full attention to the tongue (or to the pulse, for that matter), the following information, adapted from several repertories, will be useful as we develop our skills in the art of Objective Diagnosis.

These diagnostics are divided into three simple categories: Color, in which the tongue body itself is a specific color; Discolorations, in which tongue is coated with a specific color coating; and Distortions, which represent physical changes to the shape and texture of the tongue:

Tongue body color. As it does for the TCM practitioner, the color of the tongue body provides important information. The homeopathic practitioner uses these clues to identify remedies. Note that remedies listed first are best or most commonly used. "Also" remedies may be needed, but they are less likely.

• *Pale Tongue*

A pale tongue especially suggests: Mercurius. Also: Arsenicum, Natrum Mur, Sepia, and Veratrum. Also consider: Phosphorus.

If the tongue is very pale, consider: Arsenicum, Ipecac, Natrum Mur, Sepia, and Veratrum. Especially: Mercurius.

• *Red Tongue*

A red tongue especially suggests: Apis, Arsenicum, Belladonna, Mercurius, Phosphorus, and Rhus Tox. Also: Sulphur, Carbo Veg, Calcarea, Lachesis, Lycopodium, and Veratrum. Also: Gelsemium, Colocynthis, Spongia, and Nux.

If only the center of the tongue is red, consider: Phosphorus and Rhus Tox.

If only the base of the tongue is red, consider: Bryonia.

If only the edges of the tongue are red, consider especially: Arsenicum, Mercurius, or Sulphur. Also: Aconite, Gelsemium, Kali Bi, Phosphorus, or Rhus Tox.

If the tongue is red only in streaks, consider: Antimonium Tartaricum. Also: Chamomilla

If the tongue is a bright, fiery red, consider: Apis or Belladonna.

If only the tip of the tongue is fiery red, consider: Rhus Tox. Also: Arsenicum and Sulphur.

If the tip of the tongue has a red triangle, consider: Rhus Tox.

If the tongue is red and shiny, consider: Apis, Phosphorus, Rhus Tox, and especially, Kali-Bi.

If a tongue is red with a black coating, consider: Merc and Nux V.

• *Purple/Blue Tongue*

A purple tongue suggests: Lachesis.

A blue tongue suggests especially: Arsenicum. Also: Antimonium Tartaricum, Podophyllum, and Spigelia.

Tongue coating discolorations. The following discolorations suggest remedies as follows:

• *General*

If the tongue is very clean, consider: Ipecac, and Rhus Tox.

In general, for a coated tongue, consider: Bryonia and Nux. Also: Mercurius, Belladonna, Chinchona, Phosphorus, Pulsatilla, and Sulphur.

If the tongue is coated diagonally, consider: Rhus Tox.

If the coating is one-sided, consider: Rhus Tox.

• *White Coating*

If the tongue is coated white, consider: Arsenicum, Belladonna, and Pulsatilla. Also consider: Sulphur, Carbo Veg, Spigelia, Lachesis, Gelsemium, Apis, Arnica, Cina, and Chinchona. Also: Phosphorus, Mercurius, Calcarea, and Kali Bi. Also: Sabadilla, Symphytum, Lycododium, Hypericum, and Podophyllum.

A thick, white coating especially suggests: Belladonna, Bryonia, Calcarea, Kali-Bi, Mercurius, Pulsatilla, and Sulphur. Also: Arnica, Carbo Veg, Lycopodium, Natrum Mur, and Rhus Tox. A thick, white coating on a tongue that is slimy and pasty suggests: Antimonium Tartaricum, Mercurius, Pulsatilla, Sepia, and Chelidonium. Also consider: Bryonia, Calcarea, Nux, Sulphur, Lycopodium, and Ipecac.

A tongue with a white center coating suggests: Bryonia. Also Gelsemium, Phosphorus, and Sulphur.

A tongue that is coated white only on the sides suggests: Causticum. Also: Chamomilla.

A tongue that is coated white only on one side suggests: Rhus Tox.

A milky-white tongue coating suggests: Belladonna.

A tongue that is coated white only in the morning suggests: Pulsatilla. Also: Phosphorus, Chinchona, and Sulphur.

A tongue coating that is so white that it seems to have been painted suggests: Arsenicum.

A tongue coating that is silvery white suggests: Arsenicum.

A pale tongue that is coated white suggests: Arsenicum, Aconite, and Phosphorus.

• *Yellow/Brown Coating*

A yellow tongue coating especially suggests: Lycopodium, Pulsatilla, Mercurius, and Rhus Tox. Also: Bryonia, Gelsemium, Hepar Sulph, Ipecac, Lachesis, Sepia, and Sulphur. Also: Carbo Veg, Sabadilla, Spigelia, Nux, Kali Bi, Chinchona, Chamomilla, Belladonna, Natrum Mur, and Bryonia.

A tongue with a thick, yellow coating suggests: Mercurius, Pulsatilla, or Sulphur. Also Bryonia, and Carbo Veg. Also Nux.

A tongue that is coated yellow only at the base suggests: Mercurius, Nux, and Kali Bi.

A tongue that is coated yellow only in the center suggests: Bryonia, and Pulsatilla. A tongue that is coated bright, shiny yellow suggests: Apis.

A tongue that is coated dirty yellow suggests: Mercurius, Arsenicum, and Lachesis.

A tongue that is coated mustard yellow suggests: Podophyllum.

A yellow/white tongue coating suggests especially: Rhus Tox. Also: Arsenicum, Belladonna, Cocculus, Gelsemium, and Kali Bi.

A very thick yellow/white coating suggests: Arsenicum, and Gelsemium.

A yellow/white coating only at the base of the tongue suggests: Rhus Tox.

A yellow/brown coated tongue suggests especially: Carbo Veg. Also: Cina.

A brown-coated tongue suggests especially: Bryonia, Lachesis, Phosphorus, and Rhus Tox. Also: Belladonna, Carbo Veg, Nux, and Sulphur.

A tongue that is coated brown only in the center suggests: Phosphorus, Arnica, Arsenicum, and Bryonia.

If the tongue is coated brown only in the center, with sides that are shiny and moist, consider: Apis.

If the tongue is coated brown only in the center, with sides that are white and moist, consider: Arnica.

A tongue that is coated brown only on the sides suggests: Kali Bi.

A tongue that is coated brown only in the morning suggests: Rhus Tox.

A brown-coated tongue with a red tip and sides suggests: Rhus Tox, and Lycopodium.

• *Gray to Black Coating*

A gray tongue coating suggests especially: Phosphorus. Also: Pulsatilla, Antimonium Tartaricum, Bryonia.

A tongue that is coated gray only in the center suggests: Phosphorus.

A black tongue coating suggests especially: Carbo Veg, Mercurius, and Phosphorus. Also: Arsenicum, Lachesis, Lycopodium, and Nux. A tongue that is blackened only in the center suggests: Phosphorus. Also: Mercurius.

If only the edges of the tongue are darkened to black, consider: Petroleum.

Distortions of the tongue. The following distortions should be considered when selecting a homeopathic remedy:

• *Dry Tongue*

If the tongue is very dry, consider especially: Aconite, Apis, Arsenicum, Belladonna, Bryonia, Calcarea, Lachesis, Mercurius, Pulsatilla, Rhus Tox, and Sulphur. Also: Ipecac, Phosphorus, and Natrum Mur.

If the tongue is dry only in the center, consider especially: Phosphorus, Antimonium Tartaricum, and Rhus Tox. Consider also: Lachesis, Veratrum, and Aconite.

If the tongue is dry only on the edges, consider especially: Belladonna, Mercurius, and Rhus Tox. Consider also: Lachesis, Kali Bi, Antimonium Tartaricum, and Arsenicum.

If the tongue is dry on the tip, consider: Carbo Veg, Nux, and Rhus Tox. Also: Belladonna, Pulsatilla, and Phosphorus.

If the tongue is dry at the root, consider: Allium Cepa.

• *Moist Tongue*

A very moist mouth with increased saliva suggests: Mercurius.

• *Cracked Tongue*

If the tongue is cracked, consider especially: Arsenicum, Phosphorus, and Rhus Tox. Also consider: Belladonna, Bryonia, Calcarea, Lachesis, and Lycopodium. Also Mercurius, Sulphur, and Veratrum.

If the tongue is cracked down the middle, consider: Bryonia, and Rhus Tox.

If the tongue is cracked across the middle, consider: Lachesis, and Mercurius.

If the tongue is cracked down the edges, consider: Nux and Lachesis.

If the tongue is cracked on the tip, consider: Lachesis.

If a tongue has deep cracks or furrows running lengthwise on the upper part, consider: Mercurius.

• *Mapped Tongue*

If the tongue is mapped, consider especially: Natrum Mur. Also: Arsenicum, Rhus Tox, Lachesis, Mercurius, and Kali Bi. Also: Dulcamara, Chamomilla, Lycopodium, Sepia, Petroleum, and Symphytum.

• *Indented Tongue*

If the tongue is indented, consider especially: Mercurius, Arsenicum, and Rhus Tox. Consider also: Sepia, Pulsatilla, Ignatia, Kali Bi, and Dulcamara.

If the tongue is indented and flabby and moist, consider: Mercurius and Rhus Tox. Also: Kali Bi and Arsenicum.

• *Swollen Tongue*

If the tongue is swollen, consider especially: Apis, Aconite, and Mercurius. Consider also: Arsenicum, Belladonna, and Lachesis. Also: Phosphorus, Dulcamara, and Natrum Mur.

If the base of the tongue is swollen, consider: Arsenicum.

If the center of the tongue is swollen, consider: Phosphorus.

If the tip of the tongue is swollen, consider: Natrum Mur.

If only one side of the tongue is swollen, consider: Silicea. Also: Apis, and Mercurius. If the left side is swollen, consider: Lachesis. If the right side is swollen, consider: Apis. Also: Thuja.

If the tongue has the sensation of being swollen, consider: Nux. Also: Pulsatilla, and Gelsemium.

If the tongue is swollen and feels as if it has been stung by and insect, consider: Apis. Also: Aconite, Belladonna, Natrum Mur, and Mercurius.

A patient who is always biting his tongue suggests: Ignatia, and Causticum.

• *Shrunken or Shriveled Tongue*

If the tongue is shrunken or shriveled, consider: Arsenicum.

If the tongue is withered, consider: Phosphorus.

• *Bleeding Tongue*

Bleeding from the tongue suggests: Lachesis, and Mercurius. Also consider: Calcarea, Arsenicum, Bali Bi, Lycopodium, Nux, and Phosphorus. Also: Sepia, and Natrum Mur.

If the bleeding comes from the tip of the tongue, consider: Lachesis, and Phosphorus.

The Pulse as a Diagnostic Tool in TCM

This process of pulse reading in the practice of TCM dates back around two thousand years. A great deal of emphasis was placed upon pulse reading in earlier times, but some modern practitioners have come to use the process as only a method of confirming information obtained through the gathering of symptoms and the reading of the tongue.

In the past, the practitioner was said to be able to discover if any organ in the body was diseased and whether the organ was overactive or underactive through the palpation of the pulse. It is also said that it was possible for the practitioner to know whether the disease was acute or chronic and to give a prognosis by pulse diagnosis alone.

Once TCM grew and spread across the world, the number of practitioners who were able to discern such incredible amounts of information from the pulse alone dropped to just a handful. Indeed, the number of practitioners who were able to take the multiple pulses at all fell dramatically. And so the process of pulse taking was simplified.

The classical practitioner of TCM gathered information by feeling both the superficial and the deep pulse from three different positions on each wrist, each located only about a centimeter from each other. This gave a total of six pulses on each wrist: three superficial and three deep. When both wrists were considered in diagnosis, these were called "the twelve pulses."

Today, most TCM practitioners have not been trained to practice with the twelve pulses. Instead, they use what is called "pulse generalization," and take the pulse from the wrist, as is traditional in the West. The practitioner uses these readings to determine whether the pulse from each wrist is excessive or deficient, and to measure the flow the blood as well as the Chi and all the many fluids flowing through the entire body. But, without a complete understanding of the twelve pulses, practitioners can no longer diagnose the health of the organs of the body through pulse diagnosis alone. They therefore turn to the information gathered in the symptoms and the tongue reading for verification of diagnosis.

In Western medicine, of course, the pulse is only used to obtain information regarding the rate, rhythm, and volume of the heartbeat. Since homeopathy is a creation of the Western mind, if not of Western medicine, the pulse is less important as a diagnostic tool in homeopathy than it is in TCM, and there has not been much research to discover how we can make better use of the information it provides.

An earlier section in this chapter about the "four examinations" described the different pulses considered in TCM. Now, let us see what the homeopathic repertory can tell us about pulse and heartbeat.

Diagnostic Indicators in Homeopathic Medicine: The Pulse

While the consideration of a patient's pulse is not as developed in homeopathic practice as it is in traditional Chinese medicine, it still represents an important diagnostic indicator. A simple pulse reading can lead to the selection of a specific remedy as follows:

Fast(rapid/accelerated/elevated/exalted) pulse. For a patient with a fast pulse, consider especially: Aconite. Also: Apis, Belladonna, Mercurius, Ignatia, and Rhus Tox. Also: Spigelia, Nux, Natrum Mur, and Gelsemium. Also consider: Arnica, Sepia, Spongia, Silicea, Lachesis, Bryonia, Chamomilla, and Hypericum. Also: Carbo Veg, Sabadilla, Staphysagria, and Lycopodium.

Consider the following remedies for specific beats per minute:
- 80 beats: Phosphorus
- 85 beats: Lachesis

- 90 beats: Antimonium Tartaricum, and Mercurius
- 100 beats: Ignatia
- 120 beats: Ignatia, Lachesis, and Lycopodium. Also: Rumex, and Sulphur
- 125 beats: Sulphur
- 130 beats: Silicea, and Mercurius
- 140 beats: Cina. Also: Sulphur
- 150 beats: Mercurius

Specific remedies are suggested if the pulse is rapid at a specific time of day:

For the pulse that is fast in the morning, consider: Arsenicum. Also: Sulphur, Chinchona, Phosphorus, and Ingnatia.

If the pulse is fast in the forenoon, consider: Calcarea, and Lycopodium.

If the pulse is fast in the afternoon, consider: Lycopodium. Also: Gelsemium, Phosphorus, and Podophyllum.

If the pulse is fast in the evening, consider: Causticum. Also consider: Dulcamara, Lachesis, Lycopodium, Phosphorus, Nux, and Sulphur. Also: Euphrasia, Hypericum, Sepia, Silicea, and Arsenicum.

If the pulse is fast at night, consider: Dulcamara, and Nux.

If the pulse is fast in the evening and slow during the day, consider: Arsenicum, Chinchona, Ignatia, Lycopodium, and Phosphorus.

If the pulse is fast at night and slow during the day, consider especially: Sepia. Also: Silicea, Bryonia, Mercurius, and Sulphur. Also: Natrum Mur, Phosphorus, and Dulcamara.

If a pulse is fast in the morning but slow in the evening and at night, consider: Arsenicum. Also: Ignatia, Calcarea, and Lycopodium. Also: Nux.

Rapid pulse rates accompanied by certain conditions suggest specific remedies:

If the pulse seems to be more rapid than the heart beat, consider: Rhus Tox, and Spigelia. Also: Aconite, and Arnica.

If the pulse is rapid and indistinct, so that it cannot be counted, consider: Antimonium Tartaricum, Lachesis, Lycopodium, and Mercurius.

If any motion or movement makes the pulse race, consider especially: Natrum Mur. Also: Gelsemium, Bryonia, Arnica Nus, Petroleum, Sepia, Staphysagria, and Phosphorus.

If the pulse is rapid during fever, consider: Ruta.

If the pulse is rapid during croup, consider: Aconite. Also: Antimonium Tartaricum, Belladonna, and Hepar Sulph.

If the pulse is rapid with diarrhea, consider: Sulphur.

If the pulse is rapid in pneumonia, consider: Antimonium Tartaricum. Also: Mercurius, Sulphur, and Nux.

If the pulse is rapid in heart disease, consider: Lachesis, and Arnica. Also: Carbo Veg. Also: Ignatia.

If the pulse is rapid during convulsions, consider: Veratrum.

Slow pulse. For the patient with a slow pulse, consider: Gelsemium. Also: Sepia, Natrum Mur, Antimonium Tartaricum, and Camphora. Also: Nux, Kali Bi, Arnica, Arsenicum, Dulcamara, and Mercurius.

Consider the following remedies for specific beats per minute:

- 60 (at rest, 120 in motion): Arnica
- 62: Antimonium Tartaricum

Specific remedies are suggested if the pulse is slow at a specific time of day or is accompanied by certain conditions:

If the pulse is slow, but jumps to a high rate with slight exertion, consider: Arnica.

If pulse is slow during the daytime, consider: Dulcamara, and Sepia.

If pulse is slow in the evening, consider: Arsenicum.

Intermittent pulse. For the patient whose pulse is intermittent (the pulse stops and starts, and skips beats), consider especially: Mercurius,

Natrum Mur, and Chinchona. Also: Arsenicum, Spigelia, Rhus Tox, Sulphur, and Aconite.

Consider the following remedies depending upon when the intermittent beats occur:

- Every other beat, consider: Natrum Mur, and Spigelia.
- Every third beat, consider: Apis, Natrum Mur, and Sulphur.
- Every fourth beat, consider: Apis, Nux, and Sulphur.
- Every fifth beat, consider: Nux.

Intermittent pulse accompanied by certain conditions suggests specific remedies:

If an intermittent pulse is accompanied by fear of death, consider: Natrum Mur.

If an intermittent pulse is accompanied by heart disease, consider: Arsenicum.

If an intermittent pulse is accompanied by nose bleed, consider: Rhus Tox.

If accompanied by fever, consider: Mercurius.

Hard pulse. For the patient whose pulse is hard and pounding, consider: Aconite, Belladonna, Bryonia, and Graphites. Also: Allium Cepa, Lachesis, Ledum, Phosphorus, Mercurius, Dulcamara, Gelsemium, and Hepar Sulph. If the pulse is hard and fast, consider: Dulcamara.

Specific remedies are suggested if the pulse is hard at a specific time of day:

If pulse is hard in the morning, consider: Petroleum.

If pulse is hard in the evening, consider: Allium Cepa, and Dulcamara.

Hard pulse accompanied by certain conditions suggests specific remedies:

If pulse is accompanied by fever, consider: Colocynthis.

If pulse is accompanied by headache, consider: Gelsemium.

If pulse is accompanied by pneumonia, consider: Antimonium Tartaricum. Also: Veratrum.

Soft (faint/low/imperceptible) pulse. If the pulse is faint and almost imperceptible, consider: Carbo Veg. Also: Aconite, Camphora, and Gelsemium. Also: Spongia, Pulsatilla, Rhus Tox, Apis, Arsenicum, and Ipecac. Also: Ledum, and Lachesis.

If the pulse is faint and irregular (changes pace and patterns) with palpitations, consider: Pulsatilla.

Soft pulse accompanied by certain conditions suggests specific remedies:

If the pulse is faint and is accompanied by pneumonia, consider: Phosphorus.

If the pulse is faint and is accompanied by fever, consider: Arsenicum.

Irregular/changeable pulse. For the patient with an irregular pulse, consider:

Lachesis, Natrum Mur, Arsenicum, and Kali Bi. Also: Rhus Tox, Sulphur, Spigelia, Mercurius, Gelsemium, Hepar Sulph, Sepia, and Phosphorus. Also: Silicea.

If the pulse is slow and irregular, consider: Arnica, Aconite, Arsenicum Belladonna, Camphora, Chinchona, Dulcamara, Nux, and Silicea.

Specific remedies are suggested if the pulse is irregular at a specific time of day or is accompanied by certain conditions:

If pulse is irregular in the morning, consider: Causticum.

If pulse is accompanied by heart disease, consider: Arsenicum, and Lachesis.

If pulse is accompanied by fever, consider: Lachesis, and Mercurius.

Skin Color as a Diagnostic Tool in TCM (Facial Diagnosis)

Although it is not as integral to diagnosis as either the reading of the tongue or pulse, the evaluation of face color is still an important diagnostic tool for the practitioner of TCM. An evaluation of facial color as a part of the first examination can offer clues to the nature and severity of a patient's condition. Different methods of face diagnosis have developed over many years, and today the Chinese, Japanese, and Korean methods dominate.

Facial diagnosis concerns itself with five colors, each of which is related to the activity of a particular organ or system within the body. Red is related to the heart, white to the lungs, yellow to the spleen, green to the liver, and black to the kidneys.

The practitioner looks at the patient's face to see which, if any, of the five colors dominates. He then also notes the quality of the color. (Note that it is important that the patient's face be studied in natural light in both TCM and homeopathy. Outdoor light is preferable, if possible.)

The quality of the patient's face color will indicate the intensity of the illness:

If the color is bright and fresh, then the disease is still very much on the surface of the body and easily cured.

If the color is scattered over a large area of the face, then the disease is not severe.

If the color is dark and the skin looks cloudy, then the disease is moving deeper into the body and will be harder to cure.

If the color is intense and dark and gathered into one spot on the face, then the disease is deep and chronic, and will be very difficult to cure.

The five colors and their related organs. As to the five colors and the organs to which they relate:

- *Red—the color of the heart*

In TCM, red is the yang color. It is not only the color of the heart, but also of the element fire. Thus, when red is present, it represents excess. It may be an emotional excess, such as great joy, or it may be a physical excess, such as an excess of alcoholic beverages. No matter what else it represents, it always relates to an "exuberance of the heart." This is not to say that it always indicates heart disease; indeed, a reddish face may be a sign of health. When the red color moves toward purple or brown, however, it is far more likely to indicate cardiac trouble.

- *White—the color of the lungs*

The patient with a constitutionally weakened respiratory system will have a whitish complexion. These patients have the tendency toward a weak constitution and must always be concerned with the state of their health. The presence of a white complexion does not, in and of itself, suggest disease in the lungs, but when that chronically white face is overlaid with a reddish color, it is time for concern. The overlay of red gives the white complexion a peach-colored tinge, which suggests lung disease. Sick or well, the patient with the whitish complexion is said to be a worrier, and tends to sigh frequently.

106

- *Yellow—the color of the spleen*

Since yellow is the color for the element earth in TCM, and both the spleen and the stomach relate to this element, it may be suggested that yellow also relates to the stomach. Both organs carry out tasks related to the earth element. The spleen produces the blood for the body, and the stomach digests the food that supplies the body with energy. As with the other colors, the mere presence of yellow in the complexion is not a sign of illness. Indeed, the patient with a healthy and lustrous yellow-toned complexion may be said to have a strong digestion and constitution. It is the patient with a sallow yellow color, who also appears fatigued, who indicates digestive disorder.

- *Blue—the color of the liver* [Cyanosis]

Blue is the color of stagnation. While a fresh red color suggests a strong circulation, and blood that is oxygen-enriched as it is pumped, a blue-toned complexion suggests that venous blood is stagnant in the tissues, and that the blood and body are not being purified. This suggests that the heart is weak and not doing its job. In TCM, the organ that regulates the activity of the heart is the liver, so the patient with a blue complexion may be said to be "liverish." This patient is toxic, and, as a result, is overly sensitive, and susceptible to sudden anger and indigestion. Unlike red and yellow, no tone of blue indicates good health. Like white, the conditions suggested by the color blue are chronic and debilitating.

• *Blackened—the color of the kidneys*

Black is a mysterious color, the color of deep water. It relates to yin and the forces of cold, and is the opposite of red from the perspective of TCM. Patients with a blacktoned complexion are usually among our coldest patients. They will likely have a low sex drive, and are often motivated by fear. Now, some patients with black complexions can be healthy. In fact, those who are healthy are very healthy indeed, because they have been able to overcome innate weaknesses. These patients tend to have great physical and sexual energy. Note that many patients have black marks on their faces—freckles and blotches of all sorts—instead of an overall black complexion. These marks can be indicators of disease, or of hormone changes in the body, like those associated with pregnancy.

Diagnostic Indicators in Homeopathic Medicine: The Face

While the homeopathic study of the human face and complexion does not include the underlying philosophy held by tradition Chinese medicine, specific discolorations of the face are considered important indicators for guiding the selection of an appropriate remedy.

Discolorations of the face. The homeopathic diagnostic indicators are as follows:

• *Red Face*

A red face suggests especially: Aconite, Apis, Belladonna, Bryonia, Nux, Phosphorus, Rhus Tox, Lachesis, or Sulphur. Also: Dulcamara, Eupatorium, Ignatia, Arnica, Arsenicum, Camphora, Carbo Veg, and Mercurius. Also: Pulsatilla, Podophyllum, Rumex, Sabadilla, and Ruta.

A face that is dark red suggests: Belladonna, and Bryonia. Also: Sulphur, and Antimonium Tartaricum.

A face that is bright, glowing red suggests: Belladonna, and Cina. Also: Aconite, Calcarea, Coffea, Lachesis, Natrum Mur, and Spongia. Also: Sulphur, Lycopodium, Camphora, Calcarea, Bryonia, and Pulsatilla.

A face that alternates red and pale suggests: Aconite. Also: Belladonna, Ignatia, Nux, and Rhus Tox. Also: Sepia, Pulsatilla, Cina, and Camphora.

A face that is red in circumscribed patches suggests: Phosphorus, Sulphur, Chinchona, and Dulcamara. Also: Lachesis, Mercurius, Natrum Mur, Antimonium Tartaricum, Lycopodium, Silicea, Sepia, and Spongia.

A face with red spots on it suggests: Belladonna, Phosphorus, Sabadilla, and Sulphur. Also: Lysocpodium, Silicea, Mercurius, Natrum Mur, and Petroleum.

A face with one-sided redness suggests: Aconite, and Phosphorus. Also: Pulsatilla, Antimonium Tartaricum, Arsenicum, Drosera, Cina, Lycopodium, Mercurius, Natrum Mur, Rhus Tox, Sepia, Spigelia, and Sulphur.

A face that has one cheek red and the other pale suggests: Chamomilla. Also: Ipecac, Aconite, Pulsatilla, and Sulphur.

A face that has two bright red cheeks suggests: Belladonna, especially if the face feels hot and dry to the touch. Also: Phosphorus.

A face that is red across both cheeks and the bridge of the nose suggests: Sulphur.

A face that is red across the forehead, usually in spots, suggests: Sulphur.

A face that is red on the chin suggests: Natrum Mur.

A face that seems as if it is constantly blushing suggests: Sulphur.

A face with an all-over ruddy color suggests: Arnica.

If the skin is discolored a reddish/yellow, consider: Nux. Also Gelsemium, and Lachesis.

If the skin is discolored a reddish/blue, consider: Belladonna, or Bryonia. Also: Aconite, Apis, and Hepar Sulph. Also: Camphora, Lachesis, Lycopodium, Phosphorus, Pulsatilla, Petroleum, and Eupatorium.

- *White (Pale) Face*

A pale face suggests especially: Arsenicum, Carbo Veg, Natrum Mur, and Ferrum Phos. Also: Cina, Antimonium Tartarticum, Camphora, Chamomilla, and Apis. Also: Mercurius, Lycopodium, Chinchona, Bryonia, Phosphorus, Pulsatilla, Podophyllum, Rhus Tox, Silicea, Spongea, Spigelia, and Sabadilla.

A face that has taken on an ashy or pale color during illness should lead you to consider: Arsenicum, or Phosphorus. Also: Sulphur, or Kali Bi.

A face that alternates between pale and red suggests: Aconite, Camphora, Belladonna, Arsenicum, Ignatia, Nux, Pulsatilla, Rhus Tox, Sepia, and Chamomilla.

A face that is pale only on one side suggests: Chamomilla. Also: Ipecac, Ignatia, Belladonna, Arnica, Aconite, and Nux.

If the face is pale only around the mouth, consider especially: Cina. Also: Ferrum Phos, and Belladonna.

- *Yellow Face*

A face that is yellow suggests especially: Lycopodium, Nux, Sepia, and Sulphur. Also: Arsenicum, Carbo Veg, Calcarea, Natrum Mur, and Phosphorus. Also: Ferrum Phos, Cina, Chinchona, Silicea, Apis, and Aconite.

If the face has a yellow forehead, consider: Phosphorus

If the face is yellow around the eyes, consider: Nux, and Spigelia.

If the face is yellow on or around the nose, consider: Sepia, and Nux.

If the face is yellow around the temples, consider: Causticum.

If the face is yellow across the cheeks, consider: Sepia.

If the face is yellow in spots, consider: Sepia.

If the face is discolored brown, consider: Sepia, and Sulphur.

A face that has taken on a clay-colored or earth tone suggests: Mercurius, or Sepia. Also consider: Arnica, Natrum Mur, Pulsatilla, and Bryonia. Also: Phosphorus.

For the face that looks grayish in color, consider especially: Lycopodium. Also: Arsenicum, and Carbo Veg.

For the face that is grayish/yellow, consider especially: Lycopodium. Also: Carbo Veg.

• *Blue (Blue/Green) Face*

For a face that is bluish, consider especially: Arsenicum, Lachesis, Belladonna, Carbo Veg, Lachesis, and Veratrum. Also: Apis, and Nux. Also: Sulphur, Lycopodium, Natrum Mur,

Hepar Sulph, Cina, Chamomilla, Drosera, and Dulcamara.

If the cheeks are blue, consider: Chamomilla

If the area under and around the eyes is blue, consider: Nux, Lycopodium, Rhus Tox, Sabadilla, and Phosphorus. Also: Arsenicum, Aconite, Cina, Chamomilla, Cocculus, and Ferrum Phos.

If the forehead is blue, consider: Apis.

If the area around the mouth is blue, consider: Cina. Also: Sulphur, Arsenicum, and Sabadilla.

If the face is blue only in spots, consider: Lachesis. Also: Apis, Ledum, and Lachesis.

For a face that looks greenish, consider: Carbo Veg. Also: Pulsatilla, or Arsenicum.

• *Blackened Face*

A face with a black hue suggests: Chinchona. Also: Lachesis, and Camphora.

A face that is said to be "lead colored" suggests: Natrum Mur. Also: Arsenicum, Lachesis, and Mercurius.

A face that is spotted black (or black and blue), suggests: Lachesis. Also: Arnica, Phosphorus, and Rhus Tox.

• *Other Facial Indicators*

A face that has a "sickly" color suggests: Arsenicum, Calcarea, and Lycoposium. Also:

Mercurius, Apis, Carbo Veg, Chinchona, Cina, Phosphorus, Sulphur, and Nux. Also: Spigelia, Podophyllum, and Rhus Tox.

A face with a sallow tone suggests: Carbo Veg, Natrum Mur, and Sulphur. Also: Lachesis, Nux, Apis, Arnica, and Podophyllum.

A face with a dark hue suggests: Sulphur. Also: Belladonna, and Bryonia. Also: Gelsemium, Phosphorus, Apis, Arsenicum, and Lachesis.

A face that seems dirty suggests: Sulphur. Also: Apis, Mercurius, Lycopodium, and Phosphorus.

A face that is discolored only on one side suggests: Chamomilla. Also: Ipecac, Lachesis, Lycopodium, Nux, Natrum Mur, Phosphorus, and Rhus Tox.

A face that seems to continually change color suggests: Ignatia, or Phosphorus. Also: Aconite, Pulsatilla, and Nux.

A face with colored spots suggests: Rhus Tox, and Silicea. Also: Calcarea, Lycopodium, and Sabadilla.

Conclusions

In this chapter, we have taken a look at the methods by which the practitioners of traditional Chinese medicine diagnose their patients and determine an appropriate mode of treatment and some of the ways that homeopathic medicine parallels and builds upon its practice.

With more than four thousand years of history behind it, I believe that TCM has withstood the test of time. Its methods of treatment, and especially diagnosis, give us a wonderful pattern to follow as we continue to develop the philosophy and practice of homeopathic medicine.

If we can learn to apply the methods used in the "four examinations" to our practice of homeopathy, we can become more efficient in our selection of remedies and more knowledgeable of our patients. With that in mind, let us turn out attention to the classic methods by which the homeopathic case is taken.

4

Homeopathic Case Taking: Gathering and Considering Patient Information

When I first heard of Samuel Hahnemann's book *The Organon of Medicine* (also known as *The Organon of the Medical Art),* I was told it contained all that a student of homeopathy needs to know about the philosophy and practice of this form of medicine. I therefore imagined a huge volume: thousands of pages long, and filled with information, treatment tips, and antique line drawings.

When I ordered the book, what I received was a slim volume made up of 291 aphorisms (also called "paragraphs" by some practitioners). Each reveals some nugget of truth about homeopathy, health, and healing.

Upon further study, I was surprised to learn that Hahnemann chose not to write a series of books on the topic of homeopathy. He revised the *Organon* in six different editions instead. Thus, his book was a living organ, as the name implies. Almost a part of himself, it changed and evolved as he changed through years of homeopathic practice.

HAHNEMANN AND HIS ORGANON

Remember, it was Hahnemann himself who coined the term "homeopathy" and developed the principles by which it is practiced. He had no materia medica to turn to, until he himself developed a homeopathic materia medica. And he had no repertory at all. This reference work of symptoms and the remedies they suggest would not be developed for years to come. All Hahnemann had when he began his practice was his first handful of remedies, which he had himself potentized from the allopathic and herbal medicines of his day.

Hahnemann explored not only new substances that could be diluted into homeopathic medicines, but also new levels of dilution for those substances over the long years of his practice. In this way he increased the number of remedies, and added to the scale of potency available for each of those remedies.

Hahnemann revealed a profound truth in his experiments in dilution and succussion. He discovered that the more dilute his remedies became, the more deeply they acted. The science of his day accorded him no way of measuring it, but we know today that the remedies become truly powerful only when the diluted substances reach the point of totally "falling away." The energy signature of the original substance speaks to our own life's energy when no single molecule of the original substance remains.

The different editions of the *Organon* give different insights into homeopathy, as if each is a photograph of the medical art as Hahnemann experienced it at the time. It is, therefore, quite interesting to compare the different editions for their evolving opinions of how homeopathic medicine should be practiced, and just what makes homeopathy truly homeopathic.

I strongly believe that any and every student of homeopathy should read the *Organon*. For simplicity's sake, I suggest that you read either the sixth edition of the work, or a combined fifth and sixth edition. Comparing and contrasting of the different texts in the different editions can come later.

I also suggest that students pick up a particular edition of the *Organon*. It has been published in many different editions and translations, and some of these are so awkwardly written as to seem to have never been translated at all.

In my opinion, the best translation of the *Organon* available today is translated from the German by Steven Decker, edited and annotated by Wenda Brewster O'Reilly, Ph. D., and published by Birdcage Books. It is, by far, the most clearly translated and organized of the many different editions of the *Organon* on the market today. (Turn to the bibliography for full information about this edition.)

It is very important to point out that Hahnemann's *Organon* was written with the knowledge that most of its readers were either practitioners or patients of allopathic medicine. Therefore, the first seventy-one aphorisms speak not to homeopathy specifically, but to the practice of medicine in all its forms. Hahnemann himself had been trained as an allopathic doctor and had practiced this form of medicine until he came to understand the principles of healing that he named homeopathy. Therefore, he knew firsthand the pressures of practicing allopathy, as well as its goals and its treatments. He had a real respect for those who believed in their hearts and minds in the practice of allopathy. Therefore, the allopath who reads the first section of Hahnemann's *Organon* will be a better allopath for it, just as the homeopath who reads and studies these same aphorisms will be a better homeopath.

Hahnemann begins to speak specifically of homeopathy with his aphorisms on case taking. He sets aside a nice chunk of the total of 291 aphorisms in the *Organon* to discuss this important topic, first discussing the differences between acute and chronic cases in aphorisms 72 to 81, and then outlining the methods by which a homeopathic case is taken in aphorisms 82 to 104.

Recognizing the Acute Case

I have long taught the students in my classes that, to use a literary analogy, an *acute* illness is like a well constructed short story. It contains a beginning, a middle, and an end, which is to say that an acute illness is one that is self-limiting, that will end on its own without treatment.

This does not mean that acute illnesses are never dangerous. The flu epidemic of the early part of the twentieth century killed millions of people worldwide. And, as I write this, a new virus called SARS has made itself known. That virus is sweeping throughout Asia, especially China, and the numbers of cases are growing geometrically. Both influenza and SARS are examples of acute epidemics.

In his *Organon,* Hahnemann teaches that all acute illnesses are either sporadic or epidemic in nature. Sporadic acutes are those that only appear in single cases in different places at one point in time. In contrast, epidemics appear in many different cases and in many different places at one point in time. Further, all the cases of the epidemic disease present essentially the same portrait of illness. And, finally, all the cases of an epidemic illness, as with SARS, can be traced back to a single locale and a single cause.

Therefore, in treating any acute disease, we must first be sure that it *is* an acute disease, and then we must ascertain which type of acute it is. Sometimes this is a simple thing, sometimes not.

Before continuing with this discussion, we have to first consider the other category of disease: the *chronic* disease.

To return to a literary analogy by way of explanation, a chronic condition is like a soap opera. It takes some time to develop. You have to set up a locale, and develop characters and their relationships and histories, but once it is up and running, it can continue year after year, spinning on and on with no end in sight.

Chronic ailments are usually slow to develop in the same way. They will continue to exist, sometimes growing a bit better, sometimes worse, unless they are removed by medical treatment, because they usually have no self-limiting factor.

Allopathic medicines work by suppressing symptoms of illness until the body heals itself, but the overuse of this action of suppression can weaken our immune systems and our very life force. Hahnemann reminds us in aphorism seventy-four that allopathic treatments themselves can cause chronic conditions to slowly develop and appear, and that chronic conditions caused by allopathic treatments are among the most difficult to cure.

Hahnemann insists that it is very important that practitioners of homeopathic medicine try to uncover the cause of chronic conditions whenever possible. Indeed, he states that many conditions, like those caused by bad habits such as smoking, can not be successfully treated until the bad habits are eliminated.

In fact, aphorism seventy-seven concludes that diseases apparently caused by "avoidable noxious factors" are not really diseases at all, because they will fall away if the noxious factors are removed. Thus the person with rheumatoid arthritis who lives in a damp basement will feel much better if he moves to a dry attic. This person, in Hahnemann's opinion, needs to move more than he needs to be given pills for his arthritic pain.

So we must become familiar with the nature of disease if we are to treat homeopathically.

In the most basic sense, we have to be able to tell the difference between chronic and acute disease. As I said, sometimes this is easy, but sometimes it can be quite difficult.

First aid is certainly easy. When your child falls off the swing set and scrapes his knee, that is a perfect example of an acute case. The same is true for that horrible moment when you realize, as Sylvia Plath wrote, that it was your thumb instead of the onion—that you've sliced yourself in the kitchen. Or that you've had a car accident and hit your head. These are clearly all acute situations and acute cases.

Colds, flus, earaches and the like can be very tricky. While a simple cold can also be considered a simple acute case, before being sure one has to look at the number of colds a given patient is having during a year's time, the nature of those "colds," and the depth of the symptoms.

Most of us get a cold or two a year. In fact, they can almost be considered a good thing once a year. Your body detoxifies itself, and you have a chance to take a day or two of rest. All in all, this is not so bad. But, the more colds and coughs and flus you get during a year, the more you are showing signs of a deeper, chronic condition that is masking itself as several acute situations rather than one chronic one.

The same may be said if your "cold" always has the same symptoms, as if you were getting the same cold again and again instead of experiencing new and separate cases.

This is also true if your cold becomes something deeper and more threatening instead of just being an inconvenience. If your breathing becomes labored, or your fever is exceptionally high, then it is to be considered that, once again, we are not looking at a simple acute cold but at the tip of a chronic iceberg.

It is important that you seek professional care immediately for cases like these, or any time you are not sure whether you are looking at an acute situation or a chronic case. It is important that you never work out of your depth, especially when you are beginning your study of homeopathy. Treat only cases involving first aid treatments if your understanding of acute treatments extends only to first aid. As your knowledge and understanding grows, then your treatments may as well.

Remember, an acute ailment is always a new experience. Your body has met with a new virus or bacteria and doesn't quite know what to do with it. It rises to this new challenge by throwing its arsenal of weapons at the intruder, fever and mucus and the like, in an attempt to wipe out the invader.

The chronic condition, in contrast, has a "stuckness" attached to it. Rather than being a dramatic new event, it is the same old song. The symptoms are the same, the patterns are the same. The body has long ago given up on throwing off the condition, and instead seeks to contain it.

This is why Hahnemman takes a very different approach to the treatment of the patient with an acute condition and the patient with a chronic condition. Hahnemann warns that the patient with a chronic condition should not be given what he wants, because if the patient had the ability to throw off his disease he would have done so already. The chronic patient is a prisoner of his disease, and is to some extent controlled by it. Therefore, he will likely crave the very things that will contribute to the disease and not to its cure. So, if the chronic patient craves a particular kind of food or drink, one has to think long and hard before giving it to him—at least in that form. Patients who are allergic to wheat, for instance, will crave and crave it. They should be given anything but wheat.

It is quite different for the acute illness. In this case the innate wisdom of the body causes it to seek those things that lead to cure.

Therefore, if the acutely ill patient wants ice cream, give it to him. If he has very hungry, feed him. If he wants no food at all, listen to him; it may do him more good than harm to fast, as long as he doesn't go without food for a long enough period of time that it weakens his system.

To summarize, the chronically ill are chronically ill partly because they made wrong decisions, and satisfied unhealthy desires. Their wishes are not to be honored, because their treatment needs to change their life's path, if it is to make them well. The wishes of the acutely ill should be honored, however, because their bodies seek to be made well. The fact that they are acutely ill implies that they can become well again if they can only overcome the impact of their acute situation.

The Goal of Acute Treatment

The goal of the acute treatment is to restore the patient to the level of health he or she enjoyed before the onset of the acute ailment. This suggests that the patient was healthy before the onset of that acute condition. But as anyone who sees the child with a runny nose trip and fall on the playground knows, that child already had some sort of cold or allergy before his unfortunate accident.

This is important in our consideration of the differences between acute and chronic case.

In a true acute case, the patient was more or less healthy before the onset of the acute condition, and the action of the homeopathic treatment selected will perfectly match the condition itself. In other words, if the condition were a cold, the patient would feel relief of the symptoms of that cold and nothing else.

You have a strong sign that a supposedly acute condition is simply a part of an overall chronic case, however, if the treatment causes changes in the patient's system that apparently have nothing to do with the acute case at hand. For example, I once gave the homeopathic remedy Causticum to a dear friend of mine who was experiencing carpal tunnel syndrome, supposedly caused by her overuse of her computer keyboard while meeting a writing deadline. Her arm pain perfectly matched the remedy's action, and it is a common remedy for carpal tunnel, so I felt comfortable giving her a dose.

To our great surprise, the Causticum not only helped her arm pain, but also greatly relieved her chronic pattern of indigestion and headaches. She felt as if her whole life were changing based on the use of one remedy.

I had named the case acute after looking at only one symptom, and had ignored the rest of what was obviously a chronic condition. I sought to limit the action of the homeopathic remedy to what I wanted it to do. This is always a mistake.

When we take an acute case, we attempt to create two pictures of the patient: one before the onset of the symptoms, and one while the patient is under the influence of those symptoms. You are treating an acute case homeopathically when you look at the changes that have taken place from the moment of "health" to the moment of "illness," and address those changes by selecting a remedy that would cause those same changes in any other healthy person.

But sometimes—and this will happen despite your best intentions—a supposedly acute treatment will actually reveal a chronic case. All sorts of changes start to take place, and many have nothing to do with the acute case you were treating. This is a definite sign that you and your patient need to seek professional care. You need to let the practitioner know what you have given the patient, and the impact it had.

This is not to say that you did a bad thing: you many have uncovered the perfect remedy for your patient's chronic case. But you have no business treating a chronic case as a lay practitioner. This is the domain of the professional practitioner.

Keep in mind that the treatment of the chronic case involves profound changes on the part of the patient, and the case taking itself is deeper and more complex. In the same way, the treatment is deeper acting, and often quite complex. Chronic cases are best left to those with medical degrees for this reason.

The Homeopathic Band-Aid

This brings up an aspect of the supposedly acute case that I call the "homeopathic Band-Aid."

Homeopathic Band-Aids are acute treatments used to control the patient's discomfort until he or she can receive appropriate help for what are actually chronic conditions.

Good examples of these Band-Aids are acute homeopathic treatments of toothache, allergies, or headache.

Just as the use of a homeopathic remedy like Coffea will not actually cure the cavity in a tooth, but controls the ache until the patient can get to a dentist, the temporary treatments of allergies, headaches, and the like safely control the discomfort of the chronic condition until appropriate constitutional treatment can be undertaken.

I give some examples of remedies used as Band-Aids in the section of the book on the acute uses of remedies, but let me state clearly that this sort of treatment is not the cleanest form of homeopathy. It is important to be able to help your child bear his pain until you can get appropriate treatment if he wakes in the middle of the night with a toothache, however.

And, let me state clearly that homeopathic Band-Aids are *always* single remedies. Some may suggest that the combination remedies available in health food stores are appropriate for temporary use in treatment of chronic cases. Combination remedies are those that contain anything from a handful to many different homeopathic remedies in one pellet. You will find combination remedies labeled by the condition they treat, which can be for anything from diarrhea to hay fever to headaches.

I personally do not believe that these remedies are safe. Let me tell you why.

As you remember, the use of anything other than a single remedy in the treatment of any patient breaks the first law of cure: the law of Simplex. That law states that we always use one remedy at a time. In fact, Hahnemann called any use of more than one medicine *polypharmacy.* This term can relate to any treatment, whether it is homeopathic or allo- pathic, and the practice is just as dangerous in each. (You will find that two remedies may be used concurrently in some of the first aid cases described in upcoming pages. Not wishing to sound like a hypocrite, I acknowledge this now and will explain it later, when we look at first aid cases.)

As we discussed earlier, every medicine has more than one effect; it creates an entire sphere of actions in the human system. If you give one medicine at a time, you are able to clearly trace the changes made by the use of that remedy. In polypharmacy, you are giving two or more different substances, each with its own entire sphere of activity. There is no way of knowing just what medicine is doing what. Perhaps there is one remedy that speaks to the case at hand and acts curatively, but what about the other dozen or so remedies in that pellet? What changes do they cause, for good or bad? And how can we ever identify what remedy has done what?

A case treated through polypharmacy can become so confused by the actions of the many remedies that it is nearly impossible to sort out.

This ability to determine what remedy has done what has to do with the concept of *proving.* Hahnemann proved the actions of his remedies by having healthy people take a remedy and then studying its impact upon them. Sick people will prove remedies in the same way, if they take them repeatedly.

As you will remember, a remedy that does not speak to the case—whose actions do not match the symptoms—will do nothing, if it is just given once. But any remedy will begin to have an impact if it is repeated often enough, no matter how far off in its actions it is from the symptoms at hand. The power of proving comes about through repetition of dose.

So, an allergy patient taking a combination remedy until he can get to the doctor may have some initial relief from symptoms, if it contains a remedy that speaks to the case. The other remedies will begin to have an impact within the patient's system through the process of proving, however, and he will begin to experience new and different allergy symptoms. If the patient takes the combination remedy long enough, his system may be so confused by the use of many remedies that it can no longer be treated for allergies homeopathically.

This same situation can occur whenever you use more than one remedy at a time. Whether you are a practitioner or a patient, you must always use the remedies one at a time for this reason.

Taking the Case

It is important that we reconsider the idea of symptoms as we begin to look at the traditional process by which the homeopathic case is taken, because, after all, case taking is a gathering of symptoms. These symptoms are used as indicators of specific homeopathic remedies, until all of the symptoms are studied, and a specific curative remedy is found.

Remember, symptoms for the homeopath are not the same as they are for the allopath. The allopath will almost always equate symptoms with pain. They are the signs identifying the presence of disease.

Symptoms are different for the homeopath. For example, the patient who was never very thirsty before the onset of his acute condition, but now has a wild thirst for cold water, is providing important information and expressing a symptom. Therefore, in homeopathic medicine, symptoms can be indications of pain, or they can be quite benign, but they all represent a change in the patient's condition.

When gathering symptoms in an acute case, we want to determine all the changes that have taken place in the patient's life from the time just before the onset of the illness to the moment of the case taking.

We especially want to know about the onset of the disease: that moment when the patient realized that he or she was becoming ill. Where was he or she? What were the circumstances surrounding the onset? An illness after exposure to cold wind needs a different remedy from one that occurs after exposure to hot sun.

We also need to explore the patient's life at the time of the onset of the illness. The disease that occurs when the patient has been sleep deprived while studying for midterms is different from one that occurs after the patient had been lifting heavy weight while helping a friend move.

Guidelines for case taking:

- Observe the patient as a whole being.
- Let the patient speak—do not interrupt.
- Get objective as well as subjective information.
- Examine the areas of the patient's body affected by the disease.
- Keep accurate notes of the case taking.

In his *Organon,* Hahnemann stresses the importance of having a third party on hand to help with the process of case taking if possible.

This third party possesses intimate knowledge of the patient, like a parent or mate, and may have insight into the changes in the patient as he moved from health to sickness. Hahnemann's thought is that the patient has a purely subjective experience of his ailment, while the third party will be able to fill in objective information. The practitioner is also an objective party who can listen, observe, and judge the information given him, but the third party offers more than just objective information. He has an intimate knowledge of the patient that the practitioner lacks, and moreover, he offers compassion along with his objectivity.

In many cases related to this book, the practitioner will be the patient's parent or mate. From one perspective, this is a great help, because the practitioner's knowledge of the patient's condition will be much more in-depth than usual. But, on the other hand, it may make the situation more complex, because the practitioner's compassion may outweigh his objectivity. Suffice it to say that you will have to work hard in your case taking to use your unique understanding of the patient in an objective and useful manner, when you are called upon to be both practitioner and third party.

Homeopathic case taking has three levels: The practitioner must observe his patient as a whole, and gather objective information from that observation. Further, the practitioner must examine the part or parts of the body that have been affected by the disease. From this he gathers more objective information. Finally, he must have a conversation with the patient, in which he gathers that patient's subjective experience of the ailment.

In traditional Chinese medicine, each aspect of case taking follows a specific pattern. In homeopathic medicine, however, the manner in which the case is taken may change from case to case and patient to patient. The examination of the body may be the whole of the case taking, especially in some acute cases. In other cases, it may be very important to have a lengthy conversation with the patient, one in which the patient's subjective symptoms are gathered and modified. Modified refers to the process whereby the information gathered about symptoms is grouped, considered, and given order of importance.

For this reason, I will describe the different aspects of case taking in the pages that follow, but it is left for you to use them in the manner that best suits your own temperament and the case at hand.

Just be sure to include all the levels of case taking—observation, conversation, and examination—each to the degree required by the specific situation at hand.

And, after you have gathered all of the symptoms of the case, the rest of this chapter will explain how to use that information to select the remedy most likely to be curative.

Case Taking: Observation

In taking any case—acute or chronic—you must deal not just with the symptoms, but also with the person sitting in front of you. Since this book's focus is the treatment of household emergencies, the person sitting in front of you will be a member of your own family in the majority of cases and the idea of observation of the patient may seem to be a bit silly. I promise you, it is not. When the professional practitioner approaches a case, he or she begins gathering information at the very first sight of the patient, not by first examining the wound or questioning the patient. This objective gathering of information can be invaluable to the practitioner's understanding of the case.

It can also be invaluable for you if you already know the patient. If you can stand back for a moment and avoid panic, observe your child objectively, and in your case taking, match how his demeanor and physical presence has changed in his hurting himself, you will be able to choose the correct remedy for the situation all the more quickly.

Along with the valuable information it yields, this self-training of standing back a bit and learning to observe before you give your child all the loving attention he deserves, will help you to become a better practitioner. You will have trained your mind to detach, observe, and record. Those attributes, along with your loving heart, will make for a mighty practitioner.

Before you ask a question or listen to a word from the patient, observe the overall behavior of the patient. Is he tranquil or anxious? Is he excited or depressed? Is he overwhelmed by pain? Or is he just plain exhausted?

Pay attention.

Pay attention to the way he walks into the room, what chair he decides to sit in, and how he sits down. Note the mood and behavior. Note how openly he wishes to discuss the case and the symptoms. First and foremost, always note what symptom or symptoms led the person to seek help.

Always ask about that symptom first—after all, it is why the patient sought treatment—before moving on to other aspects of the case.

- **Observe the patient's movements.** Is the patient moving quickly or slowly? Is he coordinated in his motion? The movement of the body gives an overall clue to Vital Force. It will often also give you a solid indication as to the sort of symptoms you are going to be called upon to deal with.

- **Observe the patient's gestures.** Watch the hands and face of the patient. Look for any tics and/or nervous habits. Look for expressions that can uncover emotions that may have been held back. Gestures often say what words won't.
- **Observe the patient's manner of speech.** Does the person speak rapidly or slowly? Does he put words together well, or does he struggle to find the right wording? This gives a clue as to the mental strength of the patient, and can be a clear indicator of a specific remedy.

Note the following physical traits of the patient. The behavior patterns of the patient can be a great help in taking and treating the acute case. The following items are much more important in the constitutional case than they are in the acute, but I include them because it is important to have your case taking information as complete as possible.

- **Note the patient's gender.** Sexist or not, homeopathic remedies are often determined by the gender of the patient, although these hard and fast rules (such as the idea that Nux Vomica is for men, and Ignatia is for women) are beginning to fall along the wayside as traditional gender roles and behavior patterns dissolve.

Gender is a much greater issue in constitutional treatments than it is in acute circumstances. While we do want to note the gender of the patient, it is not an issue per se in the acute treatment. For example, a very macho man may require the "feminine" remedy Pulsatilla when he has a cold.

- **Note the patient's age.** This can be another clue to the patient's Vital Force, although it would be unfair to say that a very young or very old patient has a weakened Vital Force on the basis of age alone.

  Also, the patient's age is often a clue to the number of allopathic treatments he or she has undergone in the past. Practitioners have to be especially wary of older patients, and be sure to ask them what medicines they take regularly and what other medicines they have already tried for the current acute condition.

- **Note the patient's weight.** This is another clue to Vital Force.

  Also: weight can often be a guiding symptom in finding the right curative remedy. This is true much more often in constitutional cases than it is in simple acute cases, but if the patient is overweight,

140

spend a bit of time asking about other medical conditions that are often linked, such as high blood pressure. Satisfy yourself that the condition at hand is indeed acute before treating it.

- **Note the patient's clothing.** This not only includes the clothing itself, but makeup, jewelry, and anything else that humans commonly use to decorate themselves. How does the patient present himself or herself? Does she or he dress in bright or subdued colors? Is he or she neat or messy? Does the patient seem to care how he presents himself?

- **Note the patient's smell.** Use your nose to check for specific odors—sweat, breath odor, or pathological secretions. These can be clues to the remedy needed, as remedies such as Mercurius and Thuja have specific scents linked to them. Does the patient wear cologne? This can be linked with the above observation of clothing, and other such aspects in that it will yield information as to how the patient wishes to present himself. The patient clouding himself in a great deal of cologne is telling you something about the state of his sinuses, if nothing else.

Case Taking: The Examination

The examination of the affected areas of the body may actually be the whole of the case taking, or at least a major part of it, when taking an acute case.

Certainly, when your child falls from the swing and skins his knee, there is little to the case taking other than for you to look at the knee, assess the damage, and then ask, "What happened?" That concludes the case taking. The kissing of the knee and the general comforting falls under the category of parenting.

When examining the affected parts of the body, the practitioner may be looking at a wound on the skin, a red and sore throat, or a rash on the patient's leg.

During the examination, the practitioner looks for the following:

- **Discolorations.** This refers to any change in the color of the skin or of any part of the body. Discolorations may relate to inflammation of tissues or physical trauma. Most common discolorations are red, purple, blue, black and blue, yellow, brown, and green.
- **Distortions.** This refers to any change in the normal size or shape of any part of the body. Thus, you may consider swelling, shrinking, or withering to be

distortions. In addition, any body part that is normally dry and has become wet, or vice versa, may be considered a distortion. Any change in size, shape, quality, or performance of a part of the body may be said to be a distortion. The same may be said for temperature changes. For instance, an insect sting that is hot to the touch will require a different remedy from one that is cold to the touch.

- **Wounds.** In acute homeopathy, you will find yourself looking at wounds a good deal of the time. For a complete discussion of various types of wounds and their treatments, see the information on first aid in Part Three of this book.

Be sure, even while you are examining the patient, to continue to listen and observe. Make sure to note how the patient responds to your touch, and whether or not that touch is welcome. Be sure to record (in writing) anything the patient tells you while you examine him.

Remember, as Scudder said, it is important that you use all your senses during the examination, and that you stay in the moment with the patient, objectively gathering as much information as you can. In many acute cases, especially first aid cases, the examination will be the most important component of case taking, and the selection of the remedy will be made from the information gathered here.

Case Taking: The Conversation

I call the initial part of the case taking process "the conversation," but it is important to realize that the patient should have much more to say than the practitioner in this conversation. It is a conversation, but it should not be a talk show. It is not the role of the practitioner to wow his patient with his insightful and well-worded questions. Instead, the questions should be as short and as simple as possible, only challenging the patient to be as honest and as thorough as possible.

Make sure that you have already learned to listen before you seek to dig into the patient's history, dreams, aches, and pains.

Indeed, Hahnemann again and again stresses that the patient should not be interrupted. The practitioner must listen to all that the patient has to say concerning his case, without hurrying him, while carefully recording what the patient says, in the patient's own words as often as possible.

There is only one case in which Hahnemann says it is proper to interrupt the patient. That is the case in which the patient digresses, and his monologue about his condition wanders off onto other topics. In those cases, just steer the patient back to the topic at hand and then again put your attention to listening.

The patient, or those who accompany the patient, such as his or her parents, will often tell you the solution to the case (even if they have no knowledge of homeopathy) if you are listening to them. They frequently present the symptoms in the manner of a repertory or a materia medica, if only you take care to record their words as much as possible.

In opening the conversation, the appropriate first thing for you to say is, "Tell me what's troubling you." It is best to always seek information in the form of a statement rather than a question, so the patient does not feel as if he is on a quiz show.

The patient should not be interrupted until he has finished his initial statement. There will be plenty of time later to ask specific questions concerning the symptoms. Remember, the patient will nearly always begin by speaking of particular physical symptoms relating to one specific organ or part of the body. These symptoms may be the least important in your process of remedy selection, but the patient must be allowed to begin wherever he wishes when telling his tale.

Once the patient has told his story to his own satisfaction it is appropriate to start seeking more information about his case. While he has been speaking you have, in addition to keeping a close eye on him and carefully listening to his every word, been writing down his symptoms—in his own language and not in technical terms—making sure to leave plenty of room between symptoms so you can fill in the information you will need to consider for each of them.

Now it is appropriate to go back and ask for any missing information you need to fully understand the case. Be sure to do this in a manner that is as simple and straight forward as possible, without challenging the patient's interpretations of his own symptoms or their meanings. Instead, use all the information the patient gives you in an earnest attempt to understand his symptoms of pain, and how those fit into the context of the totality of symptoms and the life of the patient as a whole.

Finally, remember, it is of vital importance in case taking that the practitioner not only allows his patient to tell his story, but that he actually creates, for the purposes of the case taking, a safe place for that patient to speak. The most important job of the homeopath may be the ability to create an atmosphere in which a patient feels free and able to talk about his symptoms, and able to help the practitioner work with that information to develop it into a case.

As homeopath Richard Moskowitz puts it, "We always have to evaluate the place of the symptoms in the life of the patient."

Case Taking: The Questions

Once the initial "Tell me what's troubling you" part of the conversation is over, and the patient has related his story, the questioning process begins. Questioning the patient generally follows a standard pattern, as we are tying to gather the same information concerning each of the patient's symptoms. The most successful pattern will closely follow the method of questioning presented by Hahnemann in his *Organon*.

Move your questions from general to specific. For example, the patient says that his back hurts. Any homeopathic practitioner—lay person or medical professional—should immediately know that that information, in and of itself, is not enough to select an appropriate remedy. Indeed, if you were to open any repertory and look up "backache," you would find a listing of dozens and dozens of remedies, any of which might be the correct one for the case at hand.

So, from that very general question, the practitioner must become more specific. He must ask questions that will guide the patient to add the information he needs to select a curative remedy.

I provide a more specific list of exactly the type of information you need to open a case and lead to a curative remedy in the next chapter on symptoms. For now, let me say that the process of questioning in case taking is very similar to that used by the journalist seeking information for a story. Like the journalist, the homeopath needs to know the "who, what, when, where, why, and how" of the situation.

The specifics of a case have to do with its *onset,* or the circumstances by which the illness came on. They also have to do with the pattern of the symptoms, such as the side of the body where the symptoms began, or where they are dominant, and with how the symptoms interact with each other—whether or not there is a pattern to the symptoms. Also of significance: the exact area of the body affected by each symptom, and how that area has moved or changed over the course of the illness; how long the symptom has lasted, and the length of that symptom in comparison to the other symptoms; and the degree of pain that that symptom creates, and the sensation of that pain.

To return to the concept of a journalist researching a story, the questions for each symptom should flow as follows:

The **Who,** of course, is always the patient.

The **What** is the symptom itself—the backache, or whatever the patient is reporting. When exploring what, try to find out exactly how the patient is experiencing the sensation of the pain. What is the sensation of the symptom? A sharp backache may require a very different remedy from a dull backache. In the same way, a throbbing headache is very different from a bursting headache. "What" also relates to how the symptom changes in quality and/or intensity since its onset.

The **When** relates to the onset of the symptom, and how it compares to his or her other symptoms in a timeline. Which symptom came first, and which second? Which symptoms are still in place at the time of the interview?

The **Where** is the location of the symptom. A backache, of course, is located in the back, but where, exactly? Is it in the upper back, or the lower back, on the left side or the right? "Where" also relates to how the symptom has moved since its onset. Where is it located right now, as opposed to where it was at onset?

The **Why** relates to the situation surrounding the onset of illness. Does the patient know of any reason why his back might be aching? Did he lift a heavy box? Or did he sleep on damp ground, or a hard floor? The "Why" gives insight into the possible reason for the symptom's onset.

The **How** relates to how this symptom combines with other symptoms. Did two symptoms appear together and seem related? Do two or more symptoms alternate? Are there any other patterns for the symptoms together?

Remember in gathering this information to ask only open-ended questions that allow the patient to consider some specific aspect of his illness without guiding him to a specific answer.

While the questioning is moving from the general, during which time the patient may ramble a bit, to the more specific, it is important that the practitioner never hurry the patient along, but that he make sure the patient stays on the subject as much as possible. The wise practitioner notes that the patient is a rambler if he tends to stray, and uses that knowledge to help open the case, but it is still important that the practitioner stays in control of the question-and-answer period without strong-arming the process.

Question those things the patient has *not* mentioned. The fact that the patient does not mention an aspect of his body or health during a questioning period does not mean that he has nothing to say about it. Often, the patient can become very forgetful in his discomfort. Therefore, it is important that the practitioner also ask, "Is there anything else?" after listening to everything that the patient has to say, and after moving the information about each symptom from general to specific.

If the patient says there is nothing else, the practitioner should still ask a general question about any aspect of health that has not already been mentioned. For instance, he should ask about the patient's sleep, digestion, respiration, or any other symptoms not already reported. I cannot tell you how many times patients will say, "Oh, yes, I forgot, I haven't been able to sleep at all." Or, "Oh, no, I can't sleep, but I didn't think that that had anything to do with my backache." Assure the patient that, as a homeopath, you think that it might have everything to do with his backache, and then move the questioning concerning that symptom from general to specific.

Don't be afraid of silence. Many practitioners, especially new students and practitioners of homeopathy, feel that silence should not be allowed; that it shows a weakness or a lack of preparation on the part of the practitioner.

The truth is that a bit of silence is the questioner's best friend. Often, if there is a silence after a question has been asked and answered, the patient will feel called upon to fill that silence himself. And, in filling that silence, the patient often adds some very important information.

It has been my experience that the practitioner who knows how and when to use silence often quickly and easily gathers information that solves the case.

Remember what to ask and what not to ask. The biggest mistake that any practitioner can make is to jump to a quick conclusion concerning a case. The practitioner who, in taking the case, hears that the patient has a backache and immediately decides that this is likely a Rhus Tox case is very likely to actually shape it into a Rhus Tox case whether it is or not.

It is of vital import that the practitioner be open minded when entering into a process of case taking. It is the role of the practitioner to gather and record as much information as possible, and to be as objective about the case as possible.

The practitioner needs to observe the patient, examine the affected areas of the body and then ask questions for each symptom in the same general-to-specific pattern.

Once the case taking has ended, it is the role of the practitioner to modify and work with the symptoms in a manner that facilitates the selection of an appropriate remedy.

It is never the role of the practitioner to jump to conclusions, either based on any case he has taken in the past (each of us is a unique being requiring a unique remedy), or on any hunch.

It is therefore important that the practitioner does not ask any questions based on a previous case, a hunch, or an early conclusion, and it is also important that no leading questions be asked. In other words, the practitioner should never ask, "Wasn't this or that symptom also present?" This sort of question leads the patient to say things the practitioner wants to hear, because he fits the mold of the remedy the practitioner already has in mind. There is no place for this sort of question in homeopathy.

Case Taking: The Answers

The answers the patient provides when you are taking a homeopathic case are critical diagnostic indicators in homeopathic medicine. The practitioner must learn to pay attention to how the patient answers questions about the case, because you often can get a better indication of which remedy might be helpful by the way the patient is speaks, rather than by the words that are actually spoken. It is important that we use these indicators as the very helpful tools they are.

How the patient speaks in answering questions. The way the patient speaks when he or she responds to questions suggests specific remedies:

For the patient who speaks loudly, consider: Lachesis. Also: Belladonna. Also: Arnica, and Arsenicum.

For the patient who speaks rapidly, consider: Hepar Sulph, Lachesis, and Sulphur. Also: Mercurius, Sepia, Thuja, Ignatia, and Belladonna. Also: Camphora, and Lycopodium.

For the patient who is abrupt (almost rude) in his speech, consider: Arsenicum, Chamomilla, and Sulphur.

For the patient who is hasty (speaks without thinking, only to regret it later) in his speech, consider: Mercurius, and Lachesis. Also: Belladonna, and Camphora. Also: Bryonia, Causticum, Ingatia, Lycopodium, Nux, and Sepia.

For the patient who is confused in speech, consider: Lachesis, Nux, Gelsemium, Natrum Mur, and Lycopodium.

For the patient who is hesitating in speech, consider: Pulsatilla. Also: Mercurius, Lycopodium, Staphysagria, and Thuja.

For the patient who is forgetful in speaking, consider: Arnica. Also: Lachesis, Nux, Lycopodium, and Sulphur.

For the patient who is incoherent (his words make no logical sense) in speaking, consider: Lachesis, Phosphorus, Rhus Tox, Bryonia, Camphora, and Sulphur. Also: Apis, Belladonna, and Gelsemium. Also: Arsenicum, Coffea, Spigelia, and Mercurius. For the patient who is unintelligible (mumbling, so that his words cannot be heard and understood) in speech, consider: Belladonna. Also: Aconite, Arsenicum, Lycopodium, Nux, Mercurius, and Silicea.

For the patient who speaks as if drunk, consider: Nux, and Gelsemium. Also: Lycopodium, and Natrum Mur.

For the patient who is delirious, consider: Belladonna. Also: Sulphur, and Bryonia. Also: Coffea.

If the patient is delirious in speech during sleep, consider: Belladonna.

For the patient who cannot finish a sentence, consider: Arsenicum and Lachesis.

For the patient who answers only in mono-syllables (basically, yes and no answers only), consider: Nux. Also: Mercurius, and Arsenicum.

For the patient whose speech wanders from topic to topic, consider: Natrum Mur, Lachesis and Sulphur. Also: Rhus Tox, Phosphorus, Pulsatilla, Bryonia, Arsenicum and Spongia. Also: Arnica, Aconite, Calcarea, Chamomilla, Chinchona, Cina, Ignatia, and Dulcamara.

For the patient who speaks slowly, consider: Lachesis. Also: Ignatia, Causticum, Natrum Mur and Sepia. Also: Phosphorus.

For the patient who does not wish to be spoken to, consider: Sulphur, Bryonia, and

Chanomilla. Also: Arsenicum, Antimonium Tartaricum, Arnica, and Silicea.

For the patient who cries when speaking, especially when telling his symptoms, consider: Sepia, and Pulsatilla.

For the patient who laughs when speaking, consider: Phosphorus, Ignatia, Belladonna, Coffea, and Calcarea. Also: Natrum Mur, and Sepia.

If the patient is both laughing and crying at the same time, consider: Pulsatilla. Also: Staphysagria.

For the patient who is joking, consider: Rhus Tox, and Ignatia. Also: Lachesis.

If the patient is averse to jokes, consider: Aconite, Mercurius, and Cina.

If the patient simply can't take a joke, consider: Aconite. Also: Lycopodium, Mercurius, and Nux. Also: Natrum Mur and Pulsatilla.

If the patient is both joking and crying at the same time, consider: Ignatia.

If the patient jokes only at the expense of others, consider: Lachesis.

For the patient who is very serious in speech, consider: Arsenicum. Also: Staphysagria, Euphrasia, Ledum and Mercurius. Also: Cina.

For the patient who is inappropriate or lewd in speech, consider: Lachesis, Belladonna, and

Nux. Also: Camphora, Phosphorus, Veratrum, and Calcarea.

For the patient who screams when he speaks, consider: Camphora, and Veratrum. Also: Lycopodium, Gelsemium, Ignatia, Apis, and Antimonium Tartaricum.

For the patient who sighs when he speaks, consider: Ignatia, and Bryonia. Also: Nux, Pulsatilla, Rhus Tox, Sepia, Graphites, Ipecac, and Eupatorium.

If the patient speaks and sighs in his sleep, consider: Sulphur. Also: Belladonna, Camphora, Arsenicum, and Pulsatilla.

How the patient talks, in general. The patient's manner of speaking in general suggests specific remedies:

For the patient who talks too much, consider: Lachesis. Also: Camphora, Belladonna, Phosphorus, and Nux. Also: Aconite, Apis, Arnica, Arsenicum, Calcarea, Sulphur, Duclamara, Gelsemium, Lycoposium, and Natrum Mur.

For the patient who tends to make speeches, consider: Lachesis and Sulphur. Also: Arnica, Ignatia, and Chamomilla.

For the patient who tends to speak little, but once he gets started talks on and on, consider: Natrum Mur.

If a patient actually feels physically better after talking a great deal, consider: Natrum Mur.

For the patient who takes great pleasure in his or her own talking, consider: Sulphur, Lachesis, and Natrum Mur.

For the patient who talks to himself, consider: Staphysagria, Sulphur, Lachesis and Nux. Also: Antimonium Tartaricum, and Kali Bi. Also: Rhus Tox, Calcarea, Belladonna, and Mercurius.

For the patient who only talks to himself when he is alone, consider: Nux and Lachesis.

For the patient who talks about nothing but his aches and pains, consider: Nux.

For the patient who talks only about unimportant things, consider: Lachesis.

If the patient alternates talking and laughing, consider: Belladonna.

If the patient alternates talking and silence, consider: Ignatia and Belladonna.

For the patient who talks incoherently, consider: Lachesis. Also: Phosphorus, Bryonia, and Ignatia.

For the patient who raves, consider: Veratrum. Also: Apis, Lachesis, and Staphysagira. Also: Belladonna.

For the patient who is eager to speak about others, to gossip, consider: Bryonia, Arsenicum, and Nux. Also: Sepia.

For the patient who speaks too little, or who seems disinterested in communicating, consider: Pulsatilla, Phosphorus, and Sulphur. Also: Veratrum, Natrum Mur, Arnica, and Aconite.

If the patient seems too sad to speak, consider: Arsenicum and Pulsatilla. Also: Ignatia and Veratrum.

If all the patient's seem worse when he is talking, consider: Sulphur. Also: Calcarea and Cocculus.

If the patient seems silent over his or her sufferings, consider: Ignatia.

If the patient talks in his sleep, consider: Belladonna, Lachesis, and Rhus Tox. Also: Sepia, Silicea, Sulphur, Ledum, Gelsemium, Calcarea, Arnica, and Carbo Veg. Also: Apis, Antimonium Tartaricum, Aconite, and Bryonia.

Case Taking: Recording the Information

This is an area of case taking that I leave up to you. I am sure that with time and practice, you will find your own method of laying out the case taking on the page.

Most practitioners still take their cases in their own handwriting, working off a legal pad or other tablet of paper. Some use their computer, and spend the time case taking also quietly clicking away on their keyboards.

No matter how you choose to record the sessions, remember three things:

Record the information in the patient's own words. Many practitioners have the tendency to paraphrase the patient's words. This creates a problem in that the case has been changed: it has been put through the filter of the practitioner's mind and vocabulary.

The patient knows his case better than anyone else. He and he alone knows the subjective side of the case. Therefore, if he says that his headache throbs and you write that it pounds, you are warping the information even as you are taking it down.

Organize the information as you go. If you think that you can just write the information down on your pad in any way, shape, or form, and then make sense out of it later, forget it. Make sure to become your own most important support mechanism by writing the case down clearly, and in as neat a penmanship as possible. You will certainly find that the best taken case, if it is sloppily written, is little or no help to you later in finding that right remedy.

Do not crowd the information on the page, and avoid writing in margins or otherwise trying to cram the information into its proper place. Instead, make sure to leave plenty of room as you go. For each new general symptom mentioned in the patient's initial monologue, make sure to leave enough room for the who, what, when, where, why, and how questioning that will follow.

If you organize your material as you go, you will find that its natural flow is very helpful in working with the symptoms and opening up the case.

Pay attention to the patient, even as you record the case. In my opinion, this is the hardest part, but keep in mind that even the most timid patient will be insulted by the practitioner who spends his entire time together writing on his pad, with his head facing the paper.

The whole point of this book is to help the acute practitioner come to terms with the objective case. It is, therefore, certainly more important for our purposes that the practitioner pay attention to his patient, and observe the patient's reactions to questions and struggles with answers, rather than write down every word.

Experience will help you understand what is important to write down and what is not. An important key is to remember that we are trying to find out about the patient's symptoms, and what aspects of his life have changed from the onset of illness onward. So it is important to write down each of those changes, and then augment the general information with the specific questions that follow the patient's original monologue.

It is not important, for our purposes, to know the patient's parent's names, his political affiliation, or any other information about him that does not pertain to his health before the onset of illness and the symptoms he has experienced since that time. If you can keep yourself focused and remember your goal in acute treatment, it will help you know when to write, and when to sit bearing witness to everything the patient tells you.

Case Taking: Symptoms

In homeopathic medicine, symptoms are always good news to the practitioner, even if they represent pain and suffering (or, at the very least, unwanted change) to the patient. Symptoms are signs that the patient's Vital Force is still operating, and that it is attempting to defeat an illness, but not all symptoms are equally helpful in leading a practitioner toward a cure.

Many symptoms are simply too vague and general to be of help in finding a curative remedy. Therefore, it is important to understand that there are different kinds of symptoms, and that some are more useful than others. If we realize this, then we can learn to gather the most significant symptoms by carefully wording our questions and deciding which information to record during the case taking.

In addition to identifying types of symptoms, it is also possible to modify the initial description of a symptom to gather more information and refine a very general symptom into one that is helpful in the selection of a curative remedy.

Let's look at the types of symptoms involved in case taking, and how they can be refined and modified for this purpose.

Types of symptoms. It is important to be able to identify the type of symptom being reported during the case taking process. The types include:

- **The Chief Complaint** (also know as the **main complaint,** or **entering complaint).** This is the symptom that is perhaps the most important to the case from the patient's point of view. It is the symptom (or symptoms) that drove the patient to seek treatment, and is, therefore, the symptom least tolerated. For this reason, it is very important to the case—after all, it is the reason the patient is there to see you.

    The chief complaint can be any type of symptom. It can, and often is, very common in nature, such as a headache or backache. Or it can be very specific, and a leading keynote symptom, such as the pregnant woman who becomes sick to her stomach every time she puts her hands into warm water to do dishes.

Pay special attention to the chief complaint when seeking the remedy to treat the totality of the symptoms, whatever kind of symptom it is, and however it seems to blend or not blend with the other symptoms reported.

- **Common** (also called **Absolute) symptoms.** These symptoms live up to their type. Headache, stomachache, nightmares: all are symptoms so common to our lives that they are not helpful in leading to a curative remedy by themselves. They lead to dozens of potential curative remedies, so it is important to find some way of working with information about this type of symptom to make it usable. This is the important process of modifying information about common symptoms, because as many symptoms as possible should be modified from being simple, general statements of pain. This requires breaking down the information about common symptoms of the case so they can be identified as different types of symptoms.
- **General symptoms.** These are symptoms that speak to the nature of the patient as a whole being, rather than to specific parts or areas of the patient's body. For example,

the patient is better with heat and when he is in a nice warm room, and worse in damp weather.

The categories of general symptoms are:

1. **Mental symptoms** are often considered general symptoms because they control the patient's motivations, and they are often the "why" of the case. The mind is considered more important in homeopathic medicine than the body, because even simple mental symptoms can overwhelm the physical body.

2. **Desires and Aversions,** things that the patient especially wants or hates are important, because, again, they are motivators of behavior. The patient may crave a hot shower and may jump away from a cold washcloth, because he knows that warmth will ameliorate his condition and cold will cause pain. In the same way, food and thirst cravings are important, and are often strong indicators of a remedy.

3. **Weaknesses** in general are indicators of a breakdown in the body's physical nature. Also important are *predispositions* the patient has to specific diseases and conditions. The past number of similar conditions the patient has experienced, and known predispositions to specific condi-

tions are often strong indicators, as to whether a given condition is acute or chronic.

4. The **general physical characteristics** such as the build of the patient's body, his eye and hair color, and his general physical appearance is important, as especially in childhood, some physical types tend toward certain specific remedies more than other types. For instance, that blond-haired, blue-eyed angel may require Phosphorus more often than Sepia as a curative remedy. It should be noted that this category is not important in acute treatment, but is vital in constitutional treatment.

5. **Modalities** are the final type of general symptoms. Modalities are the things that make both the patient as a whole being and his individual symptoms feel better or worse, so they are perhaps the most important type of general symptom. See below for more information on the types of modalities that play a part in case taking.

• **Specific (or Local) symptoms** are symptoms that are *specific* to one organ or area of the body. They are perhaps most important to the case, as they are the symptoms that most often bring the patient in for treatment. Specific symptoms may also relate to the area affected by the symptom. For instance, they may include the side of the body where a specific symptom usually occurs.

- **Functional symptoms** are symptoms related to the *function* of the affected organ, as opposed to any actual pathology. In fact, functional symptoms usually precede organic or pathological changes. Functional symptoms such as acid indigestion, are often uncomfortable, but may be of little importance to the overall case unless they are accompanied by symptoms in another location.

- **Determining (or Characteristic) symptoms** are related to the chief complaint, and often are related to general symptoms as well. In fact, determining symptoms may be found within a given general symptom, once it has been picked apart.

  For instance, the patient complains about a headache that lasts a long time and leaves him weak and dizzy. This complaint may lead to a list of six or seven remedies, if only the core idea of a long-term headache is considered. But once we begin to pick this general symptom apart, we also consider that the headache leaves the man weak and dizzy. If we work with the chief complaint and the two functional complaints, we may be able to narrow that list of remedies down to just one that will be most appropriate.

Note that some texts may also refer to these as **secondary** symptoms, while others think of secondary symptoms as somewhat rarer, and consider them to be keynote symptoms.

- **Keynote (or Leading) symptoms.** Ah, keynotes. Just as the case's common symptoms give the general information as to the nature of the patient's illness, the keynote symptoms give us specific information for this particular case. These are the symptoms that are most unique and unusual, so they therefore are those that will lead us to the fewest number of remedies. It is easy to fall in love with keynote symptoms for this reason.

    One example of a keynote symptom might be that pregnant woman who becomes nauseated when she places her hands in warm water. This is keynote to Phosphorus, and the symptom, when discovered, helps lead the practitioner to that remedy. Keynotes, while helpful, should not be relied upon too much in the selection of remedies, however.

    Remember, we are treating the person, not the disease, and the keynote represents only a small part of that being. Depending too heavily upon specific keynotes leads to allopathic treatment—treatment of the parts and not of the whole. Many students of homeopathy decide to base their whole case taking on keynotes, upon learning about them. Believe me, it will not work. While there are some shortcuts to case taking—basing it on objective symptoms, for example—treating on the basis of keynotes alone is not one of them. It makes for very sloppy homeopathy.

- **Concomitant symptoms** are those that appear simultaneously with other important symptoms. The patient may, for example, never have nausea without also experiencing dizziness. The other way concomitants are considered is when one symptom always precludes another. An example of this is the patient who says, "I can always tell when I am going to get a migraine, because the vision in my left eye blurs before the headache begins."

- **Alternating symptoms.** Perhaps the most common alternating symptoms in this day and age of irritable bowel syndrome may be diarrhea alternating with constipation. But for this type of symptom we are looking for one symptom that clears entirely, only to be replaced by another symptom that clears entirely, and another symptom that replaces it and then clears, making way again for the first symptom to reappear.

Note that it is important that each symptom totally appear and complete its cycle before the next one begins for them to be considered alternating. If one does not end completely before the other begins, and the two dovetail, they are concomitant and not alternating symptoms.

Case Taking: Learning to Modify Symptoms

I know that it seems as if we have been gathering a lot of information already, but remember, in the simple acute case, the symptoms are few and easily explored and/or examined.

But there will be cases in which you, as the practitioner, are at a loss by this point in the case taking. You have so much information written down, and so much discussion of the case, and yet you don't seem to have any information that points you to a specific curative remedy. It is in cases like these, when all the information gathered seems to be so general, and so applicable to many different cases and ailments, that you need to learn to modify the symptoms you have gathered.

And modifying symptoms involves another aspect of symptoms that we have not considered until now, which is the patient's own sub-jective experience of his pain.

You see, in taking the homeopathic case, you will have to learn to deal with the *sensa-tions* along with the symptoms of the disease, especially sensations of pain that accompany the symptoms. Like good journalists, we also need to know the who, what, when, where, and how of the symptoms. As part of this process of modifying the symptoms, we also have to learn about the modalities of the symptoms, the things that make these symptoms feel bet-ter and/or worse.

Remember, you will need to gather this in-formation about each symptom to be able to clearly and completely work with that symptom.

Types of symptom modifiers. A number of standard modifiers or questions about char-acteristics of symptoms will assist in your identification of the type of symptom and the best remedy for the case. They include:

- **Duration and onset.** Questions regarding duration include: How long have the symp-toms been in place? In the case of multiple symptoms, in what order did they appear? The flow of these symptoms and their order of arrival on the scene can tell us a good deal about the patient as a whole and unique being.

Questions about onset include: What were the circumstances under which the patient first experienced the symptom or symptoms? Has he not been well since a particular bout of flu five years ago? Or, since his parents' divorce thirty years ago? The treatment for a back problem caused by anxiety and one caused by a physical blow to the back are miles apart, but simple to identify once you have determined onset.

- **Location.** This is another way to modify a common symptom into one that is helpful in finding a cure. There is a great difference in the remedy repertoire for the symptom "headache" and the symptom "frontal headache" or "occipital headache." It is very helpful in case taking to discover the specific location of the symptom.

- **Sensation.** This is where we break down the headache into a sort of philosophic notion about "What is the sensation of the pain?" Sensations are always subjective, but they are often very helpful in selecting a proper remedy. The most common sensations are cold or hot, types of pain (ranging from burning, to sharp, to dull, to cramping, and so on), heaviness, enlargement, and other such "feelings" experienced by the patient.

Note: The homeopathic research book *Sensations "As If,"* by Herbert A. Roberts, is a dictionary format collection of specific sensations of pain and the remedies they suggest. It can be a helpful tool in uncovering remedies through the use of the patient's own words concerning his experience of discomfort.

- **Specific Modalities.** Modalities are, indeed, the most helpful of the symptom modifiers. In asking about the modalities of our patient's symptoms, we are seeking to understand the particular way in which a patient reacts to his disease condition, both externally and internally. As mentioned earlier, modalities are those things that make a symptom feel better or worse. For instance, some insect stings make the patient want to cover the affected area with ice, while others make him seek a warm cloth.

  Information on individual modalities should be sought for each symptom listed by the patient, because they will help in determining specific curative remedies.

  The list of catalysts that have impact upon individual symptoms includes:

- **Time Modalities.** Ask the patient questions such as: When in the day or night is the symptom better, and when is it worse? Are there times of day when the patient's energy is high or low? Are there periods when anxiety or well being increases? Look for the rhythms of pain, energy, and weakness in the patient.

In the modality of time, also try to find out if the changes of symptoms and energy are rapid or slow. Does the patient suddenly feel faint at 4:00P.M., or does he slowly wind down to exhaustion from 2:00P.M. until 4:00P.M.?

- **Weather Modalities.** In constitutional cases, we look for the influences of the seasons upon the patient, the best and worst time of year, the easiest and hardest transitions between seasons.

  In acute cases, look for how different weather patterns and weather transitions, such as thunderstorms, damp weather, sunshine, and other climate changes affect the patient .

- **Body Modalities.** Learn how different body positions affect the patient. Is he better lying down than he is standing? Can he sleep on his back? How does he hold his head when he sits? Look at his posture and his body positions to help find the proper remedy.

- **Movement Modalities.** Ask questions relating to movement, such as: Are the symptoms better or worse when the patient is moving? On first motion or sustained motion? Check whether any specific motions increase or alleviate pain.

Both body position and movement modalities can be very important to an acute case, especially the first aid case that involves strain from lifting or physical stress. Try to find out the positions that cause the greatest pain and those that offer the greatest comfort in these cases in particular.

- **Hunger Modalities.** What foods are craved? What is the result when these foods are eaten? What food temperatures are craved, and what happens when they are eaten? Also, find out how the patient's sense of hunger has changed from the time before his illness.

- **Thirst Modalities.** Look again for craving, temperature, and the manner in which the thirst is satisfied—how often, in what amounts, and at what temperature, and what happens when the liquid is drunk.

  Again, how has the patient's thirst changed in terms of amount, temperature, and type of liquid sought from the time before he became ill?

- **Sleep Modalities.** Does sleep help or hurt the symptoms at hand? In what position does the patient sleep? What routine must be followed to get the patient to sleep?

And how has that routine changed since before his illness?

- **Temperature Modalities.** Does the patient feel cold in general, or hot? What is his vital heat? Does he wear more or less clothing than the average person for the sake of comfort? Is this patient's comfort greatly dependent upon the temperature of his environment? If so, how?
- **Emotional Modalities.** How do the patient's moods affect specific symptoms? For example, does pain follow anger? Or does the pain come before the anger?

  Often, emotions and symptoms are a chicken or the egg proposition and it is difficult to determine which came first, but it can be of great help to be able to determine how the emotions affect the symptoms.

Case Taking: Gathering Information Concerning the Patient

Now that you have concluded gathering information about the patient's disease, and its symptoms, it is important to get some information about the patient himself. For our present purposes, this means we will ignore the aches and pains in specific parts of the patient's body and again consider him as a whole being.

- **General modalities.** You have already gathered this information concerning the patient's symptoms. Now, ask the patient what makes him feel better and feel worse as a whole person. Remember not to lead him. Simply record what things he finds of comfort while he is ill, and what things present challenges.
- **Other treatments already used.** It is often very important to know about any allopathic treatments the patient has undergone before deciding to change to homeopathic treatments. Remember, allopathic medicines are suppressive by their very nature, and they may have created other symptoms. In fact, they may have caused the situation at hand.

    In the case of some patients, especially those of an advanced age or those with otherwise weakened immune systems, it may be vital that you do not attempt to treat the case at all, but instead turn it over to a professional homeopath. This is especially true if a patient has been treated with antibiotics and/or steroids, like cortisone. Remember, the stronger the allopathic medicine, the more likely it is that it will act suppressively. Patients with systems severely weakened by illness, allopathic drugs or any combination of these may not be able to handle a poorly selected homeo-pathic treatment.

We must also consider what previously taken homeopathic remedies may have done to the case. It is just as important to know what acute homeopathic treatments the patient might have already undertaken as it is to know about the allopathic treatments. If the patient tried to treat himself and has already taken one or two remedies (and neither did much good), then unfortunately some time will have to pass until he can take any other remedies. In the case of a short-term ailment like a cold, this may mean that the patient will have to suffer through his illness as best he can, drinking tea and resting. It is safe to consider another remedy only after enough time has passed for the previous remedies to have worn off.

If the patient has taken more than two remedies, or has taken combination remedies, then it is best he not be treated at all. Any other remedy will only confuse the case more, and may also create unpredictable long-term changes in the patient's health.

If the patient has already been medicated for the same acute ailment, consider the case only with the greatest care. Perhaps wisdom suggests that you learn to know when *not* to treat a case.

- **Medications regularly taken.** For the same reasons as those listed above, it is important to know what allopathic medicines the patient takes for other chronic conditions. Like medicines taken for acute ailments, those taken for chronic conditions may indicate that you should not take it on yourself to treat the case at all.

  It is also just as important to know about homeopathic remedies that are being taken regularly as it is to know about allopathic medicines. The patient under constitutional treatment should be very careful about disrupting it with an acute remedy. In fact, the patient under constitutional treatment should seek the help of the same homeopath who treats him constitutionally when he requires acute treatment. An ill-selected acute remedy can confuse or distort the constitutional case.

Concluding the Case Taking

Okay, by now you have observed your patient and have examined his wounds. You have had a conversation with him, which started out as a monologue on his part. It then became a question and answer period that let you fill in any gaps in information relating to his case. With skillful questions, you modified his general symptoms into helpful specific, characteristic, and keynote symptoms, and you have come to understand the specific and general modalities relating to his case.

Given all that has transpired, you may think that hours have passed. And indeed, a good two hours may have passed, if we were taking a complete constitutional case. But only a handful of minutes have usually gone by in taking a simple, acute case.

Perhaps your patient has a cold. It is likely he has about three major symptoms, such as a runny nose, sneezing, and a sore throat. You have done a good deal to narrow the field of possible remedies if you have modified these symptoms into a nose in which mucus flow alternates sides, so one side flows freely when the other is blocked; sneezing that is worse in the morning or when the patient is in a warm room, and better when the patient is outside; and a sore throat that started on the left side and moved to the right, so that now both sides are sore. If you have further found out that the patient is not at all thirsty in spite of the sore throat, and seems more needy and clingy than usual, then you have narrowed the list of remedies even more. And if your examination of the patient has revealed that his eyes are red and puffy, his nose is red and sore just beneath the nostrils, and his throat a dry, dark red, then you have even more helpful information.

By this time, if you know your materia medica, you may just want to check one or two remedies before you make a choice of curative remedy. If you do not know the remedies well enough, you many need the help of a household guide like this one, or of a repertory, in your selection. Either way, you have done your case taking well, and are ready to conclude the process.

The final question. You've gone through the "who, what, when, where, why, and how," and found out everything you think you want to know. The names of remedies are already dancing through your mind. You are remembering that Pulsatilla is thirstless, worse in a warm room, and better in open air. That Allium Cepa colds often feature crusty and sore noses. That both Sulphur and Lachesis, among other remedies, tend to have symptoms that begin on the left side of the body and move right.

You are chomping at the bit to get the patient out of the room so you can determine the remedy. You feel quite comfortable being finished listening to anything he has to say.

But what if he is not finished talking?

Just like those short silences that occur in case taking, the end of the conversation can often yield very important information, if you give the patient just one more chance to talk.

So, before finishing, rising, or thanking him for his time, remember to ask one last question before giving him his remedy. Tell the patient to take a minute to reflect, and ask if there is anything that he has left out, anything that you should know.

Sometimes this question will yield nothing. Everything has been said, and both of you are quite satisfied. But other times there is something the patient has been holding back, unsure if he should tell you, or whether or not he wants to tell you. This information is often the key to the whole case, but it involves information the patient is timid about, or perhaps ashamed of sharing. He may tell you if he is given the opportunity, and it may change everything about the case as you have seen it up to that point.

So make sure when concluding the case that not only you feel satisfied by the information give-and-take, but your patient does as well.

The Benefits of a Well-Taken Case

In a well kept kitchen, you can find the paprika when you need it. In a well-kept living room, you can lay your hand on the television remote on a moment's notice.

Likewise, in the well-taken case, you can find the information you need with little or no effort: for instance, the particular statement the patient made concerning a specific symptom. It is right there in front of you. The information taken flows smoothly, from chief complaint to general symptom, and from general symptom to specific, characteristic, and keynote symptoms. The symptom modifiers and modalities are right there, too. And the information on the patient is at the end: his general modalities and how they compare to the time before the illness, and the medicines he is currently taking for acute or chronic symptoms.

The information is all at hand. If it has been taken clearly and completely, it is a map of the situation that not only you can follow for proper homeopathic treatment, but any other student of homeopathy could follow as well.

And, it is a map of the territory you have covered at this moment in your study of homeopathy. This case taking will be of great help to you in the future if this patient ever needs you again, because you have already gathered so much information about him in states of health and of illness. It also will be a general record of your past case taking that you can learn from as you develop your skills.

For all these reasons, master homeopaths have said, "A case that is well taken is half cured."

After Case Taking: What to Do Next

What happens once the case is taken is determined by what has happened so far. If you have taken the case and are sure that the portrait of the patient's illness clearly matches the picture of a specific remedy in its actions, then you are ready to treat the patient.

But even when you feel sure of a remedy, I always think that it is a very good idea to return to the materia medica to reread the information about the remedy you have in mind before you begin to treat. Be sure that you feel confident that this is the curative remedy before giving it. Remember, it comes down to the symptoms and how well the patient's symptoms match those that can be created by giving a healthy person the remedy you have in mind.

Symptoms and Materia Medica

You've gathered your symptoms. And it is likely that you have formed a "disease diagnosis" along the way by giving the malady at hand a name like "toothache" or "common cold."

Now it is time to take the information you have gathered concerning the disease diagnosis and to develop it into a drug diagnosis. In doing this, you will give the treatment a name that is the name of a homeopathic remedy, so instead of being a "common cold," the case will become an "Arsenicum case" or a "Lycopodium situation."

But how do we get there?

Well, if you are like many other beginning students of homeopathy, you send the patient off to bed, and tell him that you will be upstairs in a minute with a remedy. Then you go to your bookshelf and get down this book or another like it. And never having read the section in the middle of the book (that long part on the individual remedies), you turn to the back, where it lists the remedies for each condition, and you look under "common cold." You pick the remedy that sounds best, and give the patient a dose before bedtime.

This often works, but this is the most limited way of practicing homeopathy. In fact, I am not sure that you can even consider it to be homeopathy that is being practiced—or guessed at.

You see, that section in the middle of the book on the remedies themselves is probably the most important part of the book for any student of homeopathy to read, and to read again. Often.

Homeopathy, in its true form, is always practiced from the materia medica. And while Samuel Hahnemann did not create the first materia medica—those had existed for thousands of years before him, listing herbal and natural remedies—he did create the first homeopathic materia medica. He knew that only by knowing what actions each remedy can take within the human system could we even have an inkling of what remedy to use in any given case.

Therefore, the materia medica is the source of all wisdom for any student of homeopathy. This volume has a short materia medica, listing only fifty-odd remedies, that stresses objective symptoms over subjective. It was created for use only in acute situations.

As you continue your study of homeopathy, you will soon find that this materia medica is too limited for your purposes, and it is likely that you will decide to buy another. I encourage you to do so. In fact, if you become a serious student of homeopathy, I encourage you to own as many different materia medicas as you can afford.

This is because each materia medica presents the perspective of one homeopath, and they are all different. My experience has been that each has a good deal to offer, however. The shelves in my office are filled with many such volumes, and I find that I turn to them again and again for help in times of need.

So for now, with the case at hand that you have just taken, it is fine and appropriate that you look to see what remedies are listed and which seems most likely to be curative, but don't stop there. Before giving any remedy make sure to also turn to the Objective Materia Medica section, and see what information is listed there about the remedy you think is best. In fact, check out the information on several of the remedies. You may find that, on deeper consideration, there is another remedy that may be even more helpful than the one you first had in mind.

Symptoms and the Repertory

American homeopath James Tyler Kent said, "Any man who desires to avoid this careful method should not pretend to be a homeopathic physician." Of course, he said that as one of the homeopaths who developed the repertory as a homeopathic tool in the first place.

At some point in your study it will become necessary to learn to use a repertory in case taking. When that time comes is up to you.

Certainly, home guides like this one have their place in homeopathic medicine. They provide a basic understanding of the philosophy and practice of homeopathy, and a foundation for understanding the actions of some of our major remedies as well as some minor remedies helpful in specific household emergencies. They mimic the repertory to some extent, in that they list common acute ailments, and then provide a list of remedies that are most commonly used to treat those patients with those specific ailments. They also give information on the ways in which those needing the different remedies experience the symptoms associated with a given ailment.

Household guides are fine, as far as they go. The trouble is that most can't and don't go far enough. There simply is not enough space in the guide to replicate the information contained in a repertory. So, at some point, you may want to graduate from your well-worn home guide and get yourself a repertory. But which one should you choose?

Again, that's up to you, because although each homeopathic repertory is structured in the same way, each is also very different from the other.

188

Each repertory is a dictionarylike alphabetical listing of symptoms of all types and the remedies those symptoms suggest. But each repertory is also the idiosyncratic product of one person's mind. It is organized as that practitioner thought it should be organized, so they are all quite different. One homeopathy may list a given symptom under digestion. Another may not even list digestion as a heading, putting the symptom under stomach, an area in which digestion takes place.

So look through many repertories before you select one of them. See how each is laid out, and try to understand the logic behind it. Then choose the one whose creator thinks the most like you and whose logic makes the most sense to you.

In times of emergency, you are going to have to be able to find the remedy and find it fast, so the more a book is laid out as you would have done it, the more quickly you will find the information you need.

Whichever repertory you choose, don't wait until you are faced with an emergency to open the book and then expect it to help you. If it is to be any good to you at all, you have to open it up and look through it again and again *before* you actually need it. Become familiar with the book and how to use it in times of quiet, and it will serve you well in times of emergency. Read the introductory chapter with the homeopath's suggestions as to how best to use it.

For now, back in the world of the home guide, we have looked at the various methods of case taking. Now that we have taken the case, it is important that we spend some time learning how to manage it.

5

Putting It Together: Managing the Acute Case

Case Management begins where case taking ends, and where record keeping begins. Now is the time to get out a folder and to put your patient's name on it. Place all your case taking notes inside the folder, along with your repertorization of the case, if you made one.

Now take a moment and write down your thoughts on the case. What is your disease diagnosis? What is your drug diagnosis? How did you arrive at each diagnosis?

If you narrowed the long list of available homeopathic remedies down to a short list of five or six before making your ultimate selection of a curative remedy, then make sure to write down the other remedies on the short list, and why you considered them for use. This may become very handy later.

And, after you have given the first dose of the selected remedy, make sure to note the time of that dose, and the potency of the remedy used.

WAITING

A wise homeopath from India once told me that, when it comes to treating any patient homeopathically, the formula is the same: waiting+watching=wisdom.

The first step after giving the remedy is simply to wait: to do nothing else except let the remedy act. This involves an act of trust, because you have to actually believe that well-selected homeopathic remedies have the ability to act as catalysts to change the patient's whole state of health for the better, and that as the dose of the artificial remedy acts and then fades, its symptoms will remove the natural symptoms already present in the patient's system if they are similar enough.

Once you selected the best remedy in what you think is an appropriate potency (and the always appropriate single dose) you have nothing left to do except wait—and watch what happens.

WATCHING

While you are waiting, you will, I am sure, be watching your patient. But what are you watching for?

Many new students of homeopathy are unsure about the signs or signals that might indicate that a remedy is working, and that the patient is actually improving.

Signs of Improvement

The major signs of improvement or indicators that you have, indeed, selected the correct remedy are listed below. As you look at the list, you might think that they are oddly in opposition with one another, but they share a strong common bond: each of the signs represents a strong change in the state of the patient. Any change in the patient—in his symptoms, or even better, in his whole being—is what we are watching for when we give a homeopathic remedy. But change is a hard thing to predict, and an even harder thing to control. Often the expectation is that the remedy will have one specific action, but when it is given, it instead does several other things as well, things we hadn't expected. But I have found, again and again, that there is a natural wisdom far beyond my own inherent in the healing process. The correct remedy will have the action needed to move the patient from sickness to health, whether or not it is the action I originally had in mind.

So there is not just one change that can indicate improvement in the patient, but several.

There is improvement in the patient's energy. This is the best sign that the remedy is working. The listless, exhausted, or angry patient begins to change. His eyes take on a shine that had been lacking. She seems more like her old self.

This perking up is a general improvement that involves the patient's whole being. He has more physical energy. His will seems stronger and his mind clearer. The patient with no interest in his appearance until now may ask for a mirror. That is a very good sign.

Ironically, the patient will often have this general boost in energy without any improvement in specific symptoms. The patient with a migraine may still have her headache, but she will tell you that she is "more able to deal with it now." That is a very good sign, because the specific symptoms will now fall away as well, given time.

The patient falls asleep. This is another excellent sign. You may have a patient whose discomfort keeps him from sleeping well: he may have a runny nose or a cough that keeps him awake. You give the remedy, and you see the patient begin to relax after a few minutes. His features return from the contortions of discomfort back to his normal face. His limbs begin to relax and unfold. His breathing becomes less labored.

And the patient falls into a gentle, peaceful sleep.

You may want to sit and watch the patient as he sleeps, or you may take this time to get some rest yourself. Either way, you will know that the patient will be improved when he awakens.

The patient's symptoms fall away. This is the jackpot everyone wants to see. Sometimes, when the remedy is correct and the potency is just right, something very dramatic happens. The patient's symptoms just seem to drop away, and the patient is well.

This happened to me, personally.

I used to have a weak back that went into spasm from time to time. One of those times was when I was cleaning my apartment. I had been vacuuming, or whatever, and suddenly I threw my back out by lifting or twisting. I dropped to the floor, unable to move from the pain. My home remedies were stored on the top shelf of my closet, so they were completely out of reach. They might as well have been in another building or city.

I lay on the floor in agony for a few minutes before I realized that the telephone cord was nearby. I grabbed the cord and pulled, and got hold of the telephone. I called a friend who had a key to my apartment, and told her what had happened. She got in her car and came right over.

I don't know how long I lay there while she was on her way, but the next thing I knew, I was looking up at her towering over me. It hurt to move, it hurt to breathe, it hurt to talk. But I managed to say, "Rhus Tox." She rummaged through the drawers of my homeopathic chest. "What potency?" she asked.

"1M." I answered.

The next thing I knew, I had the pellets in my mouth.

My friend sat down on the floor next to me. I thanked her for coming to my aid, and began to tell her what happened. I remember we were talking about how silly the whole situation seemed. When I started to laugh hard, picturing myself on the floor because of vacuuming, I spontaneously sat up. I didn't even realize that I had done it, and it took a moment for the two of us to realize what had happened.

The pain had simply ended. The case was closed that quickly.

That's what we all hope for when we give a remedy: that it will act, as Hahnemann promised, "rapidly, gently and permanently." It's not always the case, but when it happens, it seems like a miracle. And, in my experience, it happens most often in first aid cases. You may give that Arnica to your child, and find that the whole problem is resolved before the pellet has totally melted on his tongue.

In many cases, the symptoms do not fall away completely, but there is a fast improvement. The headache lessens. Cramps end. All of the patient's symptoms may improve at the same time, or some symptoms may recede while others remain unchanged. In any case, partial improvement of the case is another very good sign that you have selected the correct remedy.

Keep good notes about which symptoms have improved, and by how much. I usually ask for a percentage of improvement for each symptom. Even a ten percent improvement is a sign that the remedy is working. Anything at twenty percent or above is cause for celebration.

The patient's symptoms get worse. When the patient seems to become worse, this is called an *aggravation.* It is quite common in acute cases; in fact, it is so common that some practitioners actually have come to expect it.

An aggravation is a bump in the road of the acute case to the homeopath. The patient's symptoms get a little worse for a few hours before they become very much improved.

Some homeopaths think that the aggravation is the sign that the remedy selected was given in the correct potency. The artificial disease state is slightly stronger than the natural disease so the symptoms actually become worse for a time, until the symptoms of the remedy fall away and take the natural disease and symptoms with them.

Whatever the cause of the aggravation, the process holds true. The patient whose symptoms temporarily get worse will soon be much improved.

Note that an aggravation should last no longer than a matter of hours, or a day or two at most. If the patient continues to struggle with aggravated symptoms after that it may be a sign of proving rather than aggravation. Proving is an intensifying of symptoms caused by over-medicating on a homeopathic remedy. This may be the situation if the remedy has been repeated too often in too short a time. It is a temporary condition that can be avoided by following the laws of cure.

Whatever the reason, the patient experiencing an aggravation for more than two days should be taken to a professional practitioner.

Evaluating the Case

So, you've taken the case, selected and given the remedy of choice, and now you are waiting. But how long do you wait to see if the remedy is correct?

As I've described, some remedies will act in a manner that is clearly visible in only a matter of moments in some situations. This is true most often in first aid cases, from falls and spills to bee stings, scrapes and cuts.

Ironically, this is also true for cases of homeopathic Band-Aids, those cases in which you are using an acute remedy to temporarily improve a chronic condition, like allergy or toothache, until you can get the patient to the doctor. The remedy tends to act very quickly in these treatments, much to the delight of the patient, but they will not act for very long. If the patient tries to get such a treatment to hold for more than two or three days he may find himself awakened by that toothache again, and the toothache may no longer respond to the remedy.

It is the cases in the middle—things like coughs and colds, sleep disturbances, digestive upsets and the like—that may be more difficult to treat and take longer to resolve.

Colds, for instance, often take three different remedies to resolve: one for each stage of the cold. The first stage of the cold is from onset until nasal discharge begins. The second stage is the stage of clear discharge, and the third stage is the stage of colored discharge. The patient is still going to have to experience that cold, although homeopathic treatment may make the cold resolve itself much more swiftly, and make the cold itself much less taxing to the patient's system than it would be without treatment.

Remember, in homeopathic medicine, we suppress nothing. We never try to give medicine that allows the patient to pretend he is well and go out and infect everyone else. Homeopathic treatment will lessen the impact of an infectious ailment on the patient's system and greatly shorten the time it takes for him to recover, but it will not just mask and suppress his symptoms.

Since we cannot predict the change a remedy will create or dictate the path healing will take, it is of vital importance that we note the path and record the change. This is all part of case management, and case management is just as important as case taking, even in the simple acute case.

Too many students of homeopathy just want to make their best guess as to a remedy to give—and often they only know a handful of remedies to consider. These same students tend to keep no notes. They depend upon their memories to remind them when they last gave the patient a dose of the remedy, or to recall the potency of that dose.

Worse, they think that they will remember what they did, and will know what to do when such an accident or illness occurs again.

These people tend never to become better homeopaths than they were when they started.

It is my hope that you will not fall into this category, and that you will work to improve yourself as a practitioner, always honing your skills for the moment of emergency when they will be tested. This involves learning to take the case, and learning to manage it. It involves knowing what remedy to give in the first dose, and at what potency, and when and if you should give a second dose. It involves learning when and how to conclude treatment. Most of all, it involves learning: learning from the cases you get right, and, especially, learning from the cases you get wrong.

Signs of a Lack of Improvement

With the idea of something going wrong, let's take a moment to consider what you might do if you have, through you best efforts, selected and given a remedy that apparently has had no action in the patient.

The patient and his symptoms remain unchanged. If you have given a single dose of a remedy and nothing happens at all, then you have either selected the wrong remedy, or you have given the right remedy in a potency that is too low to make a change in the case.

Experience has taught me to explore a third possibility at this point, before going any further. This is the possibility that the remedy did act, but that the patient has not noticed its action. When a homeopathic remedy is given, the effects are often subtle, though powerful. The patient may often not be aware that changes have taken place, because unlike many of the allopathic medicines given for the same ailments, the remedies cause no artificial exhaustion. It is indeed quite safe to operate big machinery while under homeopathic treatment.

Therefore, get out your list of symptoms when you are not sure whether the remedy has worked or not. Starting with the chief complaint, ask the patient if he feels any difference or improvement in that symptom. Ask him for a percentage of change in the symptom.

Often the patient complaining that nothing is happening will admit that, yes, his tooth is hurting less, but may still insist that nothing is happening. Asked again, he may say that, yes, he slept better last night, but that he is sure that the remedy is doing nothing at all.

Some patients are just that way.

If there has been at least a ten percent change in some of the symptoms, it is my opinion that the remedy is the right one because it is doing something. But during my waiting and watching, I would be contemplating the possibility that the remedy should be given in a slightly higher potency next time. (To get an explanation of what I mean by "slightly higher potency," see below.)

This will happen. Patients will get you to second guess yourself many times, when you are actually quite correct in your selection of remedy. So make sure that you consider this third possibility before you consider the other two.

But say you try this approach, and the patient insists that, really, nothing has changed, and you can verify this with your own senses or a thermometer. What do you do then?

This is when you must revisit your case taking, look over your notes, and consider the case again. Open your materia medica and check each of the remedies you considered for the case before you narrowed it down to just one. Confirm your opinions, while keeping your mind open to the possibility that you simply were in error in your remedy selection.

After you have rechecked the case taking and your materia medica, it is time to make a decision. Do you stay with the original remedy, and this time give it in a higher potency? Or do you change remedies, and try a second remedy for the patient?

There is no easy answer to this question, of course, because every homeopathic case is different. There can be no simple rule of thumb. But, when faced with this question, I try to look at the patient again from all sides, from all aspects of what has changed from the time he was well until this time of illness. When in doubt, I tend to try and stress the mental and emotional symptoms, and I ask myself "What remedy is he acting like?" or "Who is he in this illness?" This is often very helpful, in that one respiratory infection, for instance, can look very much like another in terms of physical symptoms.

If this does not help, I again consider the list of remedies from which I selected the first remedy. You see, there is a difference between a list that is six remedies long, and one that has only two remedies. If I had narrowed the case down to just two remedies and each seemed to equally fit the case, then I might be more likely to try the other remedy than I would be if the list had been longer, and my original choice stuck out from the group when I narrowed down the field.

All things being equal, I tend to trust my original assessment of the case and stick with my original remedy.

How much I increase the potency also depends on many things. For instance, if I used a 30C potency only once with no result, I might dissolve several pellets of the original remedy, in that original potency, in a clean glass of distilled or filtered water. I would then succuss the dissolved remedy by stirring the liquid many times—up to two or three hundred times—with a clean spoon. (Some homeopaths refer to this as an "aqua" remedy, and add the word aqua in front of the name of the remedy to indicate that it was given in liquid form.)

This procedure will not greatly change the potency—I doubt that my stirring will change the remedy's potency even to 31C—but it will make a small change in the potency of the remedy, and often that is enough.

In fact, it is often a good idea to give aqua remedies in acute situations, and to always stir them between doses. That way, you never quite repeat the same potency, but always raise and change it slightly between doses. Often this is very helpful in clearing away symptoms and closing the case.

Finally, we have to consider the possibility that you have tried your first remedy, you have changed its potency after it failed to work, and now you have tried a second remedy with the same results. Your patient is miserable and getting no better, and you are still left with the question of whether you should change the potency again, or try a third remedy.

This is a time when you should gather your notes, bundle up your patient, and go to see a medical professional. Take those notes with you so that you can let your professional homeopath look them over, so he or she can know exactly what has already been done and why. This will be a valuable tool for your practitioner to use. It will also be a valuable learning tool for you, as your practitioner will perhaps be able to help you understand the remedies or the power of the different potencies more clearly.

If you find yourself in a medical professional's office, you should not be upset or angry with yourself for needing to ask for help. In the first place, doing so ensures that your patient, who is no doubt a loved one, is receiving the best care possible. In the second place, your humility in asking for help will ground you, and allow you to learn from your errors.

Remember, everyone, even the best of medical professionals, gets it wrong sometimes.

FROM THE FIRST DOSE ONWARD

Everything you need to know about the first dose is contained within the principles presented in the Three Laws of Cure. In fact, I have found again and again that you can't go wrong as a homeopathic practitioner if you rely on these laws. They will always make you somewhat conservative in your treatments, and therefore will always allow you to see appropriate and gentle results.

The First Law: Similar

This is the principle of homeopathy that guides us in the selection of a remedy, and in giving that remedy. It guides us as we begin homeopathic treatment, and as we end it.

The Law of Similar states, "Like Cures Like." And those three words both sum up and fully express the way healing works, and the ways in which we may be made well.

We have already explored this principle in regard to case taking. We must search for the remedy whose actions in the human system most nearly match the symptoms already at hand in the patient's system. If we give the remedy that best matches the natural ailment in action, the patient taking that remedy will be made well.

The First Law forever informs and reminds us that we can never declare a remedy to be a "backache remedy" or a "headache remedy," since the curative remedy must be the one that most closely mirrors each individual case, and there will be no such thing as a remedy that works for all backaches. If we try to cram the wide-ranging actions of any given remedy into a single slot, we cheapen the healing philosophy of homeopathy. Worse, we create the delusion that the remedies may be successfully used on the basis of "this for that." Such thinking is worse than nonsense: it is dangerous.

It is dangerous first because it means the patient does not receive the healing power of the full range of homeopathy, but instead is subject to the whim of a half-homeopath, who thinks that Rhus Tox cures any backache.

Second, it is dangerous because it makes homeopathy more allopathic. Anything that moves homeopathy toward its opposite practice makes it susceptible to the most disagreeable aspect of allopathic medicine—suppression. In homeopathic treatment, we never seek to suppress a symptom, but always to release it. In making homeopathy more allopathic by declaring and using specific remedies for specific ailments, we open the door to the possibility of suppressing symptoms, and thereby weakening the overall system—the exact outcome we object to in allopathic medicine.

The Second Law: Simplex

So simple. One remedy at a time.

Think of it this way. Hahnemann considered his remedies to be artificial diseases, in that they have the ability to create a range of changes or symptoms within the body of a healthy person. It is for this reason—the fact that the remedies have the power to create change—that they are able to bring about healing.

Now, no one remedy does only one thing. They each do many things, and create many changes, or symptoms, in the human system. For this reason, we must give only one remedy at a time. That is the only way we can measure the impact of the remedy as we wait and watch. If you give more than one remedy, you can not know just what change is being caused by what remedy, no matter how long you wait and watch. Or if, in fact, the presence of the two remedies together has created a new and un-knowable set of symptoms.

It is always safe to give one remedy. Even those healthy people in whose systems the remedies are tested and proven have remained healthy through their treatment. The results of a single remedy are knowable. If the remedy is sufficiently close in its action to the situation in the patient's system, then a single dose of the remedy will cause changes in that system.

Even if the remedy and the patient are not similar, the remedy will cause changes if it is given again and again. This process is called proving. This is the method by which the power of each individual remedy was explored and researched. Proving a remedy is not dangerous. If you have given a remedy too often to a patient and new symptoms begin to sprout, simply stop the remedy. The new symptoms will fade, and in time, the entire proving will fade.

What is dangerous is giving more than one remedy at a time. You cannot know what you will conjure up with a mix of remedies, and you cannot know what changes might occur in the patient. If not being able to predict the changes created by one remedy can cause anxiety on the part of the practitioner at times, imagine how much worse it must be when the poor practitioner is trying to sort out the changes made by more than one remedy. It can be a terrible thing.

Now, hypocrite that I am, I must admit that it may be necessary to give more than one remedy at a time in one set of circumstances, and that has to do with first aid emergencies. Certainly, if a patient has been in a car accident and is fading, it may be necessary to give Arnica and some other remedy, like Aconite perhaps, to keep the patient stable until he can get to the hospital. And in some cases of recovery from surgery Arnica may again need the assistance of another remedy, like Staphysagria, to get the patient well.

Certainly we don't want any homeopathic martyrs about whom people say, "He died, but he died a true homeopath, because he refused that second remedy." But at the same time, we can't abandon the Second Law of Cure, which is the very heart of the practice of homeopathy.

The cases that require us to break the Second Law are few and far between. For the most part, it stands as our guiding principle when giving that first dose.

The Third Law: Minimum

The Third Law, when followed, is a guarantee to the patient that his homeopathic treatment will always be gentle in its actions. Further, it preserves the beauty of the homeopathic healing process.

The Law of Minimum states two things. First, that we should give a homeopathic remedy in the lowest possible effective dose. In other words, we should tamper as little as possible with a patient's Vital Force (or, if you prefer, immune system) while creating an environment in which healing can take place. Therefore, if a simple low potency will do—a potency that will likely cause a gentle aggravation, if any at all—then we never give a higher, more powerful potency. We never want to stir up the Vital Force more than we have to.

Second, the Law of Minimum tells us to give that remedy in the fewest number of effective doses possible. If we need give only one dose of a remedy, then we give only one dose.

Our personal histories with allopathic medicine make this a hard rule to follow. We have been taught that more medicine is certainly better than less medicine. Further, we have been taught by every medicine label that medicine should be given every three to four hours.

But this simply is not true. In dosage as with all else, we are individual people and individual patients. While I may need to take a given remedy four times a day for my ailment, you many need to only take it once, or perhaps twice. Like potency, dosage is determined by the patient's unique Vital Force, and by the power of the ailment on that Vital Force.

So, how then do we know what potency of remedy to give in the first dose, and how many doses should follow that first one?

Well, to start, let's deal with dose. The perfect number of doses to start with is always the same—one. We give one dose of the curative remedy, and then we wait and watch. I tend to think that the best first dose is given before sleeping, preferably at night, and that the dose should be given the night to work. The impact of the first dose should be noted when the patient awakens. I would tend to give a first dose six to eight hours to work before even considering a second dose.

That only if nothing seems to be happening from that first dose. If, as will be usually the case, the remedy seems to have some sort of impact much sooner, you should still continue to wait and watch. See what changes occur and note when they occur. Watch to see how long the changes stay in place.

That is because each dose of a remedy has an arc to its activity. It does not progress in a straight line. The remedy begins to have an impact upon the patient, perhaps to improve his energy in general. With the arc of the remedy's action, the patient will continue to improve and the improvement may become stronger and stronger. At some point, however, the impact of the remedy will begin to lessen and to fade. If the dosage is not repeated the action of the remedy will fade completely.

The time to give the second dose of the remedy is the moment at which its effect begins to fade and its strength begins to let go. You may define this moment as the moment when the patient's symptoms begin to return, or the moment when the patient's strength begins to fade. Either way, this is the moment for the second dose.

Now, there is no way to predict the time of the second dose any more than there is a way to predict the exact action of the remedy. You may need to give a second dose in just fifteen minutes, or the first dose may hold for a day or more. In acute situations, the second dose is most commonly called for in a matter of hours after the first one to keep improvement moving forward. The second dose will begin its impact at the point in the arc where the first dose's effect ended, and it will continue the patient forward in his healing.

If the patient begins to fail again just a few minutes after taking each dose, you may well be giving the curative remedy, but in too low a potency. A higher potency dose of the same remedy, when next it is called for, may hold the patient's improvement for hours, or even days. It may, in fact, conclude the case in a single dosage.

To know just when to give the second dose, or the third or fourth, involves those two aspects of wisdom in homeopathic treatments—waiting and watching. It is important that you pay attention to your case, as it is unfolding in front of you.

Homeopathic treatments work in much the same way regarding the selection of potency as with dosage, which is to say that each of us is unique when it comes to the particular potency we need of a remedy. In fact, some patients respond better to a given potency no matter what remedy is called for, and no matter the reason for treatment. Other patients may have no particular response to a given potency, and may change potency needs with each ailment.

But, because we are attempting to find the lowest effective potency in *every* case, we have to consider the three scales of homeopathic potency, and the impact of each one.

Remember, it is a core truth of homeopathic philosophy that the more diluted a remedy becomes, the more powerful it is. Let's consider each scale of potency with this in mind:

The X Scale

This was Hahnemann's first scale of dilution, in which an amount of the original crude substance from which the remedy is taken is diluted in ten parts of water. That level of dilution is then succussed. The result is a 1X potency, which has been diluted only once, into ten parts.

If one part of that dilution is then diluted again into ten parts and succussed, we have a 2X potency. And so on; the X scale is infinite in that you can always dilute it one more level.

Because the X scale is less dilute than the other two scales, it is also less powerful. Many practitioners tend to just ignore this scale altogether for this reason. I find that, because it is very gentle in its actions, it is very good for two things. First the X scale is good for rashes and skin conditions of all sorts. You see, when working with a rash, you want to bring it forth from the body without spreading it all over the patient's skin from head to toe. If you give too high a potency, you will do just that. The rash will come forth quickly, but with the greatest possible discomfort. A rash that is treated with very low potencies, like 6X or 9X, will tend to come forth much more gently.

This low dilution scale is also helpful for cases of allergy. If, for instance, you are allergic to cat hair, and you take a remedy made from cat hair in a low potency (again, around a 6X or 9X) before seeing the cat, you will find your symptoms greatly reduced. This will be a short-term result, but it can be very helpful from time to time.

If you remember, this method of using a very low dilution of a homeopathic remedy made from the specific material that a patient is allergic to completely mirrors an allopathic approach to allergies. Often, the patient is given very dilute amounts of the material to which he is allergic, repeated over a long period of time, with the hope that these treatments will gradually make the patient less and less allergic to that material.

In the same way, low dilution doses of specific allergens, given over a period of time, can make the patient less allergic to that allergen.

The C Scale

Throughout his career, Samuel Hahnemann forever sought methods by which his medicines could become more effective. So it only stands to reason that he would test the principle of dilution as a means of making better homeopathic remedies.

The centesimal scale dilutes at each level of the process not into ten parts, but into one hundred. Therefore, each remedy is far more dilute at every level of potentization than it is with the X scale.

Think about it: that 30C remedy that you have in your home kit has been diluted into one hundred parts water and then succussed, and then diluted again, and the process has been completed thirty times.

Given that Hahnemann used a glass beaker for each individual part of dilution, it is easy to understand why he never got beyond the creation of a 30C potency in his lifetime. It was physically impossible for an individual working in a private lab to go any further.

But, in his mind, he was able to comprehend where dilution might take his remedies, and he was able to imagine a further scale. (That scale, the M scale, is discussed below.)

The C scale is our middle potency scale of dilution. It is deeper working than is the X scale, but weaker and milder in its actions than is the M scale. This is why it is our most used scale of dilution for remedies. The C scale acts deeply enough to have an impact not only on the patient's physical symptoms, but his mental and emotional symptoms as well. Because of this, many acute and chronic cases can be completely cured by C scale remedies.

Most homeopathic kits sold today are filled with 30C remedies. It is also the potency most commonly found in the average home. For the most part, it is an excellent choice, powerful enough to do some real good, yet gentle enough to not cause harm.

The M Scale

Where the X scale continues on forever, the C scale is finite. At the level of 999C, the next dilution belongs not to the C scale, but to the M scale, M representing the Roman numeral 1,000.

From the point of 1M onward, remedies are diluted to the thousands.

Because of the incredible level of dilution, the M scale remedies are by far the strongest. They reach deep in their healing action into the body and mind of the patient. They are also the longest lasting, and are usually not repeated for a month or more at a time.

Many medical professionals believe that lay persons should not be using M scale remedies in their homes at all. Indeed, some M scale remedies are by law not available to lay persons.

Personally, I don't agree. I believe that many of the remedies that are a part of the home kit should be available in both a mild mid-range potency (most often 30C) and in the higher 1M potency for more serious situations. I have seen again and again that first aid remedies should be present in the home in both medium and high potencies. Remedies like Arnica are regularly needed in high potency. The same may be said for remedies like Belladonna or Ferrum Phos, which speak to symptoms like high fevers, which are best brought under control quickly.

But by and large it is the 30C potency that belongs in the home, because it offers the benefits of its dilution without creating aggravations that can undo the benefits of the remedy. And so, for most remedies, it is 30C that will be called for.

Note, however, that the Objective Materia Medica does give information on each individual remedy and the potencies most commonly used for each of them. That should help you answer questions about individual remedies and the potencies you should have on hand.

In the same way, the Objective Materia Medica will give you information on the dosages common to individual remedies, which remedies are likely to need repeating when used in cases, and which are best in single or few doses.

Caring for Your Homeopathic Remedies

Twenty-odd years ago, when I was first studying homeopathy, remedies cost around two dollars a tube. Today, they may be seven, eight or nine dollars. But, even with such a price increase, they are still the best values available on health food store shelves today.

Also, when you select a remedy today, you have many more homeopathic pharmaceutical firms to choose from than I did twenty years ago. Whole sections of store shelves are covered with tubes of remedies, some in blue plastic, some in amber class, and some in clear glass tubes.

It can be hard to choose exactly what company's remedy to buy, but take heart, as most company's remedies are prepared in the same way. The packaging, no matter what color is used, has little to do with the quality of the remedy inside.

When you buy homeopathic remedies, make sure the tube has the letters "hpus" somewhere on it. This stands for "homeopathic pharmacopeia of the United States," and it means that the remedy in the tube was created in accordance with the laws governing homeopathy in the United States. So you need not worry.

It is true that almost all firms today have mechanized the process of creating the remedies. No one today, to my knowledge, is still making remedies by hand in the United States. And perhaps the potency of our modern remedies has suffered a bit through mechanization, a complaint I have heard many times. I don't know. But the fact that all homeopathic remedies are now completely standardized—which is to say that a 30C is always a 30C, no more, no less—is certainly a comfort to me. I'm glad that no one is still counting dilutions, and accidentally selling me a 28C instead of a 30C.

While we are looking at the label of the remedy, please note two other things. First, the label will give you some indication for the use of the remedy. Calcarea, for instance, may refer to its use in case of "indigestion." Second, each remedy will have an expiration date.

The indication of use is required by law in the United States, because homeopathic remedies are legal over-the-counter medications. They have the same status as analgesics and cold and cough medicines. Therefore, the government wants the makers of homeopathic medicines to quickly and easily sum up for the consumer the appropriate use of that remedy, in the same way instructions are provided for allopathic over-the-counter medications. The fact that homeopathy does not work this way, and that the use of a remedy cannot be summed up in just one or two words, has fallen on deaf ears. This may be because, like us, members of our government were weaned on allopathic thinking.

This is a long way of informing you that the label's indication of use is not at all helpful, and should be ignored.

You may also ignore the expiration date if you wish. It too is required by law, but homeopathic remedies, do not lose their potency when they are stored correctly. Homeopathic lore is filled with stories of homeopath's kits more than a hundred years old that are still filled with vials of potent medicines. So, worry more about how you are storing your remedies than about their expiration dates. If you want to follow those dates, that's also fine. Simply throw the tubes away as their expiration dates approach.

Storing Homeopathic Remedies

Homeopathic remedies should be stored in temperate places that are neither too hot nor too cold. Therefore, a nice shelf in a bedroom closet is great for remedy storage, while your car's glove compartment is not. I know some homeopaths who will jump down my throat for saying this, and who will tell many a tale of people who traveled the desert wastes with their remedies in their glove compartments, only to have the remedies be perfectly potent when needed. But I am giving you the best methods for storing and using your remedies and getting the most for your money, so I stand by my statements.

Too much light can also weaken or destroy the potency of your remedies, which is why most are stored in colored glass or plastic containers. Therefore, they are not best stored on a windowsill.

Strong smells may also be problematic. They should never be stored on your vanity, among your perfumes, as the perfume may interfere with the action of the remedy. Mothballs are especially problematic to remedies (and they are also poisonous to you), so you should never store your remedies anywhere near them.

Finally, radiation and electromagnetism are problematic as well. So, you should never store your remedies on top of the refrigerator or on top of the television, or near any other electronic device in your home, like the microwave, that gives off any sort of electro-magnetic pulse. When you travel, present your remedy kit to those operating the x-ray machine at the airport. Ask them to examine your remedies by hand and not x-ray them, because the radiation will distort their potency.

Giving and Taking Remedies: The Practitioner's Side

Finally, when you give and/or take a remedy, it is important to not touch the remedy with your hands before you give it to the patient. That's why the bottles of the remedies come with built-in tops, so you can spill the desired number of pellets into the lid, and then drop them onto the patient's tongue.

This is important for two reasons:

First, you cannot know for sure whether you have some substance on your hands that may undermine the potency of that dose or remedy, such as a hand cream or perfumed soap. So it is best that the pellets do not come into contact with your hands.

Second, if the pellets come into contact with your hands or with the skin on any part of your body, then you have dosed yourself with the remedy before you have dosed the patient. It is impossible to know what impact that remedy may have on your system, because without case taking we cannot know if the remedy is a similar to your own state of being. Avoid contact with your own body and remove this possible complication.

If you drop a pellet, discard it.

If you only wanted to give two pellets and a third falls from the lid, just tip it back in before giving to the patient. If the patient accidentally gets that third pellet, don't worry about it.

The whole manner of choosing just how many pellets to give at any one time is very simple. Just give enough pellets to coat the patient's tongue fully and completely with the remedy. Usually just two or three pellets will do the job nicely. (Hahnemann found over years of experimentation that the tongue was the best and most efficient entry point by which the energy of a homeopathic remedy could enter the body. He also very often applied his remedies in liquid form topically on the affected area of the body.)

Remember, when we are giving homeopathic remedies, we are giving energy, not substance. It is not like herbal medicines in which a certain amount of substance is given. No, instead we are giving energy. When giving 30C, for instance, the remedy is still 30C whether one pellet or the whole tube is given. Three 30C pellets given are still 30C—you don't add them up and get 90C. So you need not worry; just get them on the tongue and let them do their work.

This is the same reason why you don't have to worry if a young child gets into the remedies because she likes the sweet taste of them. (Homeopathic remedies are all dropped in liquid form onto pellets of milk sugar. Hahnemann selected milk sugar to carry his potencies because it is good to the taste, and is an almost inert substance that would not interfere with the actions of the medicines.) Unlike the child who takes a bottle of allopathic sleeping pills, the child who swallows the tube of 30C Sulphur is in no danger. Likely, she will prove the remedy for a time, and then it will wear off. Never hesitate to call your medical professional if your child should manage to get into your homeopathic kit, however.

Giving and Taking Remedies: The Patient's Side

When you give a homeopathic remedy, you are trying to get all the energy contained in those pellets onto your patient's tongue and into his entire system. So, as important as it is that the remedies be stored and handled correctly, it is equally important that that patient's tongue be ready for the pellets.

By this I mean that the patient needs to meet his remedy with a clean tongue, and a mouth that is as free as possible from artificial tastes, like strong toothpaste or mouthwash, and the flavors of food. Therefore, it is important that you do not give a remedy less than an hour after eating if at all possible. Let the flavors of the luncheon fade away before giving the remedy.

In the same way, give a remedy at least fifteen minutes before the patient eats a meal. This will let the remedy get into the system before the mouth is filled with food and drink.

The exception to this is water. The patient may drink water at any time before or after dosing with the remedy. In fact, the remedy may be given in water.

Now, does this mean that you cannot give your child a pellet for an hour if he has an accident right after eating lunch? Of course not. Does it mean that the remedy might not work quite as well if it is given too soon after eating? It's possible. But I certainly would not let any child of mine suffer while waiting. Give the dose, and then give it again later if it is needed.

Antidotes

This whole idea of when to give and not give remedies reminds me of one of the great controversies in the realm of homeopathy—that concerning homeopathic antidotes.

Antidotes are substances and scents that can disrupt the activity of homeopathic remedies. Among these, camphor is perhaps the most powerful antidote. The scent of camphor is so effective at blunting the actions of homeopathics that Hahnemann himself used camphor when his remedies caused aggravations he considered too powerful.

Even today, camphor remains an important antidote to homeopathics. I suggest that you keep a camphor-containing rub along with your home kit. If for any reason you need to blunt the action of a remedy, you may do so by rubbing the camphor into the pulse-points on the front of the patient's wrist. Then have the patient inhale the scent of the camphor until the action of the remedy fades.

Many homeopaths, especially lay homeopaths, tend to fear antidotes and particularly inadvertent antidotal actions. They often believe that the caffeine in coffee, or even decaffeinated coffee, will be an antidote for a homeopathic remedy. Some also believe that any strong fumes, especially artificially manufactured perfumes and petrochemicals, will be antidotes for homeopathic remedies. Some even fear that foods like garlic and onion will act as antidotes. There certainly is some truth to this fear.

I have found that the antidoting of a remedy has more to do with the life force and lifestyle of the patient then it does with the antidote itself. For instance, if a patient drinks coffee every day and is already addicted to coffee, then it can never be an antidote for him. In fact, you could dissolve the remedy in his coffee and give it to him, and it would act as powerfully as ever. It is the same with perfumes. The patient who regularly covers herself in a cloud of perfume will never be antidoted by that perfume.

Things that are a regular part of a patient's life can never overwhelm his system to the point that it acts as an antidote to a homeopathic remedy. Only things that shock the system can act as antidotes, as caffeine will in a patient who does not regularly drink coffee.

Therefore, the more sensitive and allergic a patient is, the more likely his homeopathic treatment can inadvertently be antidoted. The highly allergic patient will need to take care during treatment to avoid strong smells, spicy foods, and particularly caffeine. But patients who are not especially allergic or sensitive to their environment usually do not need to worry about antidoting their treatment.

SETTING UP YOUR HOME KIT

Finally, let's consider what homeopathic remedies should make up the contents of your home kit.

The remedies you select for that kit are those you feel will be needed most often by your loved ones in circumstances that can be called household emergencies. This means first aid situations, as well as simple acute ailments like coughs, colds, and flu. It often will also mean childhood ailments like croup and teething pains. And it may also include remedies that are related to women's health, like monthly premenstrual syndrome (PMS) remedies, and those related to pregnancy and childbirth.

Finally, you may want to have some of those homeopathic Band-Aids on hand, or any remedies that will get you through the night when a chronic condition, like allergies, suddenly appears. These remedies are not given to be totally curative, but to act as a Band-Aid until you can get the patient to the doctor.

The number and kinds of remedies in your kit are up to you, as are their potencies. There are, of course, many different kits on the market. Each contains a specific homeopath's or homeopathic pharmaceutical company's idea of what remedies you are likely to need, and the potencies you are likely to require.

I will give you a list of the remedies that, in my experience, are of the greatest help in the home in the next section of this book, the Objective Materia Medica. Take the time to study these remedies, and you may come away with some ideas as to which remedies will be most helpful to you.

There are, of course, literally thousands of homeopathic remedies to choose from, and each remedy comes in many different potencies. It may take you some time to build a home kit that suits all your needs for this reason. As you learn which remedies are most helpful to your family members, and what potencies are most curative, you will want to add them to your kit. In fact, like my own, your kit may continually evolve. As you learn more about the remedies and their uses, you may find yourself with dozens of remedies at your fingertips one day.

But where to start?

For me, the best place to start is with the remedies that are most commonly associated with first aid. Not only are first aid cases usually the simplest to work with for the beginning student of homeopathy, most are resolved with one or two of only a handful of remedies. That means that you can do a great deal of good in the lives of those you love with only ten or twelve remedies on hand.

However many remedies and potencies make up your first homeopathic home kit, it is important to understand the uses of those remedies in acute situations. To that end, the Objective Materia Medica will give you a good deal of information on the remedies and the symptoms that call for them, as well as the doses and potencies in which each of those remedies should be used.

PART TWO

An Objective Materia Medica of Common Acute Homeopathic Remedies

We neglect no source of information with reference to the origin, condition, or progress of disease, and whilst careful not to be guided by information from nurse, friends and patient, we wish to give it its true value. Attention has already been called to many sources of error. To a want of knowledge and care in observation on the part of nurse and friends, as well as their prejudices and tendency to distortion. To the want of knowledge on the part of the patient, want of language for description, and the impairment of his powers of sensation and reason from disease.

—JOHN SCUDDER, *SPECIFIC DIAGNOSIS*

Introduction

When we study materia medica, we sometimes fool ourselves into thinking that we are just learning about medicines, about things that have nothing to do with us, that are separate from us. In fact, we are learning about ourselves, in that we are studying the Vital Force—the life principle that animates each of us, and allows us to heal—and how it functions in our own and other forms of life.

The Vitalist principle that underlies homeopathy holds that all things natural to the Earth—animals, minerals, and plants alike—are alive, and partake of the life principle. Like Chi, this "life principle" flows through all natural things. When we take a homeopathic remedy, we are harmonizing our own Vital Force by applying the Vital Force of some other living thing to it. In this way, we approach our ailments with the strategy that the other life form might use in order to restore itself to health. We are using the innate wisdom of another living thing to learn—on a subconscious level—how we might better heal ourselves.

We have to learn the remedies taken from each specific form of life, and the symptoms each remedy displays as a coping mechanism, to be able to identify the remedy that might best bring about healing for a case. We have to come to understand other aspects of Vital Force. That is the function of learning the materia medica.

In the following section, I break this study down into a combination of the various possible objective and subjective symptoms that are indicators for a specific remedy. There is a distinct emphasis on the objective symptoms, in the belief that it is best to arrive at the selection of a specific remedy for simple acute situations like colds or flu through objective symptoms, which are visibly apparent. Therefore, most of this section describes the physical aspects of the patient needing a given remedy. The aspects of his face in particular will often reveal the most telling symptoms.

The subjective symptoms are those the patient may feel, but are not visible to an outside observer. These are harder to gather. They require the skill of verbal case taking, and are often harder to refine and use in the selection of an appropriate remedy. The subjective symptoms, although important in case taking, are often more important in constitutional situations. In simple acute circumstances, the physical objective symptoms are often quite enough to lead to an appropriate remedy.

While I try to avoid the deep psychological study of homeopathic types in the descriptions of remedies used in acute situations, I still give a basic sketch of the type under the topic of "Theme." The aspects of pain are listed under "Characteristics." There is also a brief sketch of the behavior pattern common to the patients of any given remedy type. "Common Causes of Illness" may give some insight into the onset of illness, and "Common Uses" lists the ailments most commonly associated with a given remedy in home use.

Keep in mind that no patient will have all of the symptoms listed for a given remedy. Indeed, he may only have a handful of the given symptoms. Select the remedy most closely matching your patient's symptoms; the remedy that, in its total picture, most closely resembles the patient's symptoms and behavior. This will be the curative remedy.

The Remedies

ACONITUM NAPELLUS (ACONITE)

Source: Wolfsbane (Monkshood)

This is a quick-acting remedy, and one whose actions pass quickly as well. Look for the symptoms of illness to start very quickly—this is especially important to understanding the remedy.

Theme: Emotionally, the theme is all about fear and anxiety. These patients fear that something bad is about to happen. They fear their own death. They fear that their illness, no matter how slight, will kill them. Physically, the theme is restlessness. The patient cannot be stilled; cannot stay still or be calm. This is a remedy for shock or panic.

About Aconite

Hahnemann wrote, "Aconite is the first and main remedy ... in inflammations of the windpipe (croup, membranous laryngitis), in various kinds of inflammations of the throat and fauces, as also in the local acute inflammations of all other parts, particularly where, in addition to thirst and quick pulse, there are present anxious impatience, an inappeasable mental agitation and agonizing tossing about..."

The Aconite Face

Eyes: It is the eyes that really give the Aconite patient away. Look for the eyes to be red, hot, and for the lids to be swollen, hard and red. The patient will not be able to stand any form of light, especially sunlight. The eyes are bloodshot and surrounded by blue rings. (This is a remedy for conjunctivitis, so think of that pattern.)

The most telling thing about the eyes is that they look dazzled and dazed. The pupils are contracted, and the eyes tend to dart about.

Ears: The external ears will be hot and red. They may also be swollen.

Nose: This is a patient who tends to be sneezing and have a runny nose. The mucus is watery and clear. The patient's nose is blocked, and he cannot breathe through his nose at all. As the texts say, "Hot water runs from nose." The nose may also bleed, and these nosebleeds start suddenly.

Mouth: Look for a black or blue tinge to the lips. The lips will also be very dry, and the skin may be peeling off the lips. The whole mouth is very dry. (All mucous membranes in the Aconite will be very dry.)

The patient may report pain in all his teeth. Healthy teeth may seem very painful. Look for the patient to grind his teeth. The gums may be red and inflamed as well.

Tongue: The patient's tongue will be red and swollen. It may have a white coating. There may be red ulcers on the tip of the tongue. Note that the patient may complain that his tongue tingles, especially the tip.

Throat: Internally the throat is red, swollen, and dry. The soft palate in particular will be red. The soft palate and back of the throat may be very red, or may be dotted by red eruptions. The tonsils are swollen, red, and dry. Look for the patient to swallow often, because his throat is so dry. The patient may have trouble swallowing food, and may report that it feels as if it were lodged in his chest, near his heart.

Countenance: This is a very serious-looking patient. The left side of the face, in particular, may droop. The patient may seem to have little control over the left side. Look for the face to have one side very pale and the other very flushed red (also consider: Chamomilla and Ipecac for this symptom), or for paleness and flush to alternate. This is particularly true when the patient rises from lying down, at which time the red face becomes very pale.

The patient will have an anxious or serious expression on his face, and a wild look in his eyes. Look for facial twitches, especially of the jaw. The patient will clench his jaw tight. Also look for saliva to drip from his mouth: an involuntary movement of the jaw, and involuntary flow of saliva.

The face is swollen, weighed down, and heavy. The face is red. The skin is hot and dry to the touch. Look for the patient to bend his head back as far as he can, constantly toss his head about, or put his hands to his head.

The Aconite Patient

Behavior: This patient is anxious, and very restless, active, manic, and fearful. This can be a very difficult patient, because he is so fearful and manic. He may even strike out with flailing limbs against those near him—not because he is angry or mean, but because he is wild and fearful.

The patient may also be confused, as if he is drunk, especially in the morning upon awakening.

Characteristics: This is a major remedy for those in pain, especially when pain starts suddenly. The pain is almost always associated with numbness, or numbness remains after pain is gone. Pains are associated with tingling, numbness, and chill. Pain drives the patient to despair. He may become violent or scream out in pain.

Ailments may develop after the patient has come into contact with a cold, dry wind.

Red is the color that flows through the symptoms associated with this remedy. This is a dry remedy—the patient is thirsty, and the skin and mouth are dry.

This is also a remedy type associated with wild alternations. The patient is manic and hot one moment; and pale, cold, and weak the next. He may rave one moment, and be passive the next. This aspect runs through all of the physical and emotional complaints of the patient.

Pulse: The pulse is very fast, full, and powerful, over 100 beats per minute. This is especially true for the patient with fever. As skin temperature rises, so does the number of pulse beats per minute. The pulse is quicker than the beat of the patient's heart. Look for the pulse to slow when the patient feels cold and weak. Cold sweat leads to a feeble pulse.

Modalities: Worse: from cold, especially cold, dry winds; from strong emotion of any sort; while sweating; in a warm, closed room; from any light or glare; from sudden noise; at night; while teething; from being touched.

Better: from resting and from sitting still; in a warm shower or from a warm sweat; in open air; from drinking a little wine.

Common Causes of Illness

Shock or sudden fright; deep fear; being overwhelmed either by a cold, dry wind, or by the heat of the sun; by taking a chill; by mechanical injury or surgery.

Common Uses

Colds, flu, croup, pneumonia; tonsillitis, otitis media (ear infection), conjunctivitis; vertigo; toothache and teething pains; measles; rheumatic pains; heart palpitations; panic attacks, shock.

ALLIUM CEPA

Source: Red Onion
The remedy theme strongly suggests the source of the remedy—an onion. Think of the symptoms you experience when you cut an onion, and you see the remedy picture. Strangely, those needing this remedy will often crave raw onions.
Theme: Think of your eyes when you slice an onion, and you will have the general theme for Allium Cepa.

About Allium Cepa

Clarke wrote: "Catarrhal conditions most decidedly lead the way to the useful employment of this remedy. All catarrhal symptoms and pains are, as a rule, worse in the evening. Lachrymation (tearing) and running from the nose, worse in a warm room. Coughs are worse in cold air."

Morrison writes: "This remedy may cure up to one third of all acute allergic rhinitis cases (hay fever), at least for that season."

The Allium Cepa Face

Eyes: The eyes are very red, with a great flow of tears. The tears are watery, clear, and bland, and do not burn the patient's face (Think of your eyes watering when you cut an onion.) The left eye will tend to be redder, and have more tears, than the right eye. Look for the patient to rub his eyes often. The eyes are very sensitive to light. The patient winks and blinks a good bit. Note that when the patient winks, he experiences a pain in his temples.

Ears: Look for a discharge of pus from the ear. The patient will be hard of hearing. This is an excellent remedy for otitis media (ear infection), when the pain in the ear extends into the eustachian tube and throat.

Nose: This is a patient who will likely be sneezing a good deal. The patient will especially sneeze when he enters a warm room. This is a hay fever remedy (especially for hay fever that begins in the high heat of August), so look for the patient to sneeze and cough at the same time. Odors will make the patient sneeze, especially the smell of flowers and peaches. As with the eyes, look for the left nostril to be worse than the right. Mucus flows constantly, watery, clear, and acrid. Look for the patient's nose to be crusted from the mucus flow.

Mouth: There is a bad odor that comes from the patient's mouth, as if he had eaten onions.

Tongue: The symptoms of the tongue are not especially guiding for this remedy, but look for the Allium Cepa tongue to be dirty, as if the patient did not follow proper oral hygiene. The tongue will be furred, especially in the morning. It may be slimy as well. Look for the back of the tongue to be dry, especially on the right side.

Throat: Look for flow of mucus in the throat. Post-nasal drip is often present in the back of the throat. Mucus at the back of the throat is viscous. The throat looks raw, red, dry, and swollen. Note that the patient may complain of a sensation of a lump or ball in his throat.

Countenance: As this is a left-sided reme- dy (meaning that the symptoms will usually be worse on the left, or will begin on the left side of the body and move to the right), look for the left side of the face to be paralyzed. The same will be true throughout the body, especially of the limbs of the body.

There is not a strong color context for the case, although things will, in general, be red—not a bright red, but raw, as if scraped into being red.

The Allium Cepa Patient

Behavior: This is a tired patient: he just wants to go and lie down. He will cause you no trouble, he just wants to rest. At worst, this is a melancholy patient. It is important to note that the patient will often fear that his pains will become unbearable.

Characteristics: A sensation of heat and a strong thirst, usually for cold water, combine in the remedy Allium Cepa. The symptoms associated with the remedy tend to cluster in the nose, eyes, throat, and bowels—all of these areas will display increased discharges.

Allium Cepa is a left-sided remedy. Most commonly, the symptoms, especially the nasal symptoms, will begin on the left side and move to the right.

The classic pain associated with the remedy is like a fine thread. It is as if that thread traced a part of the body on which that pain will run. This is especially true for cases involving injury to nerves or headache. It is also common that a sensation of glowing, throbbing heat will be centered in affected parts of the body.

Pulse: The pulse is full and hard. It also tends to be accelerated.

Modalities: Worse: from a warm room; from damp weather; from getting feet wet; from speaking or singing; from eating spoiled foods, especially fish; from eating salads or other uncooked foods; at night, especially early evening.

Better: while in cool air, especially when out of doors; from washing in cool water; from motion.

Common Causes of Illness

Contact with damp, cold winds, and damp weather in general; eating spoiled foods; getting feet wet; surgery and mechanical injury. Note that this remedy is considered especially helpful for spring colds and late summer hay fever.

Common Uses

Colds, coughs, and otitis media (ear infection); seasonal allergies; asthma; headaches; nerve pains.

ANTIMONIUM TARTARICUM

Source: Tarter Emetic

Combine sleepiness with total exhaustion and sweat for a picture of the remedy. Usually, the patient will also have a good deal of mucus that he is unable to cough up or otherwise bring out of the body. Listen for the rattling of mucus in the chest. Look for a lack of reaction to any stimulus, which becomes more and more pronounced as the patient becomes increasingly weak and exhausted.

Note: This remedy is related to and similar in action with Antimonium Crudum, which might also be a very useful remedy in the home kit.

Theme: This remedy is often associated with the picture of a drowning man—someone gasping for their last breath.

About Antimonium Tartaricum

Kent wrote, "About the first thing we see in an Ant. Tart. Patient is expressed in the face. The face is pale and sickly—the nose drawn and sunken—the eyes are sunken with dark rings around them—the lips are pale and shriveled—the nostrils dilated and flapping, with a dark sooty appearance inside them. The expression is that of suffering."

Vermeulen writes, "Defective reaction. Increasingly weak, drowsy, sweaty and relaxed."

The Antimonium Tartaricum Face

Eyes: The Antimonium patient's eyes will often appear to be sunken back into the head. They are also often surrounded by very dark circles. In the acute sphere, this is often a remedy for those with conjunctivitis, so look for a collection of mucus in the margins of the eyes (this is also true in pneumonia cases). The eyes may also be bloodshot. The lids may be inflamed, and there may be pus under the lids as well.

The Antimonium patient tends to want to keep one eye closed. Often he wants to press on his closed eyes. This patient is photophobic and cannot bear light. Look for the pupils to be contracted. The patient is also known for staring straight ahead emotionlessly.

Ears: There are no guiding objective symptoms, but the patient may complain of the sound of a rushing in his ears, as if a bird were flapping its wings inside his head.

Nose: The nostrils will be enlarged or dilated. The wings of the nose will often be flapping as the patient struggles to breathe. This is a patient with flow of mucus from the nose, much sneezing and coryza (inflammation of the membrane lining the nose). This is accompanied by chill, and by the patient losing his sense of taste and smell. If there is no mucus flow, the nose will be completely dry.

Mouth: The patient breathes through his mouth. The mouth hangs open. There may be an excess of saliva. The lips are dry and cracked. The patient's lips and mouth may be swollen. The patient will be thirsty for cold water. He will only be able to drink a little at a time, but he will drink often.

Tongue: The tongue will be coated with a thick, white cover. The tongue is swollen, with imprints of teeth visible along the edges. The tongue may have red edges, or may have a brown coating on the center. Papillae may show through the coating on the tongue. The tongue is dry in the middle.

The patient may have difficulty speaking, because it may be painful even to move the tongue. The patient will complain of a bitter taste in his mouth.

Throat: The patient has difficulty swallowing liquids. Look for a great deal of mucus in the throat, making it difficult for the patient to breathe. Listen for the rattle of mucus in throat and lungs.

Countenance: The face is cold and very pale, with a blue tinge to the skin. The face is covered with a cold sweat. The patient's jaw and chin quiver. His upper lip may be drawn up. Look for the patient's face to twitch when he coughs. Look for copious salivation, for the patient to spit all the time.

The Antimonium Patient

Behavior: This is an exhausted patient, who is having great difficulty breathing. There is a great amount of mucus and sweat. The patient is also chilly. He is weak and drowsy, and seems to be slipping away. He has a lack of reaction to any stimulus. (As noted below, however, there are times that this patient may be demanding and somewhat difficult.)

Characteristics: This is a patient who seems placid, but becomes whiny and somewhat difficult just before an increase in symptoms. The patient becomes restless just before his exhaustion increases. The patient may have difficulty breathing at these times, and suffocative attacks are common. Listen for mucus rattling in the chest. Listen for the heartbeat to become labored. It is characteristic of the remedy that the patient will have a sensation of weight in his head (especially the back of the head), the coccyx (tailbone), and the limbs.

Pulse: The pulse is weak, feeble, or thready, and is accompanied by respiratory distress. The pulse is weak and very quick. In times of distress, look for the pulse to increase to about seventy-five beats per minute. Once in distress, the pulse rate stays fast until nighttime. The pulse tends to become both stronger and quicker as the patient's breathing becomes faster.

Consider this remedy for patients with pulses that almost cannot be taken, or trusted. They are rapid one moment, fading the next, and small and threadlike the next. Motion and breathing have great impact upon the pulse. The patient may also experience sudden violent beats of the heart, without any apparent reason, that cause changes to the pulse.

Modalities: Worse: some patients will be worse in a warm room, others will be worse from cold, especially when cold is associated with damp; all will be worse from overheating, and from being wrapped up too tightly; from motion of any sort; from lying down flat; from sitting and from rising back up after sitting; from any change in weather.

Better: from coughing up mucus and from vomiting; while sitting still; while lying on the right side; from breathing cool, open air.

Common Causes of Illness

Ailments, especially cough, will greatly increase after anger and, especially, frustration.

Common Uses

Bronchitis and pneumonia; any deep respiratory infection; chicken pox; congestive heart failure.

APIS MELLIFICA

Source: Honey Bee

Consider the source of the remedy, the poison of the honey bee. The remedy picture follows the idea of the bee sting: swelling, redness, and a sensation of heat. Often, along with these physical symptoms, you will also see the patient acting like an angry bee. He tends to be irritable and jealous, and somewhat restless in his physical behavior.

Often, the patient will experience a sensation of stiffness in the interior parts of his body. There is a general sensation of soreness. The patient does not tolerate touch or any application of heat.

Theme: The theme is the sum of three things: swelling, heat, and a shiny surface. Together, they point to the picture of Apis.

About Apis

Guernsey wrote, "The pains are like bee stings, with the thirst and the burning following. Scanty urine. Shrill, sudden piercing screams while sleeping or waking, form invaluable keynotes to the use of this remedy."

The Apis Face

Eyes: Look for the eyelids to be swollen and bright red. They may become so inflamed and swollen that they curve outward instead of inward. The white of the eye may become red and swollen as well. Eyelashes may fall out during illness. The eyes tear a great deal. The tears are hot to the touch.

The patient will not be able to look at anything for very long, must keep moving his eyes. He cannot read by artificial light or bear bright artificial light for very long. The patient has to squint to see.

This is a remedy for patients whose eyes seem rather brilliant and shiny. They also have redness all around the eyes, and there will be large, baggy swellings under the eyes.

Ears: The external ears are red and swollen. Look for the patient to raise his hands to the back of his ears because of pain. The patient may scream in pain.

Patients needing this remedy tend to be either very sensitive or almost totally lacking in their sense of hearing. Those who are sensitive will be easily awakened from sleep by almost any slight noise. The other patients will be almost totally deaf.

Nose: The nose is swollen. The tip of the nose is cold to touch. Look for a great deal of mucus flowing. There may also be boils inside the nostrils.

This is a remedy associated with discharges: sudden, copious nosebleeds that start during the early hours of the morning. It is also associated with a fetid mucous discharge, which is thick and either clear or white. The discharge may also be a blend of mucus and blood.

Mouth: The inside of the mouth and throat looks like it is varnished, it is so glossy. The gums are swollen and bright red. The lips are bluish and swollen, especially the upper lip.

Tongue: The patient's tongue is fiery red and swollen. There may be raised red patches or blisters on the sides of his tongue. The tip of the tongue alone may be reddened. In general, the patient has a red, hot, and dry tongue. In some rare cases, the tongue may be yellow instead of red.

The patient will either have his tongue protruding from his mouth at all times, or will have trouble sticking it out at all. The patient may complain that his tongue feels wooden. The patient may have difficulty speaking because of his tongue.

Throat: Both the internal and external throat will be swollen. Look for the characteristic shine to the interior throat. The interior throat is puffy and glossy, with a shiny redness as if it had been varnished. In some cases, the inside of the throat may be purple. Look for a combination of dryness and heat in the throat. The tonsils may be ulcerated and pus filled. They will be very inflamed, especially the left tonsil.

The patient will have trouble swallowing solids or hot things. He may also have trouble swallowing sour substances. The patient may report that he feels as if his throat muscles are too weak to allow him to swallow. The patient will be thirsty for and will crave cold water.

The patient may feel as if he has a sharp fishbone lodged in his throat, and he may report that his throat pain extends into his ears when he swallows.

Countenance: The Apis patient will have odd emotions on his face. He may look very happy, or very much afraid, or he may show absolutely no emotion at all. His face may pass through this range of emotions.

The whole face may be swollen, red, and hot to the touch. The shiny skin may also have a waxy appearance. The right side of the face will tend to be more affected than is the left. Right-sided paralysis is possible. The patient may want to hold his right eye closed. The patient will want to wash his face with cold water, or to have a cold, wet towel on his face. This patient will have a stiff or clenched jaw.

Again, think of the bee sting: affected areas of the body are always red, swollen, and hot to the touch. They will also be better for cold applications and cold things. The color red is vital to the type, but it must be a bright, shiny red.

The Apis Patient

Behavior: This is an active, manic and angry patient. Look for the patient to have wild outbursts, to scream in pain, to be demanding and jealous, then to have periods of sudden weakness, when all he wants to do is rest.

Characteristics: Pains associated with the remedy all have a burning and stinging sensation to them—the patient may experience a sensation of hot needles. Itching may accompany burning. Pains begin suddenly. The patient is very sensitive to pain and cries out in pain. The patient may be angry while in pain.

Note that sudden bouts of involuntary diarrhea may accompany other symptoms in this remedy picture.

Pulse: The pulse is quick and very hard, yet somewhat weak. The pounding of the heart may shake the whole body. This is a pulse that can range from 100 to 150 beats per minute.

Modalities: Worse: from heat in any form, from hot applications to warm drinks; worse especially in a warm room; from touch—the patient will not even let his hair be touched; from getting wet; at 5:00P.M.

Better: from cool applications and from drinking cool water; headaches of this type tend to be better from pressure.

Common Causes of Illness

Suppressed eruptions of any sort; grief, jealousy or anger; upon hearing bad news.

Common Uses

Bee stings and puncture wounds; colds, flu, and sore throat; asthma; allergies; headache; arthritis; injuries to knees and ankles that involve swelling.

ARNICA MONTANA

Source: Leopard's Bane

A sensation of having been beaten, of everything in the environment being too hard, is thematic for this remedy. The patient seeks comfort, although he avoids touch. He seeks a soft, safe, and comfortable place to rest.

Theme: The theme is simple: trauma, whether emotional or physical, leads to the symptoms associated with Arnica.

About Arnica

Boericke wrote, "It is especially suited to cases when any injury, however remote, seems to have caused the present trouble. After traumatic injuries, overuse of any organ, strains."

The Arnica Face

Eyes: The patient's pupils will usually be dilated and enlarged, although in some cases they may be contracted. The eyes may be somewhat sunken into the patient's head. They will have a very weary look to them, and yet the patient will have to keep his eyes open. He may even sleep with his eyes partially open. Typically, the eyes are both bloodshot and photophobic.

Ears: Think of this remedy first for cases involving blood flowing from the ears, especially after a physical trauma. The ears will seem very dry.

In general, patients needing Arnica will be very sensitive to noise, especially to shrill noises. Patients may also experience a sound of rushing in their ears after physical trauma to the body, especially after blows to the head.

Nose: Nosebleed, especially after physical trauma. The nosebleed may start after fits of coughing, as in whooping cough. The nose bleeds after a tingling sensation, or after blowing the nose. The blood from the nose is very dark. There also may be nosebleeds during fever, or after over-lifting. Sneezing may also come on, along with the nosebleed or all alone, after over-lifting.

Mouth: There is bad breath. The mouth is very dry.

The lips are swollen and cracked. The lower lip will tremble while the patient eats. Look for the patient's lower lip to hang down loose.

This is also a remedy for patients complaining of toothache, or that their teeth feel sprained. Note that Arnica is a remedy commonly used after dental surgery to speed healing.

Tongue: The tongue dry and very dark in color, almost black. The tongue may have a white coating. There may be a red stripe down the center of the tongue. The tongue may have a yellow coating in the morning. The patient will also complain of a taste of rotten eggs while tongue is coated yellow.

Throat: The interior of the throat is bright red and swollen. This is a remedy for acute tonsillitis, with swelling of the soft palate.

The Arnica patient is very noisy when he swallows. The patient may report that his throat feels better after he swallows.

Face: The patient has a very hot face. The lips in particular will be hot to the touch. The face is also red and somewhat swollen. The cheeks are puffy and red. The right cheek especially may be red and swollen puffy. The patient may have bright red acne on his face.

The Arnica Patient

Behavior: These are fretful patients. They may insist that there is nothing wrong with them, they may even become violent if you attempt to touch them. They fear being touched. They may associate touch with trauma. They will want to rest, to lie down, but everything they rest on will seem too hard, too uncomfortable. They will have a difficult time finding any comfortable position. Therefore, they tend to move from place to place. They become fretful.

Because this is a remedy for those who have experienced physical or emotional trauma, the patient may also be unconscious. He may be stupefied. He may be unable to answer questions intelligently. Even if conscious, the patient may have difficulty speaking. He is slow to think, and pauses before speaking. He is easily frightened and overcome.

Characteristics: This remedy deals with both the immediate and long-term consequences of trauma, both physical and emotional. The patient suffers pains that can only be termed "bruised." The patient may feel sore all over, or only in affected parts of the body. The patient is confused by the trauma and may not believe it took place. He may also be sleepy, and somewhat withdrawn. This is a patient who may be in shock after physical trauma. He may not be aware of his injury. The patient has an unusual body temperature: with a hot head leading down to very cold feet.

Pulse: The pulse is irregular. It may also be a bit feeble. Motion has an impact on the pulse, which may be as low as 60 beats while the patient is at rest, speeding to 120 when he moves about. In general, the patient's pulse is low, weak, and rapid.

Note: Consider Arnica for cases of palpitations that develop after straining or over-lifting, for cases in which heavy breathing accompanies palpitations, and for cases in which heartbeat is accompanied by a quivering sensation. The patient may report that his heart feels strained. The patient may note a sensation of heat in his head and chest, during palpitations and chest pain, with coldness in the rest of the body.

Modalities: Worse: from any form of motion; from touch; from alcohol; after sleeping; from old age; from nightmares and bad news.

Better: from lying down, especially from lying with the head low; from gentle motion; from clear, cold, dry weather.

Common Causes of Illness

Any physical trauma, such as falls, blows, jars, bruises, sprains, overexertion; shock; childbirth or surgery of any sort; sudden financial loss; bad news; fear or anger; nightmares.

Common Uses

Physical trauma, concussion, contusions; post-surgical, especially dental procedures; eczema and psoriasis; rheumatism; arthritis; labor; flu with body aches.

ARSENICUM ALBUM

Source: White Arsenic

Along with Rhus Tox and Aconite, this is one of our most restless remedies. (Nash calls the three the "restless trio.") The Arsenicum patient is anxious and worried, and very restless—so much so that when you find an Arsenicum who wants to just lie still, you have a very sick patient indeed. The patient wants to go to bed and stay there only in the deepest illness.

Otherwise, they are fussy people. They will want to tidy and to clean; they will be certain that something bad is about to happen. They are worse after midnight, and may walk the floor in anxious fear that someone is about to break in and kill them. They are overly concerned about their own health, and may be obsessive about it. This is often the core fear in a type riddled with fears, and they may be totally controlled by their fear. They do not want to be alone. Look for their physical symptoms to grow worse when they are alone.

Theme: Fear. Whether the patient needs this remedy on an acute or a constitutional level, look for him to be motivated and controlled by fear.

About Arsenicum

Murphy writes, "Arsenicum Album is a very deep acting remedy, affecting every organ and tissue ... All prevailing anxiety, exhaustion and restlessness with nightly aggravation, are most important. Great exhaustion after the slightest exertion."

The Arsenicum Face

Eyes: The eyelids are a great clue to the remedy: they will be red, ulcerated, scabby, and scaly. Look for swelling around the eyes, but not of the eyes. Look for external inflammation. Look for tearing of the eyes. In some cases, the opposite will be true and the eyes will be so dry that it will seem as if the eyelids were rubbing right up against the eyes. Photophobia is often present.

Ears: The internal ear is red and raw. The patient has trouble hearing the human voice.

Nose: The patient sneezes and sneezes, but without relief. The nose drips constantly, the mucus is watery and clear. The patient loses his sense of smell completely, or cannot bear the smell of food. The nose will swell while nasal symptoms are present. Look for a red, swollen nose. There may be acne of the patient's nose. Nosebleed starts after anger or nausea.

Mouth: The mouth is dry. The gums are red and swollen, and bleed very easily.

The lips are swollen and cracked. They may have a black color. There may be eruptions of the lips, like black dots.

Tongue: The tongue is clean and red. It may be ulcerated, and if so, the ulcers have a bluish color. In other cases, the tongue may take on many different colors. It may be coated white, yellow, brown, or black. Often, the tongue will have a red stripe down the middle and/or a red tip.

The tongue may be swollen at the root, and there may be tooth marks along the edge of the tongue.

Throat: The interior of the throat is swollen, constricted, and very dry. The patient has trouble swallowing, especially cold things. Everything swallowed seems to become lodged in the throat. There may be internal and external swelling of the throat at the root of the tongue. Look for swelling of the submaxillary glands.

Listen for the gurgling sound the patient makes in his throat when he swallows liquids.

Countenance: The patient's face tends to look shrunken and old (especially true in children). The face typically looks haggard and distorted. The patient does not look like himself. The patient has a very serious expression, or an expression of pure pain. The face will often take on a yellow color. The face feels cold, and may be covered with a cold sweat. Look for twitching of facial muscles, especially on the right side of the face. (This is a right-sided remedy. All symptoms will either be worse on the right side, or will start on the right and move left.)

The Arsenicum Patient

Behavior: The Arsenicum patient is very fussy. He wants things just so, and may be impossible to please. This is a very cold patient, who only calms down when he is made warm enough. He wants to be covered and comforted, but once he is warm and has had enough attention, he does tend to settle down—unless you try to leave the room.

The patient does not want to be alone, especially late at night. He fears being alone. Note that the Arsenicum's symptoms are worse after midnight and when the patient is alone. This is a generally fearful patient as well. He has terrors, especially at night. The Arsenicum patient is at once restless and exhausted. Although he is truly worn down by his illness, he will fuss about and never relax.

Characteristics: It is characteristic that all of the symptoms of the Arsenicum type will have a burning sensation associated with them. (This makes Arsenicum a part of Nash's "burn trio" along with Sulphur and Phosphorus.) It is also characteristic that the patient will be chilly. This is a remedy type that wants to be warmed. He will want to be covered up. The only exception to this is in the case of headache, at which time the patient will want his head in cool air. The Arsenicum with a headache will have a blanket around him, but will sit by an open window for the sake of his head pain.

The Arsenicum patient wants to be taken care of and fussed over. He wants to have company at all times. He likes warm drinks as well as warm surroundings, and will want someone to bring him tea, which he will drink one small sip at a time. This is also characteristic—although he is thirsty, he only drinks in sips.

Pulse: The pulse may rage, with audible beats and visible pulsation. Listen for audible sounds of the heart beating, which do not agree in tempo with the pulse. This is a patient with a small, weak, and quick pulse. The pulse may be trembling in nature. The pulse may seem as if it were suppressed, in that it is so weak, while the beats of the patient's heart are so strong.

Note whether the patient's limbs are cold while taking the pulse.

This is an important remedy for patients with palpitations. Consider for cases of palpitation in which the palpitations are worse when the patient is lying down or when he climbs stairs.

Modalities: Worse: after midnight; from cold surroundings, food, or drink; from exertion; from lying down with the head too low; from being alone; on a personal cycle—some patients are worse every two weeks, some are worse at the same time every year.

Better: from warmth and warm applications, food, and drinks; From gentle motion and from walking around; from sitting up and lying with the head high; from open, fresh air; from company.

Common Causes of Illness

Eating spoiled foods, especially shellfish and meat; a long-term poor diet; taking a chill; alcohol abuse; traveling to the mountains or sea; worry, grief, and fear.

Common Uses

Colds, flu (stomach flu), coughs, bronchitis, pneumonia; allergies, especially food, environmental and seasonal; asthma; food poisoning; upset digestion, colitis, irritable bowel disorders; hemorrhoids; insomnia; anxiety and panic attacks; phobia.

BELLADONNA

Source: Deadly Nightshade

The first grand theme of the remedy has to do with congestion, especially with sudden congestion that most often includes the sensations of throbbing, heat, and burning, accompanied by redness of the affected parts of the body. Belladonna is also known as a remedy for those whose nervous system is disordered. You will find changes in the patient's five senses, as well twitching and pain. You may also see convulsions. You may also have a patient who is very excited.

This is a remedy that is sudden, in onset and in cessation of symptoms. It is very often especially curative in children.

Theme: This sudden "coming and going" of symptoms is central to the remedy's theme as is the patient's need to rest in a darkened room.

About Belladonna

Vermeulen writes, "Belladonna is always associated with hot, red skin, flushed face, glaring eyes, throbbing carotids, excited mental state, hyperesthesia of all senses, delirium, restless sleep, convulsive movements, dryness of mouth and throat with aversion to water, neuralgic pains that come and go suddenly."

The Belladonna Face

Eyes: The Belladonna's pupils will be widely dilated. It gives the remedy its name, in that the dilation was thought to be beautiful. The eyes are swollen and seem to protrude from the patient's head. The eyes are red, dry, and enlarged; his eyes seem huge. The patient's eyelids may also be swollen, so much so that they curve outward. Consider this remedy for any case involving violent inflammation of the eyes accompanied by dryness. If there are tears, they will be thick and clear, like brine.

The patient cannot bear light of any sort, including sunlight; this is perhaps our most photophobic patient. The patient will stare.

Ears: The patient has increased sensitivity in hearing. He cannot bear loud noises. He may also have roaring, ringing or other noises in his ears.

The patient may report a sudden, overwhelming earache, or a violent, tearing pain that spreads backward and forward from the external ear to the whole side of the face.

Nose: As with the sense of hearing, the patient's sense of smell will be dramatically increased. He is oversensitive in terms of smell. Some smells, especially tobacco, cannot be tolerated.

The nose is red and swollen, especially the tip, which will be a shiny red. There is swelling of both the nose and the upper lip. The patient may sneeze a good deal, but his nose remains dry. One side of the nose will be stopped up, the other side clear.

Think of this remedy for nosebleeds in patients with bright red, dry faces, or for nosebleeds in which mucus is mixed with the blood.

Mouth: The mouth is dry and hot. In the morning, the patient may have thick, white mucus in his mouth. The patient's tongue may have a morning white coating as well. The patient continually tries to swallow or to hack out his mucus. The soft palate is bright red and swollen. The lips are still and hard to move (the tongue may be hard to move as well). The top lip especially may be swollen.

Tongue: The patient's tongue is red around the edges, or the whole tongue may be the color of a strawberry. The tongue will be inflamed and swollen, with deep-red papillae. There may be a red stripe down the tongue that is wider on the tip than it is at the back. The tongue may be cracked and may have a white center with bright red sides. Red and white, in some combination, are the colors associated with Belladonna's tongue.

Throat: The throat is dry and red. The patient's tonsils may also be enlarged. The patient swallows continually, chokes easily. He must drink first in order to swallow solids. Note that the patient will drink quickly, and may tremble while drinking. The patient will be very thirsty. The thirst may be for warm or cold things. Often the patient craves lemons and lemonade.

As usual in homeopathy, the direct opposite may also be possible, and the patient may have no thirst at all. He may be totally averse to drinking anything, especially coffee or anything acidic.

The patient bends his head forward when swallowing. The patient will often clutch his throat in pain when swallowing.

Countenance: This patient's face is red—even bluish or purplish red. The face is hot, swollen, shining, and dry. Some patients' faces may alternate between very pale and very deep red.

Belladonna combines great heat with dryness. The characteristic color is a dark red. Think of a bad sunburn, and you have the idea.

The Belladonna Patient

Behavior: This is a patient who is often inappropriate in his behavior. This patient may also have wild swings of mood, laughing or singing loudly one moment, and deeply sad, crying, or violent the next. He may mistrust his caregiver. He may thrash about in forward and backward motions. As with Arnica, this patient may lose consciousness, or be unable to answer intelligently. Even those who are conscious may be forgetful and absent-minded. They may even seem to be insane, as if their words do not match their thoughts.

Because of a high fever or other cause, this patient may have hallucinations and may see ghosts, imaginary animals, insects, or hideous faces. The patient may fear to close his eyes because that brings on hallucinations.

Characteristics: This is a major remedy for those in pain, who are overwhelmed by sudden pain. The quality of the pain is cutting, sharp, and shooting. The patient may experience a sensation in his muscles as if something were moving in them, as if they were quivering. He may experience the sensation that the lower half of his body is numb. He may also experience loss of sensation on one side of his body.

Pulse: The pulse is full and very rapid. The pulse is accelerated. The pulse is large and full. At times, the pulse may slow and become somewhat softened, but in general it is hard and full.

This is a remedy filled with congestions and palpitations. Look for palpitations to appear after the slightest exertion. The blood seems to pound and throb throughout the body. The blood feels trapped and congested in specific parts of the body, especially in the head, the chest, or the uterus.

Note that the patient may experience pressure in the area of the heart, with troubled breathing and a sense of fear and anxiety.

Modalities: Worse: from the sun, from heat, from hot weather; from sudden changes in the weather, especially from hot to cold; from things that affect the head, such as a draft on the head, a haircut, or washing hair; from suppression of sweat; from company; from touch; from light, noise, or jarring movement; at 3:00P.M. (also after midnight).

Better: from resting in bed; from bending head backward; from leaning head against a support; from bending painful parts; from being covered up lightly and being in a warm, dark room.

Common Causes of Illness

Over exposure to the sun, sunburn; exposure to wind; looking at the reflection on light on water; getting hair cut or washed; eating sausages.

Common Uses

Acne; headache, especially migraine; appendicitis; vertigo; pneumonia; back pain, especially low back pain; sinusitis; tonsillitis; arthritis; sciatica; hemorrhoids; vertigo.

BRYONIA ALBA

Source: White Bryonia, Wild Hops

The theme of this remedy is one of passionate stillness. The patient, for whatever reason, cannot act, and cannot bear motion of any sort, and yet there is a passion, a restlessness underneath the surface. Therefore, the Bryonia with a headache will find that he cannot even move his eyes without pain. The Bryonia patient reminds himself again and again of all that there is to do and all the work that is waiting, but he cannot move to take action.

Theme: This is a patient who wants to remain inert. He does not want to move, to think, or especially, to speak or be bothered. To disturb this patient is to anger this patient.

About Bryonia

Boericke wrote, "The general character of the pain here produced is a stitching, tearing; worse by motion, better rest. These characteristic stitching pains, greatly aggravated by any motion, are found everywhere, but especially in the chest; worse pressure."

The Bryonia Face

Eyes: The lids are swollen and the skin around the eyes is puffy. The patient will have twitching of the upper left eyelid. The eyes tend to tear easily, especially when the patient is out in the sunshine. The right eye especially tends to water. The upper lid of the right eye especially tends to swell.

Ears: The patient wants no noise at all. There may be a bloody discharge from ears.

Nose: Nosebleeds are very common for this remedy type. Nosebleeds may occur in female patients instead of menstrual flow. There may be nosebleeds in pregnant women, or nosebleeds that start in the morning or upon rising. There may be swelling of the tip of the nose.

Mouth: The mouth is very dry, and the patient is very thirsty.

The lips are parched, dry, and cracked. They look as if they are burnt. The patient will constantly want to moisten his lips. The patient picks at his lips.

Tongue: The tongue is coated with a yellowish to dark-brown coating. (Note: if the patient has an upset digestion, the tongue often is coated white.) The tongue may be coated yellow/brown in the center and red at the base. The tip of the tongue may be moist, but the rest of the tongue is dry. White ulcers are common on the tip of the tongue.

Throat: The patient has trouble swallowing solids because his throat is so dry. The patient cannot swallow dry foods but can swallow liquids easily. Look for recurring white ulcers in the mouth and throat.

Countenance: The patient's face is dark red and bloated. The face is hot and swollen. It may also have a yellow paleness that can suggest jaundice. The patient makes chewing motions often, unconscious of his action. Look for the area of the upper lip and nose to be jointly swollen, red, and hot.

The Bryonia Patient

Behavior: This patient does not want to move, and has pain when he moves. When he drinks—and he is very thirsty—he drinks a great deal at a time, so that he will not have to move to drink again very soon. The Bryonia is called the Bryonia Bear, and for good reason. This is a difficult patient, an angry patient. He wants to lay still, rest, and be left alone, and he is better off if left alone.

Characteristics: This is a remedy filled with aching. Every muscle aches. It often is very useful for cases where Arnica fails to act. Joints ache. Muscles turn hard. The patient is filled with aches and pains, and feels bruised. Pains are also bursting and stitching in nature. The patient holds pained parts of the body: chest, head, and sides. Pains are relieved somewhat by gentle, sustained pressure. As well as not wanting to move, it is also characteristic that the patient will not want to be touched. Either action brings on bruising pain. If the patient is forced to walk, he will be unsteady and will have to sit to steady himself.

Pulse: The Bryonia patient has a slow and even sluggish pulse, when he is at rest. The heartbeat may slow to 50 beats per minute while at rest. As the patient moves, the pulse jumps to 100 to 115 beats per minute. The pulse then slowly subsides when the patient rests. The pulse is frequent during the day and slow at night.

Modalities: Worse: from any motion of any sort, such as rising up from bed, stooping down, coughing, and deep breathing; from mental or physical exertion of any sort; from touch of any sort; from dry cold or dry hot weather; from becoming heated; from lying on the painless side.

Better: from lying on the painful side; from putting gentle pressure on painful areas; from holding painful areas; from total rest; from cool air; on cloudy or damp days; from drinking cold things.

Common Causes of Illness

Drinking or eating very cold things during hot weather; suppression of discharges, especially sweat; alcohol abuse; gluttony; physical trauma; emotional trauma—anger, fright, or embarrassment.

Common Uses

Flu with body aches; bronchitis; pneumonia; appendicitis; headaches, especially migraines; toothache; arthritis, especially rheumatoid arthritis; constipation; diarrhea; backache, especially in the lower back; physical traumas of all sorts.

CALCAREA CARBONICA

Source: Carbonate of Lime

Boiron's tube of Calcarea Carbonica tells the story in a very few words: "general tonic." The theme here is one of depletion, or exhaustion. The ailments that respond to Calcarea are often a long time in coming on, being shaped by overwork and over-worry. The patient moves into a phase of feeling overwhelmed, and then succumbs to any number of acute and chronic complaints.

Fears are also a general part of the picture: fears of height, rodents, insects (especially spiders), and dogs are common. Most common, however, is the simple fear of the dark. Calcarea patients are also afraid of poverty, which often motivates them in their overwork.

Theme: Although this patient may need Calcarea only acutely, most often these apparent acute needs are covering up a constitutional weakness. This is patient whose health has been whittled away over a long period of time.

About Calcarea

Nash wrote, "If Calcarea has one symptom that not only leads all the rest, but also all other remedies, it is found in the profuse sweats on the head of large-headed, open-fontanelled children. The sweat is so profuse that during sleep it rolls down the head and face, wetting the pillow far around."

The Calcarea Face

Eyes: The time of day affects the eye symptoms. Look for the patient's eyes to water a great deal in the morning, and for the patient's eyes to be very light sensitive in the morning and at night. Look for agglutination of the eyes in the morning. Also, the eyes itch; the patient will want to rub and scratch his eyelids. His eyelids also twitch, especially the upper lids. Eye symptoms increase if the patient gets wet.

Ears: The patient will typically have a swelling in front of the left ear, which is very painful to the touch. Look for an eruption on the ear itself or behind the ear as well. A discharge from the ear can become chronic. It is whitish; it can be thick and somewhat fatty as well. It can look like chewed paper.

Hearing is distorted. The patient will hear things, especially when he is eating, chewing, or swallowing.

The patient will be very sensitive to cold around the areas of the ears and neck. **Nose:** The patient's nose will be dry and stopped up. The patient sneezes a good deal, even if he does not have a cold. The sneezing has no discharge. If there is a discharge, look for the mucus to be thick and yellow. Look for swelling at the root of the nose.

This is an important remedy for chronic nosebleeds in children following the overall pattern of the remedy.

Mouth: The gums are spongy and bleed easily. The patient grinds his teeth when he gets cold. Speech is indistinct. It may be very hard to understand what the patient is saying.

Consider this remedy for children with difficult and delayed dentition.

Tongue: The tongue is dry in the morning and at night. Because of the discomfort of dryness, the patient may not want to talk. Dryness may alternate with excess of saliva. The tongue will generally be coated white. It may also be fissured.

Throat: The exterior of the throat is swollen. There may be a goiter. The interior of the throat is swollen as well. The tonsils may be swollen. The submaxillary glands may be swollen and may be very hard. The glands are very painful if touched.

Countenance: This is a patient with a puffy and pasty face. His face may have a very pale yellow tint. He may look worn out. His eyes seem deep seated, his skin pale, moist, and unhealthy looking. There may be swelling of the upper lip. There may be dark blue rings around the eyes. Look for pimples in the beard of male patients. There may be eruptions on the chin, or pimples on the border of the lips, especially the lower lip.

The Calcarea Patient

Behavior: Calcarea patients are mild, for the most part. They tire easily, and are given to sweats after even gentle motion. They tend to smell a bit sour, a bit unhealthy, especially their heads, which sweat a great deal, especially at night. The patient will tend to be lethargic, exhausted. He is also easily frightened, and will want company.

Characteristics: A poor diet is often behind the decline in health that leads to the Calcarea patient's illnesses. The remedy tends to be most active with the skin and bones, the digestive tract and the glands. Those needing Calcarea often display an increase in sweat, especially on their head, and swelling of the glands. They also tend to have issues with breathing, and feel that they cannot get enough air into their lungs. It is common for them to feel very weak, and to feel as if they cannot walk, and cannot lift even the lightest object. They tend to be lethargic and depressed.

Their pains tend to be cramping in nature. Twitching and trembling in the muscles is common.

Pulse: The pulse is slow and often somewhat weak as well. There is an uneven pulse rate. The heart rate may tend to flutter.

This is a patient who is given to palpitations. Palpitations may occur after eating, or be accompanied by a cough at night, or upon falling asleep. Palpitations may occur when ascending in any way, especially when climbing stairs. Palpitations may be accompanied by difficulty breathing when ascending and when stooping. An audible beating of the heart may accompany palpitations.

Modalities: Worse from cooling off after getting overheated; from cold, damp weather and cold, raw air; from any change in the weather, especially from warm to cold; from physical motion, especially from ascending; at specific stages in development: for example, from teething, puberty, and menopause; in the morning, especially upon awakening.

Better: during dry, warm weather; from sneezing; from rubbing or scratching affected areas; after breakfast. Note that chronic conditions for the type tend to be improved every other day.

Common Causes of Illness

Overwork and over-worry; poor diet; being forced to go out into cold weather; getting feet cold and wet; alcohol abuse; over-lifting and straining muscles; mechanical injury, especially to the lower spine; previous illness (often flu), from which the patient never recovered; fright.

Common Uses

Exhaustion, chronic fatigue; chemical sensitivity; seasonal allergy; otitis media (ear infection); asthma; headaches, especially migraines; flu; low back pain; leg cramps, cramping pains in muscles; acne; arthritis, especially rheumatoid arthritis; anxiety and depression.

CALENDULA OFFICINALIS

Source: Marigold
While Calendula is considered to be only a topical remedy today, there is some important diagnostic data. First, because this remedy is used for patients with physical trauma, usually involving some break to the skin or some surface infection, check the site of the injury

to see if it suggests Calendula. Obviously, this remedy is available for internal as well as external use. External preparations may be used concurrently with an internal remedy such as Arnica during a recovery period following serious injury, or it may be taken internally and used externally as well. Unless otherwise indicated, the comments below relate to internal use.

Theme: Where Arnica relates to trauma, Calendula relates to wounds. Thus, both remedies may be needed together in cases of physical injury.

About Calendula

Murphy writes, "Jahr, who was in Paris during the Coup d'Etat of 1849, treated a number of cases of gun-shot wounds with comminuted bones and saved several limbs by means of Calendula. It prevents suppuration and pyemia. In some cases of carbuncle it acts with great promptitude, subduing pain and fever. In obstetric practice it is invaluable."

The Calendula Face

Eyes: For patients with injuries to the eyes, especially for the area of the eye if the wound has become infected, and if pus is present. Also used for recovery after surgery in the area around the eyes. Consider this remedy for cases of scratched cornea. It is also useful in recovery from any surgery of the eyes.

Ears: The patient will be deaf after injury. The patient hears distant sounds. Consider this remedy for cases of ruptured eardrum.

As is often the case in homeopathic medicine, the opposite may also be true and the patient may have very acute hearing, and may be startled or awakened by any sound.

Nose: Look for discharge from only one nostril at a time. The discharge is green in color.

Mouth: The patient's lips are swollen. Like the face in general, the mouth is swollen. The area between the lips and the nose is swollen.

Tongue: The tongue is dry and red, and often is cracked.

Throat: The submaxillary glands are swollen and very sensitive to touch.

Countenance: The face is pale. The patient has a nervous expression.

The Calendula Patient

Behavior: Emotionally, the theme is that the patient will seem to be in pain that is entirely out of proportion to the injury. The patient is exceedingly sensitive to pain.

Characteristics: Calendula is said to act most effectively upon the skin, muscles, spine, and liver. It is an amazing remedy that is most often used topically, but it may also be used orally, as are most other remedies. It is to be considered first for cases of lacerations of all sorts, as well as for simple cuts and scrapes. It is useful for scalp wounds and for hemorrhages of all sorts.

Calendula is most effective when the patient experiences a wound that is red, raw, inflamed, and painful. The wounded area feels bruised, as if it had been beaten. The wounded area has stinging pain.

Pulse: The Calendula patient is prone to a rapid and irregular pulse. The pulse will range from 110 to 160 beats per minute.

Modalities: Worse: from becoming chilled; from damp weather; in the evening and at night.

Better: from lying perfectly still; from warmth in general.

Common Causes of Illness

Physical trauma; lacerations of all sorts.

Common Uses

Wounds, lacerations, abrasions; incisions, especially those associated with dental procedures; infected wounds of all sorts; rashes, eczema.

CAMPHORA

Source: Camphor
The "minty fresh" quality of the remedy is something of a theme. The whole body is icy cold. But there is more to it: at the core, Camphora combines the qualities of cold, crampy, convulsive, and anxious.
Theme: Chill is the theme of this remedy. In no other patient is a state of chill so pronounced, yet he craves cold, open air. (Note that this chill state often alternates with flashes of great heat.)

About Camphora

Kent wrote, "The camphor patient is a most troublesome patient to nurse. Coldness, frenzy and heat very often intermingle ... From the shock of the suffering, the mind is almost gone, or is in a state of frenzy. Coldness then comes on and the patient wants to be uncovered, wants cold air wants the window open; but before all this can be done a flash of heat comes on and then he wants the covers on, and the register turned on, and wants hot bottles; but this stage now passes off, and while the nurse is bringing the hot bottles he wants her to throw them away, open the window and have everything cool."

The Camphora Face

Eyes: The patient stares, he tends to lock onto some object and fixate on it with his eyes. Usually his pupils will be dilated.

Consider this remedy for cases in which the patient's eyes turn upward or outward in illness.

Ears: The earlobes are hot and red. Look for a possible ulceration of the external ear, especially of the left ear.

Nose: The patient sneezes a good deal, especially during a change in the weather. The external nose is cold, especially the tip.

Consider this remedy for colds that develop during changes in the weather. Also consider this remedy for the first stage of a cold, when the nose is blocked up without discharge.

Mouth: The patient's breath is cold, as is the tongue. The patient has trouble speaking; is hoarse.

Tongue: The tongue is bluish and cold. The tongue is cold, flabby, and trembling. The patient complains of dryness in the back of the tongue, of a sensation of scraping, although there is a great deal of saliva present.

The patient has feeble speech, especially upon awakening. He seems unsure whether or not he will be able to speak. His words seem to choke in his larynx.

Throat: Listen for rattling sounds in the throat when the patient breathes or tries to speak.

Countenance: The face is pale and haggard. The patient has an anxious look on his face. The patient has a pinched expression. The face may alternate between pale and red. The face is covered in cold sweat. The patient's upper lip is retracted, drawn back.

The Camphora Patient

Behavior: This patient does not want to be left alone. He does not want to be allowed to dwell upon his own condition or symptoms. He will want to talk, or have a story told to him. And yet, look for the patient to actually have less pain when he thinks about it. Look for his pain to increase when he drifts into sleep.

Characteristics: Think of this remedy for cases that involve icy coldness, but the patient does not want to be covered up. When this coldness alternates with a sensation of internal heat, the patient may first want to be covered and then will suddenly kick the covers off.

Some patients will alternate coldness with heat, as they do paleness with redness. Remember that the temperature is the vital key here: icy coldness of the whole body. The patient is cold inside and out. Even his breath is cold. And yet, the patient does not want to be covered.

Pain, is usually cramping in nature, internally or externally. The patient may not be totally aware of his pain, or he may be overwhelmed by it. Look for the patient to become cold after the onset of pain.

Pulse: The pulse is very rapid and weak. The pulse is very small, hard to find. The pulse is also accelerated in a patient without fever. The pulse may be so vague that it cannot be counted.

The patient may also have palpitations. The patient may have palpitations after eating. Palpitations may be accompanied by a cold face, cold limbs, and body. Palpitations are accompanied by a slow, steady pulse.

Modalities: Worse: from cold in any form, such as drafts; from motion; generally, at night.

Better: from sweating or any bodily discharge; from drinking, especially cold water; from warmth; from open air, if not too cold; from discussing and thinking about his symptoms.

Common Causes of Illness

Shock associated with physical trauma; aftermath of surgery; sunstroke; chill; suppressed discharges, especially sweat; anger and irritation.

Common Uses

Physical trauma and recovery from surgery; colds, pneumonia; fainting; sunstroke; chronic fatigue.

CARBO VEGETABILIS

Source: Vegetable Charcoal

Sluggishness is key here. The whole being is sluggish, especially the digestive and respiratory systems. The patient has trouble breathing and may struggle for breath, and his digestion is very, very slow. Thus you have a patient who is slow and ill prepared for any exertion, whether physical or mental. This is also an indifferent patient who takes in information without reaction, pleasure, horror, or even thinking about what he has heard. The patient is sad and/or depressed, especially in the evening. Night fears are common. A sense of anxiety lasts all night long.

Theme: As with the Calcarea patient, the patient needing Carbo is usually not suddenly ill. Instead, his health breaks down over a period of time until he is left gasping for air.

About Carbo Veg

Boericke wrote, "The patient may be all but lifeless, but the head is hot; coldness, breath cool, pulse imperceptible, oppressed and quickened respiration, and must have air, must be fanned hard, must have all the windows open. This is a typical state for Carbo Veg."

The Carbo Veg Face

Eyes: The patient will have trouble looking upward, as if his eyes were very heavy. His pupils will not react to changes in light. Look for agglutination of eyelids every night.

Ears: The ears are dry, and yet smell bad. The ears smell of wax. There is a great deal of yellow wax in each ear. The left ear will be hot and red every evening. Look for a discharge of skin-toned, bad-smelling thick fluid from the right ear.

Nose: The nose bleeds every day. The patient is pale before and after each attack of nosebleed. The nose bleeds if the patient strains in any way. The nose bleeds every morning.

The tip of the nose is red and may be scabby. There may be varicose veins on the nose. Look for eruptions in the exterior corners of the nose. The patient may sneeze a great deal, and may or may not have flow from the nose when he sneezes.

Mouth: The gums bleed easily. The gums recede from the teeth. The gums bleed with every brushing. The lips are cracked. They may be discolored brown or blackish.

The breath may be cold. There is a bad smell from the mouth.

Tongue: The tongue is usually coated white, although it may also have a yellow/brown coating. The tongue always seems to be covered with a dirty crust. The tongue may have fissures. The tongue may have black ulcers on it. The tongue is very dry.

Throat: There is a great deal of mucus in the throat, which the patient coughs up. The throat looks raw.

Countenance: The face is pale, bluish, with a cold sweat. The cheeks may be mottled red. The nose is red. The face flushes easily, especially when the patient eats or drinks. Other possible discolorations of the face include grayish, yellowish or greenish discolorations. Look for unhealthy skin including acne, especially on the forehead. The face is puffy as well.

The Carbo Veg Patient

Behavior: This is a remedy for those whose lifestyle has broken their health. It is also for patients who never totally recovered from a severe illness. Therefore, you have an exhausted patient, unable to breathe easily.

Characteristics: These are very debilitated patients. They often have not been well since suffering through an earlier disease. Consider this remedy when the patient's head is very hot, but the body is cold (the Arnica patient also has a hot head and cold body). The hands and feet tend to always be cold. In some rather advanced cases, the patient's breath and tongue become cold, his whole body is covered in a cold sweat, and the patient loses his voice.

Pains tend to combine numbness (especially of the body part sat or lain upon) and a bruised soreness. Pains tend to increase around noon, as does weakness.

Pulse: The pulse in inconsistent, intermittent, very weak. The pulse may be so slight that it cannot be taken. Yet, the pulse is felt in the whole body.

This is a patient given to palpitations. These will be visible in the body. Palpitations will be accompanied by a great internal heat, especially when the patient is sitting. They will be accompanied by a great thirst. The palpitations will be accompanied by a sensation of anguish.

Modalities: Worse: from warmth, and especially from cooling off after becoming warm; from a diet of foods that are too rich, especially pork, butter, and other fatty foods, or from eating spoiled foods; from drinking coffee or milk; from changes in weather and in temperature, especially when nights are cold and frosty; from straining the body, and, especially, the voice.

Better: from breathing cool air, especially from being fanned; from having the feet elevated; from loose clothing; from lying down and resting.

Common Causes of Illness

A poor diet of foods that are too rich and fatty; a diet with too much salt; food poisoning; alcohol abuse; overwork, especially physical over-lifting or straining; changes in the weather; getting cold and wet; overheating and then getting cold.

Common Uses

Colds, flu, and, especially, pneumonia; asthma; indigestion, ulcers; obesity; headaches; chronic fatigue; recovery from surgery.

CAUSTICUM

Source: Caustic Lime

The Causticum patient is known for his paralysis. He is known for sensitivity to changes in the weather. He will be better when it is damp, and worse for cold. All of his many aches and pains involve numbness.

Theme: Unfairness is the key. This is a patient who feels that his illness is unfair, who also seeks justice for others, and who finds that his physical body betrays him with illness just when he needs it most.

About Causticum

Farrington wrote, "Especially suited to patients who are timid, nervous and anxious, full of fearful fancies especially in the evening at twilight, when shadows grow longer and fancies more rife. The child is afraid to go to bed in the dark."

The Causticum Face

Eyes: There are many, many diagnostic symptoms for the eyes. Note that this is a very important remedy for those with cataracts. Since this is the case, look for the patient to complain of indistinct vision, dimness of vision, and a sensation as if sand were in the eyes. The eyelids will be swollen, ulcerated, inflamed. There may be paralysis of one of the eyelids, or quivering of the eyelids. The patient may not blink; his eyes always stay open. There may be heaviness of the upper lids, as if they are stuck to the lower lids, or as if they were too heavy to keep open. The eyelids may close involuntarily. The lids may droop.

The eyes will be very sensitive to both heat and light. The patient is constantly photophobic, and will likely have one eye closed most of the time. The patient will complain that he sees spots before his eyes.

Look for the patient to constantly touch and rub his eyes.

Ears: There may be an accumulation of a great deal of brown wax in the ears. There may be a thick, gluey discharge. The exterior of the ears are red.

Nose: The patient sneezes in the morning. There may be a thick yellow or green discharge from the nose. The nose may be stopped up without discharge. Look for ulcers, crusts, or warts on the tip of the nose.

Mouth: The patient repeatedly bites the inside of his mouth when chewing. The patient swallows and hawks up mucus. There is an excess of saliva and mucus in the mouth. There may be cramps in the lips.

This is a remedy for pain in the gums and not in the teeth. The gums are swollen and bleed readily. There may be abscesses of the gums.

Tongue: The patient's tongue is red in the middle, while the sides are coated yellow. There may be painful vesicles on the tip of the tongue. Warts are possible on the back of the tongue. The tongue, palate, and uvula are swollen and red.

The tongue and other organs of speech become paralyzed. The patient cannot speak. The patient stutters when he tries to speak.

The patient may accidentally bite his tongue, or have the sensation of pain as if it has been bitten.

Throat: The patient repeatedly swallows. The patient swallows liquids the wrong way, so they come out of his nose. The throat, especially the back of the throat, is very dry. The throat is raw and red.

Countenance: There are warts on the face. The face is yellow, especially the area of the temples. The face has a sickly look. The right side of the face is paralyzed, especially after the patient becomes cold, particularly from cold water. The color that may be associated with Causticum is dirty white. The skin all over the body may be tinged with this color.

The Causticum Patient

Behavior: The sensation of tearing and drawing are important here, as they are in the physical body. The Causticum patient often feels as if a part of him has been ripped away. The emotional keys of disappointment, sorrow, and anger are also important, as they lead to this same sensation of tearing.

The patient has a sense that something unfair has happened, and fairness is very important to him. He also tends to link the future with fear, and experiences a vague sense that something bad is about to happen.

Characteristics: The action of this remedy usually centers on the muscles and joints of the body, with a slow decline in strength accompanying chronic conditions. It speaks to rheumatic and arthritic pains throughout the body, with a sensation of paralysis being quite common. Joints especially feel raw and sore, and have an accompanying burning sensation. Causticum also speaks to conditions involving the nervous system, with numbness and paralysis being the leading sensations. The remedy also acts on the skin. Look for the Causticum patient to have skin growths, especially warts. This is particularly true in constitutional cases.

Pulse: There are no guiding symptoms for pulse, although the patient's pulse will tend to become increased and excited as evening nears.

Palpitation with pain in the chest is a common symptom. The patient will become exhausted with palpitations. The patient may also complain of a burning sensation in the region of the heart during palpitations.

Modalities: Worse: from dry, cold weather; from contact with cold wind; from extremes in temperature; from suppression of sweat or any form of eruption; when stooping; at night, especially at sunset; from drinking coffee.

Better: from damp weather; from getting wet, especially from bathing; from cold drinks; from gentle motion; from the warmth of bed.

Common Causes of Illness

Tending the sick, going without sleep for a stressful reason; burns and/or scalds; lead poisoning; senility; suppressed eruptions; long-lasting grief and/or sorrow.

Common Uses

Allergies; sinusitis; cough; rheumatism; sciatica; torticollis (wryneck); arthritis, especially rheumatoid arthritis; low back pain; carpal tunnel syndrome; TMJ (temporomandibular joint) problems; constipation; acne and warts; anxiety attacks.

CHAMOMILLA

Source: Chamomile

The patient responding to this remedy will combine an almost overwhelming sense of pain with an explosive anger. Anger and pain, pain and anger. This can be played out in many different ways, but it is most often found in pregnant and nursing women, and in little children. This patient is also restless. He does not want to be held, or especially carried. He will writhe and struggle if held. The patient is thirsty at all times.

Theme: The core indication for Chamomilla is this: hot, thirsty, angry, and sensitive. No matter the condition, the Chamomilla patient is in intolerable pain. Because of its great power to relieve this pain, this remedy has been called the "opium of homeopathy."

About Chamomilla

Vermeulen writes, "The chief guiding symptoms belong to the mental and emotional group, which lead to this remedy in many forms of disease. Especially of frequent employment in diseases of children, where peevishness, restlessness, and colic give the needful indications. A disposition that is mild, calm and gentle and sluggish and constipated bowels contra-indicate Chamomilla."

The Chamomilla Face

Eyes: The Chamomilla patient stares. This is a remedy for those with inflammation of the eyes, so there is a great sensation of heat and burning in the eyes. The whites of the eyes take on a yellow tinge. Look for the patient's eyes to be swollen every morning. The eyes are agglutinated with mucus. The margins of the lower lids are inflamed and swollen. Look for the eyelids to twitch.

The patient is incredibly photophobic. The slightest light is intolerable.

Ears: The patient will be frantic from pain in his ears. The inner ears are swollen. The area of the ear is very sensitive to cold and wind, and to noise. The patient hears imaginary voices. The hearing is increased and very sensitive. The patient cannot tolerate the sound of music.

Nose: The nose is very sensitive to all smells, or has a total loss of smell.

Look for obstruction of the nose; look for ulceration of the nostrils. Look for mucus flow on cold and windy days, when the nose drains constantly. The patient will be unable to sleep because of stoppage and drainage of nose.

The mucus is hot. The eyes water during coryza.

Mouth: The patient has bad breath. His breath smells very sour. There will be a good deal of saliva in the patient's mouth. The whole mouth seems to radiate heat. Look for a deep crack in the lower lip.

The gums are swollen and hot, especially during toothache. This is major remedy for toothache and for teething. The toothache drives the patient to distraction, to fits of anger and passion. The patient strikes out in pain. In adults: toothache may occur after drinking coffee, at night.

Consider this remedy for teething children who are angry in their pain. Watery, greenish and chopped diarrhea will accompany the teething pain, as will a smell of rotten eggs. The child will be restless, especially at night, and will desire drinks, and will have a rattling sound in his breathing.

Tongue: Look for a thick white or yellow coating on the tongue, as if a rug were laid on it. The middle of the tongue may be cracked and dry. Look for blisters on and under the tongue. Look for the tongue to move in jerking, convulsive motions.

Throat: There may be an inflammation of the soft palate and tonsils. There may be swollen glands in the external neck. The patient will have trouble swallowing solid food. Symptoms of inflammation will be worse when the patient is lying down.

Countenance: Look for the patient to have one cheek red and hot, the other pale and cold. This is keynote to the remedy type. There is a hot, sticky sweat on head and face. The patient sweats especially after eating and drinking. The face is puffy, red, and hot. The patient has a hot head with a cold body.

The Chamomilla Patient

Behavior: This is an angry and difficult patient. He may be unable to be satisfied. He demands something and then doesn't want it when he gets it. Children needing this remedy may throw fits.

Characteristics: Combine the following for the Chamomilla patient: hypersensitivity, anger, thirst, restlessness, heat and numbness. This patient is perhaps the most sensitive to pain—he may literally faint from pain, or may lash out at others when he is in pain. Commonly, this remedy is helpful for cases of colic, especially when abdominal cramps are associated with hot sweat and anger.

Pulse: The pulse is small and uneven. It may at first seem to be full, but will later seem weak and contracted. Even if the pulse is small, it is usually accelerated.

The patient often suffers from palpitations. He feels sick and faint. He feels a heaviness in his limbs, and paralysis with the onset of palpitations.

Modalities: Worse: from anger; from coffee; from alcohol and/or drugs; at night; during cold, damp weather; from warmth and heat in general; from being touched; from being looked at; when lying down.

Better: when he is carried; from sweating; during warm, wet weather, and in any mild weather conditions.

Common Causes of Illness

Teething; abuse of alcohol and/or drugs; drinking coffee and use of stimulants in general; anger.

Common Uses

Teething and toothache; PMS (premenstrual syndrome), pregnancy and nursing, hot flashes at menopause; fevers; asthma; cough; colic, diarrhea; behavioral troubles with children.

CHINA OFFICINALIS

Source: Peruvian Bark

Here is another remedy with the theme of depletion, or total exhaustion, so ailments needing China tend to develop slowly. But we often see a need for this remedy in patients who have been ill for a long time, or have lost a good deal of bodily fluids, especially blood. The illness that broke their health may be past, but they have difficulty recovering their strength and Vital Force.

Theme: Loss is the theme. On a physical level, the need for this remedy usually involves a loss of fluids, especially blood, from the body.

About China

Guernsey wrote, "The chief keynote calling for the use of China is found in the sufferings caused by the loss of fluids, such as hemorrhage, galactorrhea, seminal emissions, diarrhea, etc. Debility whether much fluid has been lost or only a little ... for any disease or trouble occurring periodically, at certain definite periods ... extreme sensitiveness and irritability of nerves, or relaxation of solids."

The China Face

Eyes: The whites of the eyes are yellowed, often with black specks. This is especially true in patients with fever. There are blue colored rings around the eyes.

The patient will be mildly intolerant of bright light. Bright light causes the eyes to tear.

Ears: The outer ear is very sensitive to touch. The lobes are red and swollen. The patient will not want to have his ears touched in any way. He cannot sleep with the weight of his head on his ear. The external ear hurts, and is red and painful when it is touched in any way. Look for a foul, thick, and often bloody discharge from the ears.

The patient will have either very sensitive or very poor hearing.

Nose: Sneezing is accompanied by a good deal of discharge. The discharge is clear and watery. The patient may have hay fever with much sneezing. The nose may also alternate between being stopped up and flowing. The patient may have frequent nose bleeds, especially in the morning, or upon rising. The patient may faint from nosebleed. The patient is very sensitive to certain smells, particularly: food cooking, tobacco, and flowers.

Mouth: Look for a cold sweat around the mouth. The lips are chapped. They are dry and blackish.

Tongue: The tongue is dirty looking, with a thick coating. It is coated white or yellow, especially in the morning. The tongue may also be cracked.

Throat: The submaxillary glands are swollen.

Countenance: The Chinchona patient combines a hot head with cold hands.

The patient's face is sallow, bloated, and flushes red easily. Look for a bluish discoloration around the eyes.

The China Patient

Behavior: This is a remedy for patients who are in a state of debility. The patient is exhausted; his body aches all over. All senses are simultaneously weak and overly sensitive. Everything upsets him: light, noise, smells, and especially pain.

The patient may be unconscious. If conscious, he will not respond to stimulus, even to pain. Calling out his name loudly will bring a momentary response. The patient's words are unintelligible. The patient's voice is deep and husky when he talks or sings.

Characteristics: Most important is that this patient is debilitated by any form of discharge, whether it is blood, diarrhea, or pus from an infected area of the body. This debility often includes a loss of the senses, especially sight. The patient usually feels sore all over; his joints and bones feel sprained. The patient is very sensitive to touch in these areas, and even the slightest touch can cause a great deal of pain. The affected parts are also restless. The patient may want to move these parts, even though he does not want to move about or walk.

Pulse: The pulse is irregular. A series of strong beats will be followed by a series of weak, rapid beats. The patient's pulse will become weaker after eating.

This is a remedy type given to palpitations. Palpitations are accompanied by a rush of blood to the face. The face becomes red and hot, and the hands become cold. This is especially true for palpitations that occur after a loss of bodily fluids.

Modalities: Worse: from any discharge; from jarring motion; from touch; from sudden noise; from cold, wind, and drafts of any sort; on alternating days; from eating spoiled foods or drinking impure water.

Better: from hard pressure; from bending double; from loose clothing; in open air; when warm.

Common Causes of Illness

Loss of fluids, especially blood; taking a sudden chill; recovery from long illness; abuse of tea or alcohol; mercury poisoning; anger, and suppressed anger.

CINA

Source: Wormseed

The key to this remedy is that it is needed most often by patients, particularly children, who have parasites, especially roundworms or pinworms. Although homeopaths are never to treat disease, it is easy to understand why many will simply turn to Cina for cases of children with parasites, especially worms. The whole picture of parasites is here: restlessness, an angry and frantic nature, and an almost overwhelming need to bore fingers into ears, noses, and anuses.

Theme: This patient's whole system has been overwhelmed by parasites. Look for twitching, jerking, and pulling. The patient cannot relax, and has no idea of the cause of his woe.

About Cina

Kent writes, "The old routine of giving Cina for worms need not go into your notes, for if you are guided by the symptoms, the patient will be cured and the worms will go."

The Cina Face

Eyes: The eyebrows twitch when the patient looks closely at anything. The eyes water when the patient coughs. Look for the patient's eyes to be dilated. Look for dark rings around the eyes.

Ears: The patient will jerk on his exterior ear. He will dig into his ears, and scratch his internal ears.

The patient's hearing is reduced.

Nose: The patient is always rubbing, scratching, or picking his nose. He picks his nose until it bleeds. He rubs his nose on his pillow, or on his parent's shoulder. Or he rubs his nose with his hands. He picks his nose while awake and when sleeping.

The patient sneezes a good deal. The patient sneezes violently.

Mouth: The patient grinds his teeth in his sleep. He chews and swallows in his sleep. The mouth is dry and raw looking.

Tongue: The tongue is clean. (Note: this is important. Often the patient with the most disturbed digestion will have a perfectly clean tongue.) Look for white sores on the sides of the tongue. The tongue may also be tinged yellow or brownish-yellow, or even white, but this is a clean tongue. There may be a good deal of frothy saliva on the tongue.

Note that this is a remedy for those with chronic bad breath.

Throat: The patient will make a great deal of noise when swallowing. He will have difficulty swallowing liquids. The patient swallows constantly. Listen for a clucking or gurgling noise in the throat when the patient swallows.

Countenance: Look for bright red cheeks, or redness in perfect circles on the cheeks. The face is pale and hot, with white or bluish-white discoloration around the mouth. One cheek may be red, while the other is pale. Look for twitching of the muscles around the eyes or anywhere on the face.

The Cina Patient

Behavior: Most patients needing this remedy are children. The patient will be demanding, angry, and constantly hungry. He will want to be held, and especially rocked. He grinds his teeth. He is sensitive to touch.

Characteristics: Classically, it was thought that this remedy was needed mainly by big, fat children with ruddy complexions and infestations of pinworms. It may, of course, be needed by children (and adults) of any type, who fit the picture of the remedy. Look for this patient to be very hungry and never seem full. Look for him to grind his teeth.

Pains associated with this remedy come in sudden shocks. The patient will literally jump in pain as if he had been struck. The patient will also usually have very sensitive skin.

The patient's voice will be hoarse, or he may lose his voice altogether. Listen to a gurgling sound in the esophagus when he tries to speak or swallow.

Pulse: The pulse is somewhat small and can be difficult to find, but it is hard in nature and accelerated. The heart beats about 130 times per minute. The pulse may be trembling in nature.

Modalities: Worse: from being touched, from any form of external pressure; from being looked at; at the full moon; from being in the sun and in summer; from yawning (from anyone yawing); while sleeping.

Better: from lying down on the stomach; from motion, especially from shaking the head and from rocking; from wiping the eyes.

Common Causes of Illness

Worms and other parasites.

Common Uses

Worms and other parasites; otitis media (ear infection); colic with diarrhea; behavioral disorders.

COCCULUS

Source: Indian Cockle

This patient is experiencing spasms of one sort or another. These spasms tend to manifest on only one half of the body. It is important to note that all the symptoms shown will be worse when the patient rides in any vehicle, making it an important remedy for travel sickness.

Theme: The sensation here is one of hollowness. Affected areas feel hollow. Most especially when nauseated, the Cocculus patient will feel hollow inside.

About Cocculus

Hughes wrote, "Coldness; paralytic stiffness of the limbs with drawing pains in their bones and in the back, and sullen irritability, with anxiety, were prominent symptoms. The patient said that his brain felt constricted as by a ligature. He wished to sleep, but a frightful sensation, as of a hideous dream, came over him directly he closed his eyes, and made him start up again. He had great repugnance to food and drink. This is a frequent symptom of Cocculus, and very characteristic of it."

The Cocculus Face

Eyes: The patient tends to keep his eyes closed. You will see his eyeballs moving about under his closed lids. He has trouble opening his eyes upon awakening, although they may open involuntarily during sleep. The eyes move with jerking motions, with eyes opened or closed.

Ears: The hearing is very sensitive. The patient is troubled by noise.

Mouth: There are no guiding symptoms for this remedy.

Tongue: The tongue feels enlarged and paralyzed. The patient will have trouble speaking due to the paralysis of the tongue. The tongue is dry and rough. It may have a whitish or yellowish coat. The patient with a dry tongue may not be thirsty. He is also often averse to food.

Speech may be particularly difficult during times of vertigo.

Throat: The throat is very dry. The throat feels paralyzed, and the patient has difficulty swallowing. The patient has trouble breathing. He tends to cough a good deal.

Countenance: The patient's face tends to reflect either anger or an enveloping vagueness. This is the face of a person with not enough sleep. The patient's face is bloated, perhaps to the extent of distortion. His face is cold to the touch. The patient may be too weak to hold his head up, to stand, or even to speak.

The Cocculus Patient

Behavior: These patients are slow to notice anything. They are slow to answer questions, or to acknowledge you, and are vague in their answers. This is a remedy for those who are exhausted. It is often needed by those who have been keeping watch on a sick person, and those who are in great need of sleep. It is also needed by those with motion sickness.

The patient may look and seem drunk. He tends to seem a bit distracted.

Characteristics: This patient feels sudden spasms in his body. The sensation of pain is cramping in nature. These are also known as shuddering patients. Shuddering and trembling of the jaw, head, and muscles in the abdomen are most common.

Vertigo runs throughout this remedy. The patient has heart palpitations with vertigo, or vocal paralysis with vertigo. He feels faint, and may actually faint if he does not support himself. He has trouble reading, thinking, or speaking during the attack of vertigo. This difficulty may last for days after the attack. You may also find paralysis in the patient, especially in the tongue and face. He may be unable to speak or hold up his head. Numbness and tingling may accompany other symptoms in these areas.

Speaking will aggravate all of the patient's symptoms, especially those in his head. His voice has a whimpering quality and may be tremulous.

This patient often cannot sleep, and is much worse from lack of sleep.

Pulse: This is a small, accelerated pulse. The pulse is 90 to 100 beats per minute. There may be an irregular pulse with a heart murmur.

This is a remedy type also prone to palpitations. These palpitations will be linked to vertigo. The patient will suddenly have to grip something to support himself during palpitations. He may feel as if he will faint, or may actually faint.

Modalities: Worse: from motion, especially the motion of a car or boat; from swimming; from touch; from jarring motion; from coffee or tobacco; from talking and laughing.

Better: from sitting still; from warmth; from quiet.

Common Causes of Illness

Travel, especially in a vehicle; lack of sleep; sun; abuse of tea and coffee; mental or physical overstraining; anger, anxiety, disappointment, grief.

Common Uses

Travel sickness; headache, especially migraine; nausea; vertigo; chronic fatigue; anxiety attacks.

COFFEA CRUDA

Source: Coffee

This remedy combines oversensitivity, especially of the senses, with nervousness and restlessness. This is a manic patient. Just think about how you feel when you drink too much coffee, and apply that to the case.

Theme: Oversensitivity is key. The patient's senses become too acute. His vision improves, his hearing improves to the point that he cannot bear noise.

About Coffea

Murphy writes, "The great characteristics of Coffea are exaltation of the senses and sensibility in general. Sight is improved, fine print can easily be read, hearing is more acute and noises are intolerable and are accompanied with fear of death. Mental activities are exalted. Great sensitiveness to touch or contact."

The Coffea Face

Eyes: The eyes are bright, reddish, and shining. The pupils are dilated. Look for the patient to hold his eyes half open during sleep and to move them convulsively when awake.

The patient actually has improved vision, and can read fine print easily. Vision is especially good when the patient is in open air.

Ears: The hearing is very sensitive. The powers of hearing are greatly increased, to the point that noise can bring on physical pain. Or, hearing may be dulled. Either way, noise equals pain for the Coffea patient.

Nose: The sense of smell is very sensitive. Nosebleeds are common.

Mouth: Tooth pain dominates (this is another remedy for teething children). The patient moves his head about in jerks when a toothache begins. The toothache is soothed by cold liquid. Look for the patient to spit out liquid as soon as it becomes warm, as the warm liquid makes the pain return.

The sense of taste is increased and is very acute. The patient eats very quickly.

Tongue: There are no guiding symptoms for this remedy. But look for the patient's sense of taste to be enhanced, as are his other senses. Patient will be especially sensitive to sweet tastes.

Throat: The patient swallows constantly.

Countenance: The patient's cheeks are dry, hot, and very red.

The Coffea Patient

Behavior: This is a remedy in which the behavior of the patient often tells the whole tale. The patient is manic, antic, like someone who has drunk too much coffee. He cannot rest or sleep. The other key is the enhancement to all of the senses. This is truly the oversensitive patient, overwhelmed by his sensory intake. The patient cries or laughs very easily. He is talkative, and filled with ideas. He is interested in doing anything except sitting quietly or sleeping.

Characteristics: Symptoms tend to cluster around the joints, muscles, and kidneys. This is an important remedy for both children and older patients. This is also a good remedy to remember for cases that involve exhaustion following a long journey, especially if the trip takes place in hot weather.

Pulse: There is a rapid, irregular heartbeat. The pulse may be full and frequent, becoming less vigorous and even weak.

There also may be nervous palpitations of the heart. Heart palpitations are initiated by sleeplessness, overthinking, and the overexcitement of hearing good news.

Modalities: Worse: from overeating; from drinking alcohol and coffee; from any sensory stimulus: noise, smells, touch; motion; strong emotions.

Better: from sleep; from lying still; from warmth; from holding ice in the mouth (especially for cases of toothache).

Common Causes of Illness

Jet lag after a journey; abuse of alcohol, especially wine and beer; abuse of coffee and tea; abuse of drugs; excessive emotions, good or bad: fear and fright, joy, surprise, very good or very bad news; disappointment in love.

Common Uses

Headache, especially migraine; toothache; insomnia; jet lag; chronic fatigue.

COLOCYNTHIS

Source: Bitter Cucumber

Colic and Colocynthis go hand in hand. It is most often called for in cases of abdominal colic, but it is also used when a patient is beset with kidney stones and gallstones. The keynote here is that the patient bends double with pain. The sensation of pain is cramping in nature. Colocynthis is also linked to times of seasonal change, especially when the change involves cold air and a hot sun. The patient is given to staggering pain, especially in the left side of the body. These may be rheumatic pains, made worse from changes in the weather.

The remedy speaks especially to the digestive tract and to sciatic pains.

Theme: While there is no poetic emotional key to this remedy, Colocynthis is a wonderful little remedy that is so helpful in nearly all cases of colic that match its physical picture.

About Colocynthis

Tyler wrote, "I suppose we have, all of us, witnessed the wonderfully prompt action of Colocynth in spasm and colic relieved by bending over and pressing hard into the abdomen; 'til Colocynth has come to mean, for us, just this and nothing more. But Colocynth stands for a great deal more than 'the intestines as if ground between hard stones, the pain relieved by doubling up and by hard pressure.' It has frightful nerve pains, in spine, in limbs, in head, in ovaries, especially if cause by anger and indignation."

The Colocynthis Face

Eyes: Look for twitching of the patient's eyelids, which are somewhat swollen and pronounced. This is a major remedy for glaucoma. The patient's eyes become stony hard.

Ears: Look for the patient to dig his finger into his ear, especially the left ear, in order to scratch as deeply as possible.

Nose: There will be a great deal of mucus flow from the nose, especially the left nostril. The flow is increased when the patient is in open air.

Mouth: The patient will complain about a bitter taste in the mouth.

Tongue: The tongue is rough, and looks as if it has been scalded. It is red and clean. The tip especially looks burned. The tongue may be coated yellow or white.

Throat: There is much belching in the throat. The belching often accompanies palpitations.

The throat looks dry and raw.

Countenance: The left side of the patient's face is swollen. The face shape is distorted. Look for the patient to have a relaxed expression on his face; the muscles in the face look relaxed. The face is pale. The patient's eyes look sunken into the head. The face itself looks distorted, as if the left side were being ripped from the right. Pain runs from back of the left ear to the eye and the mouth, all on the left side.

The Colocynthis Patient

Behavior: This is an angry remedy and an angry patient. The patient is made worse by his outbursts of anger and becomes ill after them. This is one of our most important remedies for those who cannot bear contradiction, and those who become ill after their own explosive bouts of anger or after feeling humiliated.

Characteristics: The quality of pain in the classic texts is said to be "atrocious." The pain is sudden, griping, cramping, and tearing. The patient cannot help but suddenly bend double to relieve the pain even a bit. He will cry out in pain. The patient will press something hard—often his fist—into the area to bring relief. Thus, this is a remedy for many cases of digestive distress and diarrhea that follow this "bend double" pattern.

While this remedy is usually needed by those with intestinal colic, it is also useful for those with rheumatic pains, even those that are long lasting. It is helpful for those with sciatica. It is also helpful for cases of premenstrual syndrome (PMS) that follow the given pattern.

Pulse: There is a strong, throbbing heart-beat. The pulse may race to 130 beats per minute. This may be accompanied by a great thirst. Look for the pulse to become slow and weak during periods of colic. It is difficult to find, yet it still races.

Look for palpitations that begin with belching or hiccoughs.

Modalities: Worse: from anger or any strong, negative emotion; before and after urinating; from eating or drinking; from cold and drafts; from rest, especially in bed; at night.

Better: from hard pressure; from bending double; from heat; from gentle motion; after passing stool or gas; from lying on the stomach; from drinking coffee.

Common Causes of Illness

Anger and humiliation; grief; upon catching a cold.

Common Uses

Colic, especially in young children; abdominal pains that follow the pattern; irritable bowel syndrome; kidney or gallstones; sciatica; PMS.

DULCAMARA

Source: Bittersweet

Dulcamara relates to the time of oncoming autumn, when the days are hot and the nights are cold. It is a small, mostly acute remedy that helps primarily with hay fever and the rheumatic pains related to this time of year. In addition to its helpfulness with acute allergies, think of Dulcamara as a remedy for those with backache and neck pain related to late summer, and for aches and pains that develop in damp weather.

Theme: No other remedy is as linked to seasonal change, especially that linked with the change from summer to autumn weather, as is Dulcamara.

About Dulcamara

Hahnemann wrote, "A very powerful plant."

Tyler wrote, "Dulcamara affects the entire length of the respiratory mucous membrane. Nose—dry coryza, or profuse discharges. Nosebleed of clear hot blood, worse after getting wet. Throat—tonsillitis from every cold change; hawking up tough mucous with rawness. Chest, cough a long time in order to expel phlegm. Great oppressive pain in the whole chest, especially on inspiration and expiration."

The Dulcamara Face

Eyes: Colds settle into this patient's eyes. Look for yellow or greenish discharge from the eyes. Look for granular lids. This is an important remedy for those with hay fever: Look for a profuse and watery discharge from the eyes. This becomes worse in open air. The patient's eyeballs will twitch when they are out in cool air. The eyes move in jerking motions. The pupils are dilated. Look for an eruption of yellow vesicles under the patient's eyes. Also look for the patient's cheeks to turn reddish-blue.

Ears: Cold air causes earache. This is an excellent earache remedy when the symptoms match the patterns and timetable of Dulcamara. The earache pain will keep the patient up for the entire night. Look for swelling of the parotid glands.

Nose: There is complete stoppage of the nose, especially when the patient comes in contact with cold air. The nose becomes blocked when there is a cold rain. The patient wants to keep his nose warm. The nose flows when the patient is in a warm place. The mucus is thick and yellow, with blood in it. The nose has bloody crusts in it. For patients with hay fever: nasal symptoms are worse around the smell of newly mowed grass.

Mouth: Look for saliva that is thick and ropy. The mouth and tongue are dry. The lips twitch. Look for herpes or cold sores on the lips. The whole mouth may be drawn to one side. It can look distorted. Look for the mucous membrane of the mouth to be red and very swollen. The mouth may be filled with raw and excoriated spots, which make talking, chewing, and swallowing very painful.

Tongue: The tongue becomes so swollen that it is difficult for the patient to speak. The tongue and the jaw both become stiff in cold air or rainy weather. The tongue is dry and rough. Look for an increase flow of saliva. The patient will be very thirsty.

Throat: There is swelling of the interior throat. Tonsillitis recurs with every change of weather.

Countenance: There is a brown or yellow discoloration of face. There are moist yellow crusts on the face, especially on the forehead and chin. The face looks sickly and pale, although there may be redness on the patient's cheeks.

The Dulcamara Patient

Behavior: This is a confused patient. He seems unsure as to what he is talking about.

He asks for something, and then doesn't want it. He has trouble talking and making sense. The Dulcamara patient can become delirious with pain. He may also become very depressed.

Characteristics: The action of this remedy is more or less specific to the mucous membranes and to the skin, glands, and digestive organs. It is associated with increased secretions of the mucous membranes at the given time of year—what we would call hay fever, and for the colds that develop during the change of season. The remedy is also associated with increased urination. The patient often has the urge to urinate whenever he gets cold.

Pains associated with the remedy include stiffness and soreness (think of how you feel after having sat on cold, damp ground for a long time), and with tearing pains. The remedy is associated with stiff necks, backache, and bone pain.

The patient's speech is inarticulate due to his swollen tongue, and yet this is a patient who talks incessantly. His voice sounds rough and hoarse.

Pulse: The pulse is slow during the day. It may seem slower than the beating of the heart. The pulse speeds at night, becoming hard and tense, although it is still small and may be difficult to find.

The patient may experience palpitations at night.

Modalities: from getting cold after being overly warm; from any sudden change in temperature; from cold and damp; from eating or drinking cold things; from getting cold feet; from damp cellars; before the onset of storms; from sitting still.

Better: from moving about; from moving painful parts of the body; from warmth in general; in warm, dry weather.

Common Causes of Illness

Late summer and early autumn; getting wet, especially in cold, damp conditions; suppressed sweat; mercury poisoning; physical trauma.

Common Uses

Allergies and hay fever; asthma; colds, sinusitis, bronchitis, pneumonia, otitis media (ear infection); rheumatism and sciatica; lower back pain; headaches.

EUPATORIUM PERFOLIATUM

Source: Thoroughwort
This remedy used to be known as "boneset" and it lives up to that name. Its keynote symptom is pain that digs deep into the pa-

tient's bones. Yet the patient is very restless in his pain, and can't keep still. In the acute context, it is used for flu that causes bone aches. In short, bone aches and more bone aches.

Theme: It's all about the aches that the patient feels deep in the bones. They motivate his every behavior and direct his movements.

About Eupatorium

Morrison writes, "Eupatorium Perfoliatum is famous for its use in influenza but also covers recurrent febrile conditions and malaria. We are guided to this remedy by the tremendous bone pains which accompany the febrile conditions. The patient often complains of unbearable pains in the limbs or the back, sometimes in the muscles but most typically felt directly in the bones. The pain is often described 'as if the bones are broken.'"

The Eupatorium Face

Eyes: The margins of the eyes are red. The whites of the eyes become yellowed. Look for an increased tearing of the eyes, especially when the patient coughs.

The patient is very sensitive to light.

Ears: There are no guiding symptoms for this remedy.

Nose: There is a great deal of sneezing and flow of mucus. Each sneeze makes the patient's whole body ache. As is often the case in homeopathy, the opposite may also occur, and the nose will be very dried up and stopped up.

Mouth: There are cracks in the corners of the mouth. The patient is very thirsty.

Tongue: The tongue is coated yellow. It may also be coated white. In this case, the coating may be very thick, and it may resemble yellow or white fur.

Throat: The patient has a sore throat that is worse in the morning. The patient is hoarse in the morning.

Countenance: The patient looks older than he is. He looks worn out. There is a look of long suffering on the patient's face. Often you will find that the patient feels his head is so heavy that he must literally lift it off his pillow with the help of his hands. You may also see the patient letting his head fall backward because it is too heavy to lift.

The Eupatorium Patient

Behavior: This is a very restless and anxious patient. His mood is somewhat driven by his pain, making him irritable and somewhat fault finding. He is not an easy patient to care for.

Characteristics: The pain characteristic involves violent aching. The patient will cry out or moan in pain. The pains feel bruised, sore and aching. The pain tends to center in the chest, the back, and, especially, the limbs. Remember, this remedy is taken from thorough-wort, which was also called "boneset," because of its ability to reduce pains in the limbs and muscles. A sensation of weight or heaviness runs through this remedy as well. All affected parts of the body feel heavy, pressured, and shrunken. This is also a restless, chilly, and nauseated patient.

Pulse: There are no guiding pulse symptoms, although the patient will usually feel a constriction in the chest, as if the area in which his heart is seated is too small. He will feel as if something is pressing against his heart, weighing it down. His chest feels heavy.

Modalities: Worse: from motion; from cold air; from coughing; from the smell of food; on a periodic cycle, most often every third or fourth day; between 7:00A.M. and 9:00A.M.

Better: from conversation, which takes his mind off his pain; from sweating; from lying face down; vomiting.

Common Causes of Illness

Being chilled in cold, open air, air conditioning, or an icehouse.

Common Uses

Flu; fevers; fractures.

EUPHRASIA

Source: Eyebright
The key to the theme is present in the remedy source once more: the herb from which the remedy derives is called "eyebright," which quite concisely suggests that the most important symptoms cluster in the eyes. Since this is a remedy that speaks mostly to the eyes, consider it for conditions including seasonal allergy and colds, as well as conjunctivitis. This is truly an acute remedy.

Theme: While Euphrasia has several uses that involve symptoms running through the whole body, central to all other symptoms are those of the eyes. If the eye symptoms are not present, then this not the remedy.

About Euphrasia

Boericke wrote, "Manifests itself in inflaming the conjunctival membrane especially, producing profuse lacrymation. Patient is better in open air. Catarrhal affections of mucous membranes especially of eyes and nose. Profuse acrid lachrymations and bland coryza; worse, evening. Hawking up of offensive mucus."

The Euphrasia Face

Eyes: The eyes provide the most important indications of the remedy. The patient will have eyes that water constantly, with an acrid and hot discharge. The patient will want to wipe his eyes constantly. Scalding tears accompanied by sensitivity to light. The eyelids will swell from the discharge. The patient blinks all the time. The cornea may take on a bluish color.

As this is a major remedy for cataract, there may be patches of opacities on the eyes. As this is an acute remedy for conjunctivitis, the discharge may be thick, but it remains copious and acrid and hot.

Ears: The ears feel blocked and pressurized, as if the eardrum would burst. The patient may have trouble hearing. There may be ringing in ears, or earache.

Nose: There is profuse discharge from the nose. Nasal discharge is bland. The discharge increases at night. There is a violent tendency to sneeze.

Mouth: Cough, at times constant coughing, brings up a great deal of mucus.

Cough is worse in the daytime, and better when the patient lies down at night.

Tongue: The tongue is stiff, as is the whole of the interior of the mouth, especially the cheeks. The patient may have difficulty speaking because of his tongue.

Throat: The patient must hawk in order to bring up mucus. The patient gags when he tries to clear his throat, especially in the morning.

Countenance: The cheeks are red and hot. There is a stiffness of the upper lip, as if it were made of wood. The left cheek may also seem stiff and the tongue may also be stiff. The face becomes red and burning hot when it is washed. A rash may cover the whole face, itching, red, swollen, and hot.

The Euphrasia Patient

Behavior: This is an indifferent patient. He seems to not care about his own case, or about anything else, for that matter. He may be quite melancholy and withdrawn. He will not want to talk, or answer any questions. He may have difficulty speaking because of paralysis of the tongue.

Characteristics: The fact that the patient's eyes water all the time is important to understanding the remedy. But the action of the remedy includes the eyes, the nose and the chest. Think of this remedy when a patient suddenly starts sneezing; when there is a great deal of nasal discharge for no apparent reason; for the early moments of a cold, when the sneezing comes out of nowhere, but the cold is not yet apparent.

There is not so much a sensation of pain associated with the remedy as a sensation of itching. If there is pain, it tends to be stitching in nature. A sensation of weight may also be felt, especially in the chest.

Pulse: There are no guiding symptoms for this remedy.

Modalities: Worse: sunlight; wind; from being indoors; from touch; in the evening and at night.

Better: from winking or wiping eyes; from drinking coffee; from being in open air; from being in a dark place.

Common Causes of Illness

Seasonally (usually in the spring); from contact with wind, especially the south wind.

Common Uses

Allergies; colds; conjunctivitis; measles (especially in the early stages).

FERRUM PHOSPHORICUM

Source: Iron Phosphate.

On the acute level, look for this remedy to reflect the midpoint between the very yang response of a Belladonna or Aconite patient and the very yin Gelsemium patient. This patient, while obviously ill, is neither overwhelmed by a freight train of illness that renders him weak, nor fighting off a demon of illness with a wild response. Instead, this is a patient with common symptoms of illness, such as fever, but nothing to show or report that adds up to a strong diagnosis. Therefore, Ferrum Phos is often identified by what it is *not* rather than what it *is.* It is a great general remedy for the onset of colds and other respiratory ailments. It is also for fever in which the patient is flushed. A keynote is bright red blood from any wound, so it is also a remedy used to stop bleeding after operations.

Theme: Theme? What theme? It is almost the lack of theme that suggests this remedy. This is a general remedy helpful in cases of simple fever.

About Ferrum Phosphoricum

Schussler wrote, "The pains which correspond to iron are increased by motion, but relieved by cold. In the muscle-cells iron is found in the form of phosphate, we should therefore in therapeutics use Ferrum Phosphoricum."

The Ferrum Phos Face

Eyes: The patient's eyes are red and inflamed.

This patient is also photophobic and cannot bear bright light.

Ears: The external ears are red and swollen, as are the mastoid glands. The internal ear is also red, and the eardrum looks angry, red, and swollen.

The patient is hard of hearing.

Nose: This is an important remedy for the first stage of a head cold. This stage can be measured from the first attack of sneezing to the onset of nasal flow. This is a remedy for patients with nosebleeds that have bright red blood, especially children.

Mouth: The mouth is hot. The interior of the mouth is red and inflamed.

Tongue: There is inflammation of the tongue. The tongue is swollen and dark red.

Throat: The internal throat is very red, and inflamed. There is an ulcerated sore throat. The tonsils are red and swollen. The eustachian tubes are inflamed. Consider this remedy for cases of sore throat in singers and public speakers.

Countenance: The face is flushed, and the cheeks are very hot to the touch. The complexion is florid. Paleness may alternate with redness.

The Ferrum Phos Patient

Behavior: This patient usually will want to be alone, and will have no desire for company. He certainly will not want to have strangers around him, or to be in crowds. He fears crowds. This patient will want to talk and talk, and may be quite animated when talking. He may laugh and laugh, and become hysterical as well.

See if things in which the patient usually finds great pleasure now seem quite indifferent and unimportant. That is an indication of the remedy.

Characteristics: Situations needing Ferrum Phos tend to cluster in the chest—colds, bronchitis, and the like. Fever is almost always present. Hemorrhages are very common, indeed, look for almost all discharges to be blood-streaked at least. (This is an important blood remedy, and one often called for with cases of nosebleeds. Perhaps only Phosphorus speaks more to issues of blood.) The patient will also have pains in the muscles that leave him feeling sore and bruised. Headaches are also associated with the remedy, and may appear with any of the other symptoms. These are overwhelming headaches in which the pain is so great that the patient cannot even bear to have his hair touched.

The patient's voice is hoarse. This is a remedy for those with laryngitis, or an over-strained voice. It is also a remedy to strongly consider for cases of bronchitis, especially in children.

Pulse: There is a short, quick pulse. The pulse may have a very soft nature. There may be an accelerated pulse, most especially when it is accompanied by fever. The pulse may race to 150 or 160 beats per minute.

Modalities: Worse: from motion, especially from jarring motion; from being touched; from noise; from cold air; early morning, especially from 4:00A.M. until 6:00A.M.

Better: when bleeding; when lying down; from cold applications.

Common Causes of Illness

Physical trauma; suppressed sweat, especially on a hot day.

Common Uses

Fever; colds, flu, otitis media (ear infection), pneumonia; tonsillitis; bursitis; nosebleeds; anemia.

GELSEMIUM

Source: Yellow Jessamine

The general idea of this remedy is weakness that extends to all levels of being: body, mind, and spirit. The weakness itself may be the complete picture of the illness, or it may accompany another set of symptoms. This is a remedy in which many symptoms dominate on the left side. Gelsemium is also a remedy picture for the patient who anticipates all sorts of terrible things. This apprehension (most especially of test taking or public speaking) leads to an assortment of responses, from trembling, to fainting, diarrhea, and a sudden need to urinate.

Theme: This is a patient who is overwhelmed by something in his life—a test being perhaps the most common—and that "something" is often the cause of the illness. This patient is future-oriented, and sure that something bad will happen soon.

About Gelsemium

Clarke wrote, "Gelsemium is a great paralyzer. It produces a general state of paresis, mentally and bodily. The mind is sluggish, the whole muscular system is relaxed: the limbs so heavy he can hardly move them. The same paretic condition is shown in the eyelids, causing ptosis; in the eye muscles, causing diplopia; in the esophagus, causing loss of swallowing power; in the anus, which remains open."

The Gelsemium Face

Eyes: Look for the patient's eyelids to be heavy, for the patient to be hardly able to open them. It is a symptom unique to this remedy that the patient will have one eye with the pupil dilated, and the other eye with the pupil contracted.

The patient may complain of double vision. He lacks the muscular power to bring his eyes together for a single image. Gelsemium is useful in cases of detached retina, also for retinitis.

Ears: The patient will be very sensitive to sound. The patient experiences a sudden and temporary hearing loss. The hearing loss may be accompanied by a pain that travels from the middle ear into the throat.

The patient may have earaches that are brought on from contact with cold.

Nose: There is watery discharge from the nose, alternating with total dryness of the nose. The watery discharge is acrid. Typically, the left nostril floods with a scalding stream of watery discharge, while the right nostril is stopped up. Look for the patient to sneeze violently in the morning.

Mouth: The lips are dry and coated with dry mucus.

Tongue: The tongue is numb, thick, and has a yellow coating. Look for the tongue to be yellowish-white. It may also have a thick brown coating. The tongue will tremble when it is extended.

The patient has trouble speaking and sounds drunk.

Throat: The patient has difficulty swallowing, especially warm food. This is a dry throat and mouth. Look for swollen tonsils. Look for a crimson flush of color for both the tonsils and the face.

Countenance: The patient's face is hot and heavy. The complexion flushed, red, may be a bright crimson. The patient looks exhausted, or drunk. The patient's face is hot to the touch. The patient's face is filled with tremors and twitches. The chin quivers, and the lower jaw is dropped and wags from side to side.

The Gelsemium Patient

Behavior: This is one of our most exhausted patients. The patient is dull, drowsy, and trembling. He does not want to speak or to be spoken to. He does not want anyone near him, even if they are totally silent. When spoken to, he answers very slowly, or he may not answer at all.

The patient wants to be alone and in total quiet.

Characteristics: The patient feels achy, tired, and very, very heavy. Pains tend to run throughout all the muscles of the body, and combine a sensation of weakness with an ongoing soreness. Parts of the body always seem to be twitching, especially the chin and the face muscles. The patient will often fear falling, or have to hold onto furniture to keep from falling or fainting.

Strongly consider this remedy for all cases of summer colds. The patient sneezes in the morning. The edges of the nostrils are red and sore. There is inflammation of the throat, with pain on swallowing. There may be earache, moving into the throat. The hands and feet are cold.

Consider this remedy for the patient who becomes ill with every change of weather. Consider this remedy as well for the patient who has lost a loved one and is trapped in an overwhelming sense of grief.

Pulse: There is a weak, slow pulse. The pulse may be very faint, especially in older patients. The pulse has a flowing nature. The patient's pulse is slow and soft. The patient may complain of pain in the region of the heart, especially when he rises, for example, from a seat. The pain and weight in the area of the heart is worse when the patient thinks about it, or from a feeling of grief. In some cases, the patient may feel that his heart will stop beating if he does, not keep moving. Consider this remedy for patients whose heart's actions seem weakened or depressed. Consider also when the patient's hands and feet are constantly cold, the pulse is irregular, or there is a marked decrease in the frequency of the pulse.

Modalities: Worse: from motion; from surprise of any sort; from foggy weather; from humid weather; in spring; in summer; from the heat of the sun.

Better: from sweating or urinating; from continued, gentle motion; from bending forward; in the afternoon; from resting with the head propped high.

Common Causes of Illness

Anticipation of upcoming events; physical or emotional shock, loss, grief; thunderstorms; damp weather; alcohol abuse; bad news; anger, depression, or fright.

Common Uses

Fever; flu; allergies and hay fever; headache, especially migraine; vertigo; insomnia; diarrhea; chronic fatigue; anxiety; stage fright.

HEPAR SULPHURIS

Source: Sulphuret of Lime
Something (often a physical infection) has hit this patient hard, and has made him feel extremely vulnerable mentally, physically, and emotionally. On the emotional plane, look for the patient to seek security, and to want to constantly know that all is well for himself and all those he loves. The patient will become angry and even violent if he feels he is being threatened.

Theme: In a word, the theme of this remedy is vulnerability. Physically, this is a patient who is vulnerable to everything in the environment. Like the Mercurius patient (with whom this patient is often confused), he will be very sensitive to changes in temperature. Like the Phosphorus patient, he will be sensitive to changes in weather patterns.

About Hepar Sulph

Tyler wrote, "Hepar—sensitive beyond all bounds of reason: irritable—impetuous. Sensitive to draughts; to air; ulcers so sensitive that they cannot bear the lightest touch (also:

Lachesis); sensitive mentally—even to sudden murderous impulses."

The Hepar Sulph Face

Eyes: There is always some sore of inflammation of the eyes present. There may be a general inflammation of the eyes, always with discharge. The patient will open and close his eyes over and over again in the morning. The eyes and lids are red and inflamed. This area is sore to the touch, with burning pains. The eyes tear a great deal. Consider for those with ulcers of the cornea or those with pus coming from the eyes. Look for a profuse discharge, a discharge that can combine tears and pus.

Here's an odd keynote: listen for the patient to complain that everything looks as if it were red. The patient may also feel a sensation of blindness when rising or standing up after sitting bent over.

Ears: Look for eruptions on and behind the ears. Look for a wax buildup in ears. The eardrum may be perforated. The ear is very sensitive to touch. The patient's reaction to being touched is out of proportion to any actual pain.

Nose: The nose becomes totally blocked whenever the patient goes outside into cold air. The patient sneezes every time he goes into cold, dry wind. Nasal discharge is thick and offensive. The nose is inflamed and swollen, with a bloody and offensive discharge. The bones of the nose are sore to the touch. There is a chronic discharge from nose, chronic catarrh (inflammation of the mucous membranes). The nose is filled with crusts and scabs. The interior of the nose is sensitive to air and to touch.

The sense of smell is either lacking entirely, or is very sensitive.

The patient will typically complain of heat and burning in his nose. He may also complain of a pain that lasts far into the night.

Mouth: The gums bleed easily. There are white, ulcerous patches on the inside of the lips and cheeks. There is an abscess at the root of filled teeth. There are ulcers on the soft palate. The middle of the patient's lower lip will be cracked.

This is an important remedy for toothache that is worse when in contact with anything warm, or when the patient bites his teeth together or is in a warm room.

Consider this remedy for patients with offensive odors of the mouth. The odors will be so bad that the patient himself notices them.

Tongue: Look for the tongue to be coated either white or yellow. The tongue looks dirty. It may be very swollen, even to the point of showing teeth marks on the sides. Look for white sores or pustules on the inside of the lips and cheeks, and on the tongue. The tongue, especially the tip of the tongue, is sore.

Throat: Consider this remedy for cases of tonsillitis, especially chronic tonsillitis. Look for swollen tonsils and hard glandular swelling on the patient's neck. There may be a sore throat, with increased saliva. The throat looks raw and red. The patient's saliva has terrible odor. The patient will be very thirsty from morning until evening.

The patient will complain of a terrible pain in the throat. A pain is if a splinter or fish bone were sticking in his throat.

Countenance: The face has a yellowish complexion. There are blue rings around the eyes. The patient's upper jaw projects forward. The upper lip is swollen and very sore to the touch. There is swelling of the patient's face, especially his cheeks, which are hard and swollen. The face is hot and red.

The Hepar Sulph Patient

Behavior: These are patients who speak quickly, and answer questions very quickly. They are given to sudden impulses. Sudden thoughts drive them. They are given to anguish and deep distress during the night. They may have thoughts of murder or suicide at this time.

This is an intense type who is pain and sensitivity driven. In the classic texts, these patients are said to be "vehement." Note that pain is an important feature of this remedy type. The patient, typically, will react to any pain in a manner that is out of step with what he actually feels. The patient acts as if the pain were far greater than it is. He is very, very sensitive to pain.

Characteristics: In almost all Hepar cases there will be fever and some sort of infection. The patient seems to have an aura of unhealthiness. He is weak and overly sensitive to everything. His skin looks unhealthy, and every slight wound to the skin seems to become infected. Indeed, the ease in which various conditions lead to infection is a hallmark of the remedy. Pus formation is quite common. Discharges from the ears, nose, and even eyes often contain pus. In short, every inflammation of any sort leads to suppuration. Note that the Hepar patient's skin tends to be sweaty. Patients with dry skin contraindicate this remedy and tend to indicate Belladonna.

Pain sensation is sticking in nature. The patient feels that there is some sort of physical object or block in the affected area. He will, for instance, feel as if there is a stick caught in his throat when he has a sore throat.

Patient may have sudden attacks of suffocation, during which their face turns dark red, and their lips bluish. The patient will bend backward in trying to breathe. Attacks last for some minutes and then end with a whistling or crowing sound from the patient.

Pulse: The pulse becomes weaker and shallower as the patient moves into deeper and deeper illness. The patient may experience chest pains, after which he may experience neck pain and an inability to lie down flat.

The patient may feel palpitations, which are accompanied by stitching pains in the area of the heart.

Modalities: Worse: from being uncovered; from being cold; from contact with cold, dry air; from any physical or mental exertion; from touch; from noise; at night.

Better: from being wrapped up tight; from heat; in warm, damp weather; after eating (this is especially characteristic of the type).

Common Causes of Illness

Physical injuries; mercury poisoning; contact with cold, dry wind.

Common Uses

Colds, flu, croup, bronchitis, otitis media (ear infection), pneumonia, laryngitis, tonsillitis; sinusitis; skin conditions: acne, eczema, abscesses, warts; allergies; asthma; depression, phobia, anxiety.

HYPERICUM

Source: St. John's-wort

Hypericum is our great remedy for nerve damage and injuries to nerves. There are, therefore, few indications for the countenance; most indications are in the body, especially in the back and limbs. This is also a homeopathic remedy that will heal puncture wounds of all sorts, and it is used after operations to relieve pain. It is an extremely good remedy after dental surgery.

Theme: Along with Arnica and Rhus Tox, Hypericum is one of our best pain remedies. In this case the pain has a tendency to run along or be associated with a nerve or nerves. This gives Hypericum its general theme.

About Hypericum

Tyler wrote, "Hypericum, St. John's Wort. Thrice blessed herb for the relief of pain."

The Hypericum Face

Eyes: The Hypericum patient stares at people, often with a disturbed look. His pupils are dilated. This is a remedy for those whose eyes have been injured, perhaps up to several years earlier. It is a remedy for eyes that are irritated and painful. Also, this is a remedy for the patient with styes, most especially for a stye on the left lower eyelid.

Ears: There are no guiding symptoms for this remedy, although some patients experience an increased sensitivity of hearing. The external ear is hot to the touch.

Nose: The bridge of the nose is very sensitive to touch, especially when the patient first awakens.

The sense of smell is increased.

Mouth: The patient is very thirsty. Both the mouth and lips are dry. The lips feel hot to the touch.

Tongue: The tongue is coated white at its base, but is totally clean on the tip. The tongue may be white or yellow. The tongue may be very sore, as from lacerations.

The patient may not be able to speak because of the extreme pain and soreness.

Countenance: The face looks hot and bloated. The face is red.

The patient wears an expression of sadness.

The Hypericum Patient

Behavior: The Hypericum patient is said to be in a fog. He is vague, distant, and even sleepy. The patient will make mistakes in writing; for example, he will omit letters. In the same manner, he will tend to become confused as he speaks. He will forget what he meant to say.

These patients tend to be overwhelmed by their pain, and associate numbness with their pain.

They are aggravated by and cannot bear foggy weather.

Characteristics: The pains characteristic to this remedy tend to run along a nerve. Its actions are especially pronounced in the hands—the fingers, fingernails, and fingertips—as well as the toes. It is also helpful for pain in the coccyx (tailbone). It is said to prevent lockjaw and to be more helpful than morphine in the treatment of pain after surgery. Also, it is said to be a wonderful remedy for the breathing spasms associated with asthma, if that asthma attack develops during a weather change with a storm approaching.

Consider it for puncture wounds and any sort of laceration in which the sensation of pain is intolerable and shooting in nature, such as shooting pain down a leg or up an arm. The pain carries with it an aftermath of soreness, especially in the occiput (the back of the head) and coccyx. In short, this remedy has been called "the Arnica of the nerves."

Pulse: There is a rapid and hard pulse. The patient may suffer from a violent beating of the heart with a quick, hard pulse following physical injury.

Modalities: Worse: from jarring motion; from exertion; from touch; from pressure; from changes in weather, especially before a storm; during foggy weather; from being in a closed room; at night.

Better: from being still and quiet; from rubbing; from bending head backward.

Common Causes of Illness

Physical trauma; concussion; injury to the coccyx; animal bites; lacerations and puncture wounds; shock.

Common Uses

Treatment of injury to body parts that are rich with nerves: fingers, toes, tongue, teeth, eyes, genitalia; injury to coccyx; any contusion, laceration or puncture wound; injury to the spine; recovery from surgery; post labor recovery; whooping cough, pneumonia; asthma.

IGNATIA AMARA

Source: St. Ignatius Bean

The emotional symptoms are most often dominant over any physical symptoms in the case of the Ignatia patient. The patient seems deeply troubled and emotionally erratic. This remedy is for those trapped in grief, who cannot move on from grief, which in their mind is combined with betrayal.

Theme: It is often too simple to simply call Ignatia a remedy for grief. Certainly it can be a wonderful remedy for those trapped in an unhealthy grief, but it can be called on in many other cases as well. Therefore, center your selection on the wide changes of mood and symptoms so associated with Ignatia, and not simply on grief. Note that Ignatia and Pulsatilla patients both have mood swings, but Pulsatilla patients lack the sheer intensity of Ignatia patients. Make sure that both mental and physical symptoms are present before using Ignatia.

About Ignatia

Nash wrote, "A remedy for paradoxicalities."

Guernsey wrote, "Anyone suffering from suppressed or deep grief, with long-drawn sighs, much sobbing, etc., also much unhappiness, can't sleep, entirely absorbed in grief;

for recent grief, as at the loss of a friend; affections of the mind in general, particularly if actuated by grief; sadness; hopelessness; hysterical variableness; fantastic illusions."

Hahnemann wrote, "It is best to administer the (small) dose in the morning, if there is no occasion to hurry. When given shortly before bedtime it causes too much restlessness at night."

The Ignatia Face

Eyes: Look for spasms of lids and eye muscles. The eyes, especially the eyelids, are dry.

This patient is photophobic and cannot bear any glare. Sunlight, especially, causes a headache.

Ears: One ear will be red and hot, the other normal.

The patient can't hear anything very well, except the human voice.

Nose: A keynote symptom is a cold nose and hot knees. The nostrils are swollen. Many things make him sneeze. The patient sneezes while breathing in.

The patient is very sensitive to smells, especially tobacco.

Mouth: The patient bites the inside of his cheek when talking or chewing. The patient works his jaw continuously. The lips dry, cracked and bleeding. **Tongue:** The tongue is moist, with a white coating.

The patient may bite his tongue or the inside of his cheek when he talks or eats. Although he will insist he does not mean to do so, he will bite his tongue an inordinate amount of the time. The Ignatia patient will also tend to bite the same spot over and over, and usually will only bite one side of the cheek or tongue, and not the other.

Throat: The patient has a tendency to choke easily. There may be inflammation in the throat and tonsils, which are ulcerated. Look for swelling or goiter of the exterior throat.

The patient has pain in submaxillary glands when he moves his neck.

Countenance: Look for twitching of facial muscles. (Nux is also a remedy for this symptom.) The face will change colors frequently. The face flushes with emotions. One cheek may be pale, the other red. The patient's face sweats when he eats.

The Ignatia Patient

Behavior: This remedy is given much more on the basis of emotional symptoms than it is based on physical indicators. It is a grief remedy, a remedy for those who feel they have been betrayed. The patient is hysterical, emotionally changeable, and physically and emotionally overreactive. Nighttime can be very difficult for the Ignatia patient. He may be unable to sleep, or may walk in his sleep. He is very restless at night. The patient's eyes tear during the night, and there is pain in his eyes. He has headaches at night. He has palpitations at night, with the heart beating wildly.

This can be a very difficult patient. In fact, it may seem as if he is doing everything in his power to not get well.

Characteristics: The contrary nature of the symptoms is often helpful. For instance, the patient is very thirsty when he is chilly, but is not thirsty during times of fever. He can be very contrary emotionally as well, and move from laughing to crying in seconds. The wild swings in mood leave those around the patient confused and often frightened.

This patient will also have a characteristic lack of physical coordination. Other common symptoms are a tendency toward facial tics, and tics and spasms throughout the body. The patient often suffers from hiccoughs as well.

Pain sensation often carries with it the sensation of a lump somewhere in the body. Twitching, trembling, and shuddering accompany pain and emotional upset.

These patients are often suffering from long-term grief. They may be trapped in grief long after it has ceased to be a healthy response to loss. They tend to be sad, to sigh frequently, and to feel both physical and emotional emptiness. Yet, this is a patient who wants very much to be alone.

Pulse: The pulse is throbbing. Generally, the patient's pulse will be hard, full, and frequent.

The patient may feel a throbbing of his pulse in the blood vessels throughout his body. The patient's pulse will be quick and full in the daytime, and becomes less frequent, slower, and smaller as night comes on. Note that the Ignatia patient's pulse can be as variable as is his emotional state.

Note that the patient will often experience palpitations at night, and will feel a pain as if being stabbed in the heart. These palpitations may also occur in the morning while the patient is still in bed.

Modalities: Worse: from any strong, negative emotion; from worrying too much; after losing anything, especially a beloved object; from any contact with coffee or tobacco; from odors; from open air, cold air; in the morning; at the same hour daily.

Better: when alone; from breathing deeply; from changing positions; from lying down on the back; when in a warm room; while eating.

Common Causes of Illness

Grief at the loss of a loved one; betrayal; disappointments in love; injuries to the spine.

Common Uses

Headaches, especially migraines and congestive headaches; low back pain; cramps, tics, and spasms; hiccoughs, cough; arthritis; asthma; chronic fatigue and environmental allergies; recovery from grief.

IPECACUANHA (IPECAC)

Source: Cephaelis Ipecacuanha

Consider this remedy for cases of nausea, especially long-lasting nausea accompanied by vomiting. This remedy relates to digestive disorders and nausea more than anything else. The tongue gives a very important clue: the very clean tongue combined with the vomiting and nausea leads directly to this remedy.

Theme: Very simple: nausea. Other remedies may have a clean tongue, and others may be nauseated, but when nausea is central, simple symptom, no other remedy—not even Arsenicum Album—will be as helpful as Ipecac.

About Ipecac

Boericke wrote, "The principal feature of Ipecacuanha is its persistent nausea and vomiting, which form the chief guiding symptoms. Indicated after indigestible food, raisins, cakes, etc."

The Ipecac Face

Eyes: The patient's eyes are sunken, with blue marks around them. This is a remedy for patients experiencing profuse watering of the eyes which is accompanied by nausea. The patient may complain of severe shooting pains in the eyeballs. Look for the patient to have dilated pupils. Look for the patient's eyes to tear when he looks directly and steadily at anything.

Ears: The ears are cold to the touch during fever.

Patient cannot bear the slightest noise.

Nose: The patient has nosebleeds, especially when he gets cold. The blood is bright red. There is a stoppage of the nose, or thin discharge. Nausea accompanies discharge.

Mouth: The mouth is moist, and there will be a good deal of saliva. The patient's teeth chatter when he is chilled. Patients, especially children, may thrust their fists in their mouths during times of nausea, vomiting, and/or diarrhea. The patient's mouth commonly will be filled with saliva, making him swallow constantly.

Tongue: The tongue is clean, and may be pale yellow or white. The tip of the tongue may be red.

Countenance: The face is pale, with a blue tint around eyes and on the lips. The eyes are sunken. The patient's face is pale and puffy. His body is cool and shrunken. One side of the patient's face is hot, the other is cold. The face carries a look of distemper.

The Ipecac Patient

Behavior: The Ipecac patient holds everything in contempt, and wants others to do so as well. This is a patient who does not wish to speak. When he speaks, his voice sounds hollow.

Characteristics: The action of the remedy centers on the chest and stomach. This is a remedy for cases involving vomiting, diarrhea, or hemorrhages. All discharges are very profuse, and have a foamy quality. This is accompanied by nausea and shortness of breath. The patient is weak and averse to all food. He does not want to eat.

Consider this remedy for cases of severe headache: of migraines that involve indigestion, with nausea and vomiting; semilateral headaches; headaches located over the left eye. The headache may extend into the occiput (back of the head) and the nape of the neck.

Pulse: The pulse is accelerated, and yet weak. It may be hard to find.

Modalities: Worse: from eating, especially ice cream and other dairy products, also: pork, veal, and other meats; worse from eating raw or cold things, fruits, and salads; from hot and from cold; from motion; in damp weather; from vomiting.

Better: from lying still.

Common Causes of Illness

Poor diet; suppressed eruptions; abuse of pain killers, especially morphine; loss of blood; physical trauma; anger, and displeasure.

Common Uses

Nausea and vomiting; abdominal colic with nausea; fevers, especially recurring fevers; labor and postpartum recovery; miscarriage; asthma; bronchitis; migraines; nosebleeds; blood loss.

KALI BICHROMICUM

Source: Bichromate of potash

The Kalis are a large group or remedies all based on the substance potassium. Kali Bi is the most commonly used remedy from this group, and is the best one to have on hand in your home kit.

Theme: In the acute sphere (and in the constitutional as well) the theme of the remedy is glue. The discharges from the patient's nose all tend to be thick, ropy, and gluey. (In constitutional cases, you will see that the patient's personality tends to be rather gluey as well.)

About Kali Bi

Morrison writes, "Often the patient gives a five paragraph answer when a simple sentence would suffice; he seems to cling to your attention. It is unusual for a Kali Bichromicum patient to complain of mental or emotional problems, instead he focuses on his physical pathology. However, when the patient feels his material needs are not being met, he may become irritable and gloomy."

The Kali Bi Face

Eyes: The eyelids are swollen. There is a common yellow/green discharge from the eye. The patient may have conjunctivitis, with only slight irritation to the eye. There may be ulcers on the eye, but there is no discomfort or photophobia. Note: photophobia to daylight will begin only when scabs or crusts are removed from the nose.

Keynote is that there is only slight pain with severe inflammation.

Ears: Outer ears swollen. Look for a thick, yellowish, and stringy discharge from the ears.

Nose: Look for a stringy, yellow/green discharge from the nose. This discharge will be acrid with blockage of the nose. There is much sneezing. The patient's nose is very dry. The patient blows and blows his nose, but without result.

Also, the patient may experience a discharge of large masses of thick, clean discharge that alternates with a headache that extends from occiput to forehead.

The patient has elastic crusts and scabs in the nose. His nose is very raw if they are removed too soon. If they are allowed to stay for a period of days, they may be removed without pain.

The patient's sense of smell is greatly diminished.

Mouth: The patient has a dry mouth. The mouth may contain drying, viscid saliva. Look for ulcers with hard edges on the roof of the mouth or on the mucous surface of the lips.

Tongue: The patient's tongue is red, shining, smooth, and dry. The tongue may also be enlarged, and thickly coated with a lemon yellow. This enlarged tongue may be accompanied by deafness. Also look for white ulcers in the mouth, inside the lips, and on the tongue.

Throat: The throat is red, raw, and dry. There are white ulcers in throat. Expectoration is tough and stringy. The patient coughs up mucus that must be wiped away. Look for the patient's soft palate to be slightly reddened. Look for red tonsils. Note that swollen and red tonsils may be accompanied by a sensation of deafness, most especially in children. Look for dryness and burning in the throat every morning. The patient will likely not be able to breathe through his nose, and will have to breathe through his mouth.

Countenance: The face is flushed, with a blotchy red complexion. There may be acne on the face. Look for the bones of the face to be very sensitive to touch. Look for sweat on the upper lip.

The Kali Bi Patient

Behavior: This is a listless patient, who does not want any mental, emotional or physical challenges. He will want to be pretty much left alone, to rest. He may become ill tempered if bothered, especially by strangers.

Characteristics: In home use, this remedy will most often be called for at the last stage of a cold, when the discharge is yellow/green and very thick and gluey. Mucus tends to come out only with a good deal of effort and will be like a long, strong rope.

The patient's voice has a strong nasal quality because of the blockage. This will also be true in more chronic conditions like postnasal discharge and sinusitis, both of which are well treated with this remedy.

Kali Bi has impact upon the mucous membranes of the body, specifically upon those in the air passages and the stomach and bowels. It also has impact upon bones and connective tissues.

A keynote is that pain appears only in small spots. If asked, the patient can point to the specific spot of the pain. This will be especially true of sinus headaches that are treated with this remedy.

Pulse: In general, the pulse is weak and somewhat accelerated. The pulse becomes contracted and even weaker in times of nose-bleed.

Modalities: Worse: in the spring, and during cold, damp weather at any time of year; in the morning; while undressing; from alcohol, especially beer; when sitting or stooping; from any suppression of mucus flow.

Better: from heat; from pressure; from motion.

Common Causes of Illness

Seasonal: spring, especially, and autumn; abuse of alcohol, especially beer.

Common Uses

Colds, croup, pneumonia; sinusitis; sinus headache and migraines; allergies and post-nasal drip; low back pain; sciatica.

LACHESIS

Source: Venom of the Lance-headed Viper
While there are many remedies based on venoms, Lachesis is the most commonly used in the home.

Theme: The true theme of this remedy does not relate well to its acute uses. Like any snake venom, Lachesis acts on the blood, making it clot less easily and flow more quickly and easily. Thus, this is a remedy that speaks

81

 chronic conditions, like high blood pressure.

In the acute sphere, we look at the patient who reacts as if he had been bitten. Ailments occur very quickly, seeming to strike out of nowhere. The patient rapidly becomes very ill. The patient is exhausted.

About Lachesis

Kent wrote, "Self consciousness, self-conceit, envy, hatred, and cruelty: an improper love of self. All sorts of impulsive insanity: with face purple and heat hot: perhaps choking, and the collar feels tight."

The Lachesis Face

Eyes: The whites of the eyes may appear yellow or even orange. The eyes are watery, from pain.

The patient will have trouble focusing on any object; the eyes tend to move about vaguely. Look for the patient to have photophobia only in the morning after sleeping.

Ears: The ears are dry, with a buildup of white wax. The buildup may cause partial deafness. The patient's ears feel stuffed up. He may have hearing loss, especially in the left ear.

The Lachesis patient will be very sensitive to sounds. He may hear sounds in his ears, such as rushing, thundering, or cracking.

Consider this remedy for cases of earache that occur in the right ear during the night. The pain will be improved by external applications of warmth and by lying on the right side.

Nose: Think of this remedy for those with nosebleeds, especially when the nostrils are very sensitive. The blood will be very dark and thick. This is also a major remedy for those with hay fever, especially with wild sneezing accompanied by stiff neck. Like every other symptom, the sneezing is worse after sleep.

It is keynote of this remedy that both blood and pus come from the nose. The patient experiences discharge from his nose with every cough, every sneeze. This is a mixture of blood and mucus. The mucus discharge may be watery. It is worse on the left side. Look for bloody scabs in the nose.

Mouth: The gums are spongy, and bleed easily. The mouth filled with thick, pasty saliva. Look for chattering teeth. The interior of the mouth looks dry and raw, and may have white ulcers.

Consider this remedy for the patient with bad breath.

Tongue: The tongue is swollen, making for difficult speech. It tends to loll in the mouth.

Listen for the patient to complain that his tongue feels as if it will peel. It will be particularly sore on the left side. The tongue is red and dry on the tip; the tip may be cracked as well. The tip of the tongue sticks to the teeth. There may be white ulcers on the tongue. In general, the patient's tongue is dry, red, swollen, and cracked on the tip. The tongue may have a white coating on it, but look for the tongue to be bright red under that coating. Look for the patient's tongue to tremble.

The patient will also characteristically allow his tongue to dart in and out of his mouth as he speaks.

Throat: The patient cannot bear to have his throat touched. He does not want tight clothing around his throat (and usually not around the waist, either). He also will not want his nose or mouth touched. Often, the patient will feel that there is constantly something in his throat that he must swallow. There may be a constant tickling in the throat. It is a keynote of this remedy that the patient will have a more difficult time swallowing liquids than solids.

Countenance: The Lachesis patient commonly has a pale face that looks swollen and puffy. It may take on a purplish tint. The patient's face goes through periods of heat as well, when it takes on a dusky red tone. At these times, his lips swell enormously.

Look for an expression of pain or stupor. The face will look distorted and haggard.

The Lachesis Patient

Behavior: The patient will want a good deal of attention and be very talkative. He will want to laugh and have company.

It is keynote of the remedy that the patient sleeps into aggravation of his symptoms. Everything will be worse after patient sleeps.

Characteristics: Lachesis is one of our most important remedies. Its actions flow through the entire being. It is a left-sided remedy, which is to say that the symptoms of the person needing Lachesis tend to originate or cluster on the left side of the body.

The patient's voice tends to be rough and/or nasal. The voice tends toward hoarseness in the evening. Note that this is a remedy for those who have chronic hoarseness or laryngitis. It is used when something hinders the patient's speech, when he is constantly clearing his throat. The patient typically feels as if there were a button in the pit of his throat. The button seems as if it can be cleared away, but it cannot.

The patient will not be able to bear extremes in temperature, either hot or cold. Both tend to exhaust him in short order.

Again, think of the patient as someone who has been poisoned in a traumatic manner. He feels toxic. He trembles in his exhaustion. His sensation of pain tends to be throbbing. His muscles feel weak.

Pulse: This patient has an irregular pulse. The pulse may be slow, intermittent, or weak.

The patient is restless and trembling. He speaks quickly and with effort during periods of suffocation and racing pulse. At these times, the pulse is around 160 beats per minute.

Often, the patient will be forced to sit up in bed and to loosen his collar and waistband in order to breathe and quiet his racing heart. He may lean to the right, because the pain is in the left chest.

This patient may well suffer from palpitations, accompanied by a pain in the region of the heart and a feeling of great anxiety. Palpitations may also be accompanied by pain in the left arm and a sensation of choking. These symptoms may be improved sitting down, or, especially, by lying on the right side. Look for the pulse to accelerate at night. Upon falling asleep the patient suddenly awakens, with a suffocative constriction around the heart. He struggles to breathe. The patient's face will be reddened and covered by a warm sweat.

Modalities: Worse: from sleep—it is keynote of this remedy that the patient will sleep into aggravation of symptoms; in the morning; from heat; in the summer; from cold; in the winter; from pressure, especially from the pressure of tight clothing; from touch, even a slight touch, especially to the area of the neck; from liquids, especially hot drinks; from motion; from standing or stooping; from alcohol.

Better: from the free flow of discharges; when in open air; from hard pressure; from cold drinks; from loose clothing; from bathing; from eating, especially eating fruit.

Common Causes of Illness

Physical trauma, especially puncture wounds; effects of poisoning; alcohol or drug abuse; high heat in summer; direct sunlight; drafts of cold air; strong emotion: anger, fright or grief; disappointment in love.

Common Uses

Physical trauma, especially puncture wounds; diarrhea, constipation, colitis; bleeding hemorrhoids; colds, sore throat, otitis media (ear infection); asthma; allergies; headaches, especially migraines; sciatica; menopause with hot flashes; alcoholism and drug abuse; angina, arrhythmia; high blood pressure; nose bleeds; paranoia, phobia and behavior issues.

LEDUM PALUSTRE

Source: Marsh Tea

Historically, the leaves of the marsh tea have been used to cure lice, and to soothe bee stings and bites from mosquitoes, wasps, and even rats. This herbal use is mirrored in the remedy Ledum.

Theme: The classic texts tell it: "there is a general lack of animal heat." This theme runs through the remedy no matter the causation, from puncture wounds and ankle injuries to poison oak.

About Ledum

Tyler wrote, "If tetanus comes on after punctured wounds, think of Hypericum; but give Ledum at once, and prevent tetanus. Torn nails, or lacerated parts rich of nerves, and here Hypericum is the remedy. For bruising, however extensive, and sensation of bruising, the remedy is Arnica. Open lacerations and cuts, think of Calendula. He (Kent) says, for local causes, use local remedies, for internal causes, treat with internal remedies. (But, as we have seen, Ledum internally in potency is amazingly helpful and comforting to external injuries.) He says also if a wound, carefully dressed, does not heal by first intention, look out for the constitutional cause, and ferret out its remedy."

The Ledum Face

Eyes: There is bruising in and around the eyes. Think of this remedy for cases involving black eyes. This is a remedy for those with contused wounds. The patient's pupils are dilated. The patient is photophobic. There is much watering of the eyes, with acrid tears that inflame the lower lid and make the cheeks sore. Note that these symptoms often begin in the left eye and move to the right eye.

Ears: The patient is hard of hearing, especially if his head is wet or his hair is cut.

The patient suffers from noises in the ear, either ringing or whizzing.

Nose: Consider this remedy for the patient with persistent nosebleeds. After the bleeding stops, the nose—especially the top of the nose—is very sore. Look for small pimples to break out on the root of the patient's nose.

Mouth: The mouth is dry, with a sudden flow of watery saliva. This is a patient with bad breath.

Tongue: There are no guiding objective symptoms for this remedy, although the patient may complain of a stinging sensation on the front of the tongue.

Throat: Check for swollen glands under the patient's chin.

Countenance: Look for red pimples on forehead and cheeks. These are painful when touched. Look for crusty eruptions around the nose and mouth. Look for a mottled complexion that alternates between red and pale. The whole face is bloated.

The Ledum Patient

Behavior: In general, the patient will be very chilly, yet he will want cold applications to his wounds.

This is a peevish patient who is never satisfied. He wants to be left alone, and is a difficult enough patient that you will be happy to comply.

Characteristics: Ledum affects many different areas of the body, especially the skin, ankles, heels, tendons, and joints. It is especially characteristic that there will be a sensation of weakness, numbness, and chill in the affected parts. Ledum is also said to be an excellent preventative for black-and-blue marks and bruising after a mechanical injury.

The sensation of pain associated with the remedy is bruising.

Pulse: The pulse is full and strong. As a keynote, the pulse often will only be able to be found in one of the patient's arms.

Modalities: Worse: from motion; from warmth, especially from warm covers or any warm application; from alcohol, especially wine; at night.

Better: from cold bathing and cold applications on affected parts; from putting feet into cold water; from resting.

Common Causes of Illness

Wounds, especially puncture wounds; insect stings; mechanical injury; abuse of alcohol.

Common Uses

Wounds; stings and bites; bruises; sprains; rheumatism; alcohol abuse.

LYCOPODIUM

Source: Club Moss.

Historically, club moss was ground into a powder that was used to coat pills to make them easier to swallow. It was Hahnemann who tested the substance, and, in doing so, created one of our best remedies.

Theme: The fact that this remedy is taken from club moss gives a good indication of its characteristics. Like the moss, the acute or chronic stage Lycopodium type tends to be very threatened by change. He yearns for things to be under his control and to stay exactly as he is. This resistance to change often leads the Lycopodium type into a rut, where many unhealthy habits develop. Therefore, this remedy is often associated with ailments that are very chronic in nature and take years to develop. It is also among our most useful acute remedies, however, especially for dealing with digestive and respiratory complaints.

About Lycopodium

Tyler writes, "Lyc. Is one of our most constantly used drugs. It does not always stare you in the face as the patient walks in, but a few questions will generally have you hot on the trail. Ask early as to time of day. The patient says, 'worse afternoon, or worse 4:00P.M. to 8:00P.M.' and you look to see that he conforms to the Lyc. Type, and inquire further."

The Lycopodium Face

Eyes: The eyes are ulcerated and the lids are red. This is a common remedy for styes, especially when they are found only in the right eye. The eyes may be so dry that the patient has trouble opening them. The eyes are glued together with yellow mucus every morning, but the eyes are not red. The patient must wipe mucus from his eyes in order to see.

The patient will have day-blindness, or more commonly, night-blindness. Vision issues increase as the sun goes down. There may be pronounced vision problems at night.

Ears: There is a thick and very offensive yellow discharge from the ears. There is eczema behind the ears.

The hearing is either reduced or very sensitive.

Nose: The nose is stopped up every night. There is chronic stoppage of the nose, and the patient blows his nose all the time. The patient snuffles and sniffs constantly in order to breathe. The sides of the nose twitch as the patient tries to breathe. When flow begins from the nose, it begins from right nostril.

The sense of smell is very acute.

Mouth: The patient's gums bleed every time he brushes his teeth, or even touches them. His teeth are yellowed. The patient has bad breath.

The patient stammers. The patient speaks with an indistinct speech.

Tongue: Typically, the Lycopodium tongue is covered with either a yellow or gray coating. The tongue is dry, cracked, and swollen. The patient will move his tongue back and forth in his mouth. Look for possible blisters on the tongue.

Throat: The throat is dry, yet the patient is not thirsty. The throat is inflamed. There is ulceration and inflammation of the tonsils, beginning on the right side. Inflammation either begins on the patient's right side, or is worse on the right. Look and listen for constant swallowing, hawking, or clearing of throat.

Countenance: The face looks shriveled, withered. The patient looks older than his years. His expression is full of weight and cares. There are blue circles around the eyes. The patient lets his lower jaw drop. He breathes through his mouth.

Yellow and gray are the two colors associated with Lycopodium. Hair grays prematurely. The teeth are yellow. The skin of the face often takes on a gray or yellow tinge.

The Lycopodium Patient

Behavior: This patient can be difficult. He likes to be alone, and yet he is afraid to be alone. He will want to be in his room alone, but to have the sounds of the family drifting in to him. He may be a very demanding patient, always wanting things, and then criticizing them when you bring them. These patients tend to crave cool air. They tend to feel better in the late evening, especially before midnight. They will be much worse if they skip a meal. They will demand their meals on time.

Consider this remedy, along with Gelsemium, for those suffering from stage fright. Also consider this remedy for cases of long-lasting grief after the loss of a loved one.

Characteristics: Lycopodium is a true polycrest, so it has an impact upon every cell of the body. In most cases, however, expect the symptoms to involve either the urinary system or the digestive tract.

You should also expect to see the symptoms either dominating on the right side or beginning on the right side and moving toward the left in any Lycopodium case. It, along with Arsenicum, is one of our great right-sided remedies.

Lycopodium is also quite specific in terms of time of day, and the patient will be worse around 4:00P.M. or between the hours of 4:00P.M. and 8:00P.M.

Lycopodium is certainly used in the treatment of patients with many different acute complaints, but it is possibly even more useful for patients with long-standing ailments and ailments that develop very slowly over a long period of time.

The pains of the Lycopodium patient tend to be raw in nature and almost always also involve a chill—the patient has either a general chill or a sensation of cold in the affected parts of the body. This is an overly sensitive patient who reacts quite strongly and quite poorly to pain. This is also a gassy patient. He tends to have a great deal of abdominal gas and bloating, even after eating only a small portion of food. In fact, the whole process of digestion is difficult for this remedy type, and some digestive discomfort will be associated with almost every case needing Lycopodium. Many of the Lycopodium patient's other symptoms also become worse after he has eaten, during digestion.

Two odd characteristics may help you to identify this remedy: patients tend to have a left foot that is of normal temperature and a very cold right foot; and they tend to have a sensation of pain like hot coals between their scapulae (shoulder blades). (They share this last symptom with Phosphorus.) Look for either or both of these characteristics to confirm your opinion that a patient needs Lycopodium.

Finally, in terms of speech pattern and voice, the Lycopodium patient tends to speak with a rather feeble voice. He may also be hoarse from dryness in the windpipe. This is a patient who may clear his throat often, or who coughs as he speaks. The patient may also have spells of suffocation at night.

Pulse: The pulse is fast, and becomes even faster after the patient has eaten. The pulse also quickens in the evening. Look for the patient's face and/or feet to become cold as his pulse races.

This is a patient with palpitations. Palpitations occur at night, especially after turning over in bed. The patient may also have palpitations after eating, during the long and difficult process of digestion.

Modalities: Worse: from pressure, especially the pressure of tight clothing—Lycopodium must loosen his pants after eating; in wet weather, especially stormy weather; from warmth, especially a too-warm room or warm applications; between 4:00P.M. until 8:00P.M.; from eating poorly: onions, oysters, beans, bread, pastry, cabbage and all raw vegetables tend to be problematic.

Better: from warm drinks (which soothe the throat and the stomach); cold applications; cool air; from uncovering; from motion; from urinating; after midnight.

Common Causes of Illness

Food poisoning, especially from shellfish; poor diet; overstraining and over-lifting; fever; motion sickness; abuse of alcohol or tobacco; strong negative emotions, especially grief, anger and impatience.

Common Uses

Colds, fever, sore throat, otitis media (ear infection), sinusitis, bronchitis, tonsillitis; colic; irritable bowel syndrome, Crohn's disease; allergies, especially food allergies; chemical sensitivities; asthma; migraines; skin conditions: eczema, warts, rash; kidney stones, kidney infection; blood sugar problems; chronic fatigue; anxiety and panic attacks.

MAGNESIA PHOSPHORICA

Source: Phosphate of Magnesia.

Cramps are generally the key to the Mag Phos patient. This remedy is most often recognized, not from diagnostics, but from the keynote symptom: colic pains that are radiating in nature and better from any application of heat to the affected area of the body. This can even be a very high heat—some patients have been known to use hot bricks to relieve pain. Therefore, it is a very useful household remedy for patients with abdominal colic and for women with premenstrual syndrome (PMS), either of which are improved by applications of heat.

Theme: Look for the combination of pain, cramps, and paralysis. When all these are present, and the pain is relieved by warmth, and especially when the patient doubles over from pain, think of Mag Phos.

About Mag Phos

Boericke wrote, "The great anti-spasmodic remedy. Cramping in muscles with radiating pains. Neuralgic pains relieved by warmth. Especially suited to tired, languid, exhausted subjects. Indispostion for mental exertion."

The Mag Phos Face

Eyes: Watch for twitching eyelids. Also, the patient squints in order to see.

This is a photophobic patient, very sensitive to any form of light.

Strabismus (the turning in of either eye) and nystagmus (involuntary rhythmic rapid eye movements) are both possible in this remedy type. The patient may also see double. Look for headaches to be caused by visual defects.

Ears: The patient loses his sense of hearing.

Mouth: Look for swelling of glands in face, throat and neck. Look for cracks in the corner of the mouth.

Listen for spasmodic stammering in speech.

There may be an extreme toothache that is better with hot liquids. A keynote of this remedy is that the patient suffers from severe pain in filled teeth. Toothache pain tends to be felt on the right side of the mouth.

Tongue: The tongue is clean, especially during colic pains. The tongue may be swollen.

Throat: There is stiffness of the external throat, especially on the right side. The throat is swollen, puffy. The patient chokes easily due to constriction of the throat.

Countenance: Look for spasmodic twitching of the facial muscles. Look especially for twitching and jerking of the jaw. The patient attempts to "work" the jaw to loosen it and to relieve pain. Look for spasmodic yawning to loosen the jaw. The patient's face is distorted due to pain. He has an expression of extreme agony.

Most pains will cluster on the right side of the patient's face, so look for distortion of the right side. Pains suddenly shoot through the right side of the face. Pains are improved by warm applications.

The Mag Phos Patient

Behavior: This patient is completely exhausted. The old texts refer to him as "languid."

He cannot think clearly; he does not want to think.

The patient may cry from pain. The patient may sit and talk to himself.

Characteristics: This pain shoots like lightning; it is sudden and very sharp. The pain is in both nerves and muscles, and is improved by heat. The pain may also be boring or constricting in nature. The patient cries out in pain. There may also be twitching and muscular tics.

This is a chilly patient. He wants to stay covered up. He will experience a chill that runs up and down his back (Gelsemium also has this symptom).

The action of the remedy tends to be right sided and is especially suited to the head, the face, the ear, the chest, the sciatic nerve, and the ovary.

Pulse: This is an irregular, "irritable" pulse.

The patient may also suffer from palpitations that start suddenly, or from attacks of chest pain that are equally sudden in onset.

Modalities: Worse: from cold air, drafts of any sort; from touch; at night, when the patient is exhausted; from uncovering.

Better: from warmth, from a hot bath; from bending over double; from pressure; from rubbing.

Common Causes of Illness

Cold winds; getting wet and cold; teething and tooth decay; over-studying.

Common Uses

Premenstrual syndrome (PMS); cramps, including writer's cramp; abdominal colic; whooping cough and spasmodic coughs; toothache and teething pains; migraines; sciatica.

MERCURIUS VIVUS

Source: Quicksilver

Like the mercury in old-fashioned thermometers, the Mercurius patient is highly sensitive to changes in temperature. He will be comfortable in only a very narrow range of temperature, and will respond very negatively to variations, either hot or cold. (Note: There are several mercury-based remedies grouped in the family Mercurius. The remedy listed here is called Mercurius Vivus in some materia medica, and simply Mercurius in others. As there are several mercury-based remedies, it is important that you find the right one.)

Theme: Again, sensitivity is the key. But in the case of this remedy, it is sensitivity to temperature that is central to the remedy. Like the mercury in an old thermometer, the patient responds to even a slight change in temperature

About Mercurius

Tyler wrote, "Merc. is notable especially for its foulness and offensiveness—of breath—of its profuse saliva—of its drenching sweats: but, curiously enough, stool, urine, menses, leucorrhea are not especially offensive."

The Mercurius Face

Eyes: The lids are swollen into thickness. Look for the lids to be red, and for profuse watering that is acrid and irritates the eyes. Look for the eyes to close involuntarily. This is a remedy for those suffering from conjunctivitis accompanied by a cold, and especially for chronic conjunctivitis. Look for agglutination of the eyelids every morning.

The patient struggles to see anything clearly. He cannot bear light, especially light associated with heat, such as firelight or candlelight. He cannot bear glare in any form.

Ears: Look for a thick, yellow, and possibly bloody discharge from the ear. Look for boils on the external ear canal.

The patient will have trouble hearing if he becomes overheated. Hearing is better as a result of the patient blowing his nose or swallowing.

Nose: This patient sneezes a great deal without relief. The nose is stopped up, and the nostrils are raw, without flow. The patient sneezes in the sunshine.

When there is nasal discharge, it is yellow-green and thick, as if pus were coming out of the nose.

The nose bleeds at night, in the dark. The patient may also have nosebleeds from coughing. The blood is dark and stringy, and hangs from the nose in strings.

Mouth: Keynote of the remedy is the great increase in salivation. The patient wets the pillow with saliva while sleeping. The patient's mouth has terrible breath, which can be smelled throughout the room. Look for white ulcers on mucous membranes, that are themselves bluish-red and spongy. The gums are swollen, receded, and bleed very easily. They are very sensitive to the touch. This is also a remedy for tooth decay. The teeth may be black with decay.

Tongue: The tongue is thick and swollen, with the impressions of teeth running along the side. The tongue is so flabby that it may be difficult for the patient to talk. The tongue may be coated yellow; in this case, look for a dirty-yellow coat on the top of the tongue and gray patches on the sides and edges. The tongue is moist; the whole mouth is very moist.

Throat: The patient will experience pain on swallowing, but will have to continually swallow saliva. The internal throat is very red or bluish-red, and very swollen. The redness and pain are worse on the right side of the throat, or the sore throat begins on right side and moves left.

While the mouth is very moist, the throat will often be very dry. Look for the greatest moisture in front of the mouth, and for the mouth and throat to become drier as you move back. Thus you may have a patient who is very dehydrated and thirsty, although he is almost drowning in saliva.

In the external throat: look for glands to be swollen in the throat, neck, and the ears.

Countenance: This patient will have a pale face with earthy, almost dirty tones. Look for swelling under the eyes. Look for the patient's cheeks to be swollen, red, and hot to the touch. There may be pustules on the patient's face. The bones of the face are extremely sensitive; the patient will not want them to be touched. The patient's face will be paralyzed by cold. Look for the jaw to become immobile.

The Mercurius Patient

Behavior: There are several keynotes for Mercurius, but none is more important than the fact that the patient is intolerant of both heat and cold. He will be better from rest, but worse from the heat of his bed, so he spends a good deal of effort trying to get comfortable.

It is also important to note that this is an exhausted, trembling patient, who often seems to be slipping away. High fevers are possible; indeed, they are rather common. This is a remedy for severe sore throats (those known a hundred years ago as "quinsy"). It is also an important remedy for ailments that involve trembling.

The Mercurius patient has a very weak memory, and forgets everything. When he is asked a question, he pauses for a long time before answering. He may forget the question before answering. He seems incapable of intelligent speech. Yet he easily becomes embarrassed at his apparent lack of intellect.

Listen to this patient: he will often say how he wishes to travel, to be anywhere other than where he is. Or he may simply mutter to himself. Listen for delirious ravings, especially from the patient with fever.

Characteristics: This is a very powerful polycrest, so it has an effect that is felt throughout the whole body. It is especially helpful within the lymphatic system and on the membranes and glands in the body. Look for all symptoms to be worse at night and when the patient sweats. He will also be worse from resting. This remedy is also known for the powerful odor of illness that emanates from the patient: both his sweat and his breath have a potent odor of illness and decay.

Pains tend to be sticking in nature and centered in one point or small area. The pains tend to recur each night when the patient tries to sleep, and may prevent sleeping.

Pulse: This is an intermittent pulse. It is irregular, at times strong and at other times weak. Most of the time the pulse has a trembling nature. The pulse will race and the patient will have palpitations after even a very slight physical exertion.

Modalities: Worse: at night, especially when trying to sleep; from air, from drafts; from sweating; when overheated; when cold, especially when damp and cold; during changes in weather and during weather with damp, cold nights and hot days; from lying on the right side; from artificial light; before and during stool, during and after urination.

Better: when at a moderate temperature; from sexual intercourse; from rest; in the morning.

Common Causes of Illness

Infection; suppressed discharges; fright.

Common Uses

Infections of all sorts, abscesses; upper respiratory infections, cold, flu, otitis media (ear infection), sinusitis; seasonal allergy; colitis and ulcerative colitis; acne; phobia.

NATRUM MURIATICUM

Source: Chloride of Sodium

Another of our major polycrest remedies, Natrum Mur speaks to such a wide range of symptoms throughout the body that it is difficult to know where to begin. We might start with the theme of the remedy, which carries through on both the emotional and physical levels, and holds true for both acute and chronic conditions. This theme combines retention (as noted above, both physical and emotional) with denial. Something is being held within the Natrum Mur patient's secret self: it is neither being dealt with, nor resolved and released.

With the exception of Sulphur, there is perhaps no more useful remedy than Natrum Mur. It will be used by those with colds, allergies, digestive disorders, vision disorders (especially eyestrain), headaches, thyroid disorders, and so on.

Theme: Retention. The Natrum Mur patient retains water, just like salt, but also retains emotions, thoughts, and especially on a constitutional level, old hurts.

About Natrum Mur

Blunt wrote, "Nat Mur is the last remedy I would part with. I have more Nat Mur cases than any two other drugs put together. When I get worse from heat and cold, and better in open air, then I ask early, 'How does wind affect you?' 'Eyes water.' 'You say you weep? From what?' Nat Mur will answer 'from admonition and pity.' Is worse consolation. These people hide their tears for fear of pity and consolation. If asked, how are you? Nat Mur will answer, 'Better, thank you,' when he is not. Lachrymation with laughter is pure gold. As for 'fond of salt; aversion to fats; greasy skin; crack lower lip'—I have found the remedy in Nat Mur when all these are absent."

The Natrum Mur Face

Eyes: This is a remedy for those with eyestrain. Look for the patient's eyes to give out when he reads or write too much, and from close work. The eyes water. The patient will appear to be crying when he is not. His eyes will water when he laughs, coughs, or sneezes. The patient will have to constantly wipe his eyes. His eyes will also itch; he will want to rub or scratch his eyes. The margins of the eyelids will be inflamed, red, and irritated, and they often will be agglutinated in the morning.

Ears: Look for swelling and heat in the external ear. The patient will have itching behind his ears; he will have to scratch behind his ears.

Nose: The patient's nose will run a great deal. The mucus will be like raw egg white, thick and clear. Discharge may alternate with stoppage, making breathing very difficult. There will be violent sneezing (Nat Mur is said to be the best remedy for colds that begin with a lot of sneezing).

There may be nosebleed when the patient stoops, or after he coughs. The nosebleeds are most common at night. The blood clots very easily.

Look for fever blisters on the wings of the nose.

Nasal symptoms involve the loss of both taste and smell. The patient will speak with a very nasal voice.

Mouth: The lips and corners of the mouth are dry and cracked. The patient suffers from a deep, painful crack of the lower lip. The lips are pale. The patient may feel that his mouth is dry when it is not. This patient is thirsty: very, very thirsty for cold water. This is perhaps the leading remedy for those suffering from white ulcers in their mouths or on their tongues. The ulcers are very sore.

Tongue: There may be a frothy coating on the tongue. The tongue is mapped with raised red patches (consider also: Rhus Tox for this symptom). The tongue is striped along the edges.

The patient may report that the tongue feels dry, and yet it is not.

Throat: The patient hawks up mucus. The patient has a chronic dry, sore throat. There is a nagging cough. The throat glistens, yet the patient reports that it is dry. The patient is very thirsty for cold water. The patient can only swallow liquids and has trouble swallowing solids. Often, the patient will report that he feels as if a lump or a ball were trapped in his throat.

Countenance: The patient's face will be shiny, as if it is oily and unwashed. Both the hair and the face may seem greasy. The face is sallow. Look for a dark complexion. Look for redness and swelling of the left cheek. The upper lip may be swollen. Look for a deep crack in the center of the lower lip. Look for vesicles at the corner of the mouth and white, pearl-like vesicles on the lips. Look for white ulcers inside and outside the mouth.

The patient has a benign or blank expression. He is pleasant, but rather emotionless in his responses and awkward in his speech.

The Natrum Mur Patient

Behavior: The Natrum patient will want to lie down, especially if he is in pain. He will want darkness and quiet, and to be left alone. Nothing will make him angrier than for you to fuss over him or tell him that you know just how he feels. He does not want to be consoled, and is much worse from consolation. Most commonly, he feels great weakness in the morning when he is still in bed.

Characteristics: For the characteristics of this remedy, think of the drying effect that happens when a person's diet contains too much salt. So, in the persons who need Natrum, you may expect to see dry mucous membranes throughout the body, a dry throat with a great thirst, a dry mouth, and so on. And you may expect a good many conditions to be caused by digestive disturbances, as in the case of the person who has eaten too much salt.

The pains associated with this remedy all contain an element of numbness. The patient is awkward as well; slow, weak, and weary. He will tend to want to be left alone.

The Natrum Mur patient is somewhat awkward in his speech, and may be a bit forgetful. Or he may seem absent minded, and make frequent mistakes of speech. He is easily made nervous when questioned, particularly about himself and his symptoms.

The patient's voice will tend to be weak and faint, as if speaking exhausts him or as if he were a child just learning to speak.

Pulse: The pulse is irregular. It tends to be full, slow, and rather weak, with a rapid, hard pulse on every third beat. The pulse increases with the patient's every motion. Commonly, this patient will feel a strong pressure below the area of the heart each evening.

This is a patient with palpitations. These tend to occur from emotional causes such as sadness or anxiety. Palpitations are made worse from any motion, and are improved if the patient lies quietly.

Modalities: Worse: from heat, and, especially from the sun—symptoms rise and fall with the sun; when by the seashore for physical symptoms; in summer; from 9:00A.M. until 11:00A.M. daily; on alternating days; from reading too much; from talking too much; from noise and music; from touch; from consolation.

Better: when in open air; from bathing or sweating; from lying down and resting—especially when lying on the right side; from deep breathing; when by the seashore for emotional symptoms; before breakfast; from rubbing; from tight clothing.

Common Causes of Illness

Mechanical injury to the head; loss of body fluids; eating too much salt; poor diet, especially from breads, fats, and sour foods; alcohol abuse; from strong negative emotion, especially betrayal and grief.

Common Uses

Colds, sore throat; fever; allergies; asthma; irritable bowel syndrome and colitis; blood sugar problems; backache; hemorrhoids; insomnia; premenstrual syndrome (PMS); anemia; headaches, especially migraines; herpes, eczema; depression.

NUX VOMICA

Source: Strychnos Nux Vomica

Nux Vomica is one of our greatest homeopathic remedies, and it speaks to a huge number of common complaints, most often those involving colds and flu and those related to digestive distress. The rallying cry of the remedy is emotional, however, as the core indication of Nux is anger. This is an irritable, grumbling patient. The mere fact that a patient is not angry or difficult contraindicates its use, although he may display all the physical complaints related to the remedy.

Symptoms tend to both develop and go away slowly in the Nux case. Colds take days and days to arrive, and then never seem to go away, and the Nux patient is in a bad mood the entire time.

In the acute context, Nux is also used for toxic states, especially as a hangover remedy for those who abuse alcohol.

Theme: Anger+chill=Nux, especially when grouped with digestive distress and constipation.

About Nux

Tyler writes, "Nux affects body and soul, and that always in an extreme manner. Not only mind, head, brain, special senses, but the whole of the digestive system; the liver and portal system; the urinary and genital systems. It affects nerves, muscles, skin, and sleep. It is a great fever medicine—if symptoms agree. No wonder the homeopaths of what may be called the middle period of homeopathy who indulged in low potencies and got their best results in acute disease, made such great use of Nux. They had the polycrests at their fingertips."

The Nux Face

Eyes: Photophobia is the primary guiding symptom for the eye. This is, along with Belladonna, our most photophobic patient. He simply cannot bear light, especially sunlight and glaring light of any sort. Photophobia is worse in the early morning.

Also look for inflammation and swelling of the eyes (this is a remedy for those who get conjunctivitis every spring), with red streaks in the whites of the eyes.

Movement of the eyelids is difficult for this patient. There is stiffness of the muscles in the eyelids. Look for twitching of the muscles in the eyelids, and in the muscles surrounding the eyes. Such tics are an important symptom of this remedy type. Also look for bloodshot eyes in those who have used tobacco and/or alcohol.

Ears: The patient is very sensitive to sound, and cannot bear noise. Noise makes him angry, especially if it awakens him from sleep.

Irritation in the ears awakens the patient every night.

Nose: The nose is stuffed up, especially at night. There is a chronic stoppage of the nose. The patient has snuffles, especially in cool, dry atmosphere. Snuffles become worse in a warm room, but the patient is worse when he gets cold. Nasal discharge is watery, and tends to alternate between the nostrils.

There may be nosebleeds in the morning (consider also: Bryonia). Nosebleeds may also start during sleep. The blood will be very dark. Nosebleeds will often be preceded by headaches and by a reddening of the patient's cheeks.

In spite of the blockage, the Nux patient's sense of smell is very acute, especially to smells that trouble him. The patient will be sensitive to the smell of flowers and perfumes, and may actually faint from perfumed smells.

Mouth: The gums are swollen, white in color, and bleed very easily. Look for painful vesicles on the tongue and gums. The saliva is bloody. The Nux patient has foul breath in the morning.

The patient's mouth is dry, but he is not thirsty.

Tongue: The tongue and soft palate are slimy. The tongue may be coated white, yellow, or brown. In some cases, the first half of the tongue is very clean and very red, and the back half is covered in a deep fur.

The tongue feels heavy and thick to the Nux patient. It interferes with his speech, causing him to lisp or become inarticulate.

Throat: There are small ulcers and vesicles in the throat. The throat dry, but patient is not thirsty.

Countenance: Look for swelling in the area of the cheeks, especially when the patient lies down, drinks alcohol, or smokes tobacco. Look for the left side of the mouth to droop or turn down. The patient's jaw is stiff, and snaps shut. He will hold his jaw very tight. Look for acne on the face of the Nux patient who uses alcohol. This can also be caused by eating cheese or any dairy product. There may be pimples on the chin.

The Nux patient will have a tense or angry look on his face.

The Nux Patient

Behavior: This is one of our angriest remedy types. The Nux patient always seems to be angry and critical of others.

This is also one of our chilliest remedy types. The Nux patient cannot bear to be cold and becomes very angry if he gets cold. He will not be able to bear the slightest draft or movement of air. He will cover himself up to the chin when he is in bed.

This may also be the patient who has the hardest time getting to sleep. He may suffer from chronic insomnia, and lie awake rehashing the day's stress, thinking of things he should have said or done. Many Nux patients will lie awake for hours before falling asleep. Therefore, they become very, very angry with anything or anyone who awakens them once they are sleeping.

Characteristics: This is a very yang type in constitutional terms; these patients correspond largely to the "Type A" personality. Even in acute cases, you will see a person who is usually mild and calm getting wound tighter and tighter and becoming more and more irritable. They make for crabby, difficult patients.

This is a remedy known for its oversensitivity. This patient is oversensitive to noise, light, smells, and especially cold. This is a very cold patient who can never get warm. This is also a remedy known for its addictions. These patients may easily become dependent upon coffee, tobacco, and/or alcohol. They may also turn to recreational drugs for relief of their stress.

The pain associated with the remedy is cramping and bruising. Body parts feel sore. Patients tend to have many tics and twitches, especially in the muscles of the face. Look for jerking and shuddering throughout the whole body.

Pulse: The pulse is tired and labored, or it may race and become irregular, missing beats.

The patient may also experience palpitations when he lies down. During these palpitations, the patient may report that he is very tired; that he feels his heart is tired. He may have palpitations with belching, indigestion, nausea, and vomiting.

This is a leading remedy for chest pains (angina pectoris). Pain is worse at night and reaches down the left arm to the anterior neck, lower jaw, lower back and kidneys. During severe attacks, the patient will kneel on the floor with his body bent backward in attempting to find relief. Attacks can be from emotional causes, indigestion, or from use of alcohol or tobacco.

Modalities: Worse: from cold, drafts, wind, or cold air moving in any manner; from touch; from noise, especially music; from light, especially glaring artificial light; from smells, especially tobacco; from the pressure of clothing around the waist; from alcohol and tobacco (even though the patient may crave these things); in the early morning.

Better: from sleeping, if it is a deep uninter-rupted sleep; from hot drinks; after eating, especially dinner; from stretching; from sweating and from other bodily discharges.

Common Causes of Illness

Alcohol abuse; drug abuse; tobacco abuse; coffee abuse; "high living"; sexual excess; insomnia; overwork; lack of exercise.

Common Uses

Constipation, irritable bowel syndrome, colitis, Crohn's disease; colic; colds, coughs; asthma; low-back pain; headaches, especially migraines; allergies; sciatica; alcoholism.

PETROLEUM

Source: Petroleum

Three areas of the body share the effectiveness of this remedy—the skin, the mucous membranes and the digestive system. But in acute situations, most people narrow down their consideration of the remedy to the symptoms associated with motion sickness.

In this case the patient is worse from traveling in any vehicle but is also worse from open air, so he is unable to seek relief by opening a window or walking out on a ship's deck. He shivers when in contact with open air.

(Internal itching is) a common symptom. It will be a part of the symptom portrait no matter what part of the body is affected.

Theme: As this is most often an (acute) remedy, don't seek a deep emotional "theme." Sweat and nausea, especially when associated with motion sickness, suggest Petroleum.

About Petroleum

Boericke wrote, "Very marked (skin) symptoms, acting on sweat and oil glands. Ailments are worse during the winter season. Ailments from riding in cars, carriages, or ships; lingering gastric and lung troubles; chronic diarrhea. Long-lasting complaints follow mental states—fright, vexation, etc."

The Petroleum Face

Eyes: The patient will have to rub his eyes often, because they are itchy. The skin all around the eyes will be dry and crusty. In some cases, look for the patient's eyelashes to fall out.

The patient will not be able to read fine print; he will have to hold papers far in front of himself in order to see them. He will squint in order to see near things. Typically, he is far sighted.

Ears: Discharge of pus and/or blood is possible, as is a large quantity of hard and dry brown wax in the ears. Look for rash, especially eruptions like eczema, behind the ears.

The patient will either have deafness or very sensitive hearing. Most often, the patient will have hearing that is very sensitive to the sound of the human voice. He will be unable to bear the sound of more than one person speaking at a time.

Nose: The tip of the nose itches, and the patient repeatedly rubs his nose. The nostrils are ulcerated and cracked.

Mouth: The patient's breath smells like garlic.

Look for swelling of the gums and increased saliva in the mouth. Petroleum should be considered for cases involving abscess at the root of any tooth, especially when accompanied by external swelling of the mouth and jaw. The patient will be unable to chew because of pain in his teeth. The lips are cracked. Look for eruptions at the corner of the mouth; also look for swelling of the submaxillary glands.

Tongue: The tongue will have a white center with dark streaks along the edges.

Throat: The throat is dry, except for mucus in the back of the throat. The patient coughs up this mucus in the morning. The patient avoids swallowing because of pain and tickling in his throat.

Countenance: The Petroleum patient's face will be white or pale yellow. The face becomes hot to the touch after the patient eats. The jaw is the most vulnerable part of the face. It dislocates easily. The patient is very careful of his jaw, and protects it. He does not want it touched.

The Petroleum Patient

Behavior: This is an emotional patient. He is both angry and afraid, and he is worse from his emotions. Look for the patient's physical symptoms to increase when he becomes emotional.

This is a patient who wants instant results, who demands help. He may also seem quite confused about his case. He is also worse from being in the presence of strangers, who confuse, irritate, and frighten him.

Characteristics: The bodily discharges associated with Petroleum are thick and yellowish green. Any discharge of blood tends to be bright red. The patient will complain of a sensation of coldness in his chest in the area of the heart and in his abdomen.

Rather than the traditional sensations of pain, the Petroleum tends to feel weak and heavy. Nausea is combined with this heaviness and exhaustion. Pain, if any, is clustered in the occipital area at the back of the head.

Pulse: The patient's pulse is elevated by every motion and slows when he lies still.

This patient is likely to experience palpitations. He may have wild palpitations that can be felt through his clothing. The palpitations may cause the patient to faint. Look for cold hands during palpitations.

Modalities: Worse: motion of any vehicle: car, boat, train; from changes in weather, such as before or during a thunderstorm; in cold weather; while eating.

Better: while at rest with the head supported high; in dry weather; at noon.

Common Causes of Illness

Motion of a vehicle; mechanical injuries, especially sprains; anger.

Common Uses

Motion sickness, nausea, diarrhea; vertigo; headache; otitis media (ear infection), and the aftereffects of ear infection; deafness; eczema and psoriasis.

PHOSPHORUS

Source: Phosphorus

Sensitivity is the key to this remedy. The Phosphorus patient is in a state of increased sensitivity and is having trouble with boundaries, both emotionally and physically. These patients are very responsive to every catalyst. Emotionally, they are very open to the feelings of all those around them. They are emotional sponges. Physically, they respond strongly to everything in the environment. No one, for instance, is more sensitive to weather change than the Phosphorus patient, who has earned the name "human barometer."

The symptoms of Phosphorus tend to start suddenly—the patient is suddenly faint, or has sudden pain. These are also very sensitive patients: sensitive to light, sound, odors, touch, and changes in the environment. They are especially sensitive to electrical changes and to thunderstorms.

Another important keynote of this remedy is the tendency to hemorrhage. The patient will bleed a great deal from every little cut. The blood will be bright red. It is difficult to stop the bleeding in the Phosphorus patient. The remedy was used in homeopathic hospitals to control bleeding after operations.

Theme: As with Arsenicum, burning pains are an important indication of this remedy. Along with the fact that the patient is overly sensitive both physically and emotionally. This is also a fragile patient.

About Phosphorus

Kent wrote, "The complaints of Phosphorus are most likely to arise in the feeble constitutions—born sick, grown up slender, and grown too rapidly—persons emaciating, rapidly emaciating—who have the seeds of consumption fairly well laid."

The Phosphorus Face

Eyes: The odd thing about the Phosphorus patient is that he will usually, even when very sick, have quite beautiful eyes. The white of the eye is very white. The eyes are surrounded by long, curved lashes. You will sometimes see blue rings around the eyes, but the symptoms that can be associated with the eye are internal and cannot be seen by the physician.

You may look for the patient's eyes to tear when he walks in the wind, or you may also notice that the left eyelid twitches, or that the patient will want to shade his eyes with his hand in order to see, but, by and large, you will have to count on the case-taking conversation to get usable symptoms, as they are often not visible to the naked eye. Among these are double vision, fatigue (with burning pains), and a sensation of a veil over the eyes. As Phosphorus is often used for those with cataracts, this last symptom can be common.

Ears: The patient will have great itching inside his ears. He will want to scratch, and will dig with his fingers into his ears in order to scratch and clear his hearing. Look for an enlargement of the mastoid.

This is one of our most used remedies for middle ear infections. The patient will have a difficult time hearing, especially the human voice.

Nose: This patient, like the Sulphur patient, will have to move his nostrils in a fanlike motion to try to breathe. The Phosphorus patient has chronic stoppage of the nose. Look for an ongoing problem with small hemorrhages. The patient's Kleenex will always have some blood on it. The patient's nose most typically will alternate between dry blockage and fluent discharge, which is watery and mixed with blood. The nostrils often alternate between discharge and blockage.

In women patients, a nosebleed may appear instead of menstrual flow.

Also consider this remedy for young patients with frequent nosebleeds. The blood will be a vivid, bright red.

The patient will be overly sensitive to smell (along with Nux), especially to floral smells and to smoke. The sense of smell is especially strong when the patient has a headache. This is also a patient who complains of imaginary odors.

Both the internal and external nose will be swollen. Externally look for the nose to be swollen, red, shiny, and painful to the touch. Internally the nose is swollen and dry, with scabs in the corners of the nostrils.

 It is keynote of this remedy that the patient will have symptoms from putting his hands in water. In this case, look for the patient to sneeze when he puts his hands in water.

Mouth: The gums are swollen and they bleed very easily, with bright red blood. This is a remedy for those who bleed a great deal after dental surgery or tooth extraction. The patient's breath will be sweetish. There may be a rack in the center of the lower lip. The whole mouth may be characteristically drawn to the left. The patient may get a toothache from putting his hands in water, for example, when washing clothes.

Speech is difficult. The patient may stutter.

Tongue: The tongue is dry and smooth. Usually, the tongue is red on the sides with a colored stripe in the center. The stripe may (most commonly) be yellow or gray, or may be brown. The tip of the tongue may be swollen, with enlarged papillae. The patient may complain that his tongue feels burnt.

Throat: The patient has a dry throat, day and night (he is very thirsty for cold things). There is pain from coughing. The tonsils are swollen. The throat looks rough and scraped.

Countenance: The Phosphorus face may have an appearance of transparency, as if the face were carved from ivory. The skin may seem as if it is drawn too tight across the bones. One or both cheeks may be red. The face is pale. Blue rings around the eyes. Lips, too, are blue, and dry. The face may be swollen and puffy.

The Phosphorus Patient

Behavior: This patient wants a great deal of attention. He is better for company, and for being touched. He wants to be rubbed, to have his back scratched. He wants sympathy and laughter. In fact, look for the Phosphorus patient to react by laughing at serious things, and at things that scare him. Weeping may alternate with laughter.

This is also an exhausted patient, so you will find that some needing this remedy are apathetic and refuse to talk or answer questions. If the patient answers at all, it will be slowly, and after a great time. His mind is clouded and not working quickly. His powers of speech are likewise exhausted. Speech is slow and difficult, and stuttering is common.

Yet, remember, this is a patient who is wide open emotionally. He will appreciate all of his caregiver's work and will be touched by it. He will tend to cooperate in his recovery.

Characteristics: As a substance, phosphorus irritates and causes inflammation. The conditions requiring the remedy Phosphorus will also show inflammation. Symptoms begin suddenly in response to external catalysts, such as weather. The symptoms may suddenly change as well.

The Phosphorus patient bleeds a good deal. Even the smallest wound will bleed a lot. He is given to chronic nosebleeds, and hemorrhages of all sorts.

Along with Arsenicum and Sulphur, Phosphorus is part of Nash's "Burn Trio," in that all the pains the Phosphorus patient suffers will have a burning sensation attached to them. Along with burning pains, look for itching, especially internal itching.

Pulse: The pulse is rapid, full, and hard. The pulse rate is about eighty beats per minute or more. In some cases, however, there may be a small pulse that is hard to find, although it is racing.

This is a patient who will be given to palpitations, especially during fits of anxiety, or while lying on the left side. Palpitations are made worse by any motion. They may awaken the patient during the night. They cause great anxiety, and a peculiar sensation of hunger. Palpitations may occur in young adults.

Modalities: Worse: from negative emotions; from talking; from seemingly slight causes; from cold, especially cold air; from changes in the weather, especially thunderstorms; from lying on the left side; at sunset.

Better: from sleep; from eating; from drinking cold water, or washing the face with cold water; from being rubbed or touched; from resting; from lying on the right side.

Common Causes of Illness

Emotional upset; negative emotions: anger, grief, fear, worry; mental strain; changes in weather: thunderstorms, lightning; sexual excess; tobacco abuse; overwork, over-lifting, straining; mechanical injury that involves bleeding; recovery from surgery; strong odors, especially flowers.

Common Uses

Any upper respiratory infection: colds, sore throats, flu, bronchitis, otitis media (ear infection), croup; vertigo; ringing in the ears; nosebleed, hemorrhages of all sorts; recovery from surgery; headaches and migraines; chronic fatigue, environmental illness, chemical sensitivity; phobia, anxiety, and panic attacks.

PODOPHYLLUM

Source: American Mandrake (Mayapple).
This remedy is taken from a plant native to North America. Indian tribes used this plant to cure everything from worms to deafness.
Theme: This is such a slight remedy that I don't know that it even has a theme. I just know that it is probably the best remedy for cases of acute diarrhea that I have ever seen.

Podophyllum is sometimes considered to be "vegetable mercury," in that it will show the same portrait of symptoms as Mercurius, but it is taken from a plant, the Mayapple.

About Podophyllum

Murphy writes, "Notable Podo symptoms are: Thirst for large quantities of cold water.

Intense desire to press the gums together. Viscid mucus in mouth, coating teeth. Diarrhea while being bathed or washed, (consisting of) dirty water, soaking through napkin, (accompanied) with gagging.

"Patient is constantly shaking and rubbing region of liver with his hands. Great loquacity during chill and heat. Podo is mainly right sided, throat, hypochondrium, ovary."

The Podophyllum Face

Eyes: Look for the patient to hold his eyes half open, especially during teething and bowel disorders. The eyes have a yellow tint.

Ears: There is pain in the right ear only, which travels into the eustachian tube.

Nose: Look for little pustules in the nose.

Mouth: Look for white, sticky mucus in the mouth and on the tongue. Look for the patient to grind his teeth.

Tongue: The tongue is enlarged, and seems broader than usual. It is coated yellow, as if mustard had been smeared on it.

The patient experiences a loss of taste. Everything tastes bitter, sour, or rotten.

Countenance: The patient's face is yellow. The face and especially the cheeks become flushed and hot during nausea and particularly during diarrhea.

The Podophyllum Patient

Behavior: This is a restless and fidgety patient who talks a good bit. Look for a tendency to stretch. Look for patient to roll his head, especially in his sleep. Look for alternating fever and chill. Look for the patient to be very talkative during periods of heat. He will be conscious during periods of chill, but will have difficult speaking and will forget what he is saying.

Characteristics: The actions of this remedy center in the small intestine, the rectum, and the liver. It is mostly used for cases of diarrhea accompanied by colic and vomiting.

Pains are jerking in nature, and tend to develop in sudden shocks. The patient is drowsy and tends to want to stretch to feel better.

Pulse: This patient is all but pulseless. The pulse is slow and barely perceptible. The patient will feel as if his heart is literally rising into his throat. He will complain of a stinging sensation in and around his heart.

The patient may suffer palpitations from mental exertion, deep emotions, or physical exertion. During palpitations, the patient will again feel as if his heart were rising into his throat. He will have troubled respiration. He will feel rumbles in his ascending colon.

Modalities: Worse: from eating; in hot weather, in summer; from teething; from motion; first thing in the morning.

Better: from rubbing, especially the area of the liver; from lying face down; from bending forward; from warm applications.

Common Causes of Illness

Diarrhea associated with teething; diarrhea associated with pregnancy; summer; over-lifting or straining.

Common Uses

Acute diarrhea, associated with teething, pregnancy, or that occurs after eating fruit in summer; irritable bowel syndrome; colitis.

PULSATILLA

Source: Wind flower
Taken from a form of the anemone, the wind flower is also known as the "pasque flower" in that it blooms at Easter. It also flowers in colors.
Theme: This remedy is taken from the windflower, and like a little flower blowing in the wind, this remedy type has the theme of changeability. Both physical and emotional symptoms change constantly, without rhyme

or reason. Note that no one cries as much as a Pulsatilla type.

About Pulsatilla

Morrison writes, "Though Pulsatilla is well-known to all homeopaths, we often have some difficulty in recognizing a Pulsatilla case, especially if we expect always to see the typical blond, blue-eyed, mild, and tearful patient. This is true because greater psychological 'sophistication' teaches people to compensate or hide their natural tendencies."

The Pulsatilla Face

Eyes: Pulsatilla is known for its discharges, which are rather thick and yellow/green in color. As this is a remedy for those with conjunctivitis, look for this yellow/green, thick and sticky discharge from the eyes, especially at the end of a cold. The eyes also tend to tear a good bit. The discharge may be a mixture of tears and mucus, and will be worse when the patient is in a warm room. The patient will want to rub his eyes a good bit, because they are itchy and burning. Look for swelling of the upper lids.

Ears: The external ear will be swollen and red. It is characteristic of the remedy that the earlobe will be swollen. Look for the characteristic yellow/green discharge from the ear as well. This discharge will have an offensive odor.

This is a major remedy for ear infections. Pain in the ear will be worse at night and when the patient is in a warm room. The patient will be better for being carried or rocked, and from cold applications to the ear. This is very commonly a remedy for childhood earaches that follow the pattern of symptoms put forth here.

The patient will be hard of hearing.

Nose: Again, look for the characteristic discharge: yellow/green, thick, and bland. The discharge is abundant, especially in the morning. It pours out of the nose and surrounds the nose like a cloud as it is discharged. Also look for green scales inside the nose. The patient's nose and the bones of the nose will be sore. The nasal symptoms will improve if the patient goes outside, and worsen when the patient is inside, especially if he is lying down.

This is an important remedy to consider when the patient is in the third stage of a cold, from the moment the mucus is colored until the end of the cold.

Mouth: The patient's mouth is dry, but the patient has no thirst. If there is saliva in the mouth, look for it to be thick and frothy. For cases of toothache, look for the patient to hold cold water in his mouth to get relief (The Coffea patient also does this).

As with the ear, there will be an offensive odor from the mouth, especially in the morning.

Tongue: The tongue is covered in thick, sticky mucus. It is usually yellow, but sometimes is white. There may be blisters on the tip and sides of the tongue.

Throat: The interior throat is dry or covered in a thick mucus, especially in the morning. There will be a sulfur odor when the patient coughs.

Countenance: As this is a remedy for mumps, the glands under the jaw may be very swollen. The patient's lips will be very dry. Look for him to lick his lips often. Look for a crack in the center of the bottom lip. The right side of the face will be more affected by symptoms than the left, but look for the left eye and ear to have more discharges. Look for the skin of the patient's face to be very sensitive, especially to touch.

This is a patient whose face will reflect pain and suffering easily. Look for the patient to cry when he talks about his suffering or symptoms.

The Pulsatilla Patient

Behavior: This is a highly emotional patient easily given to tears, either from joy or sorrow. Often, in the case taking, the case may seem to make no sense: symptoms and especially pains jump from one part of the body to another without rhyme or reason. The patient will often only answer your questions by shaking or nodding his head, and will not speak aloud.

The patient is better in open air in every way, and worse in a warm, closed room. He may faint in a warm room. He also is better from moving: either from walking, or, especially, rocking. These patients often rock when in pain.

Morning is a difficult time for these patients. They may feel weak in the morning and be unable to get out of bed. All symptoms are worse in the morning.

Although this is a remedy often used for those with fevers, the patient is thirstless, even when he has a dry mouth and a fever.

Characteristics: This remedy is often prescribed on the basis of the mental and emotional symptoms rather than the physical symptoms. This is a remedy for those who contradict themselves, who seem rather timid and soft, but who can become quite peeved (as opposed to actually angry) or very sad and crying at a moment's notice.

The Pulsatilla patient is thirstless (even in fever), chilly and rather short of breath. He is especially chilly when he is in pain. Pain carries with it a sensation of numbness and burning.

Pains may also be scraping, tearing, or jerking in nature. The patient also usually feels very heavy when ill, and will feel like he cannot breathe. Therefore, even though he is chilly, he will not be able to bear a warm, closed room. It is important to remember that contradiction is the key here. The patient's symptoms will change for no apparent reason. No two attacks will be the same. Pains tend to appear suddenly, but leave gradually.

Note that Pulsatilla, like Lycopodium, has the strange characteristic of having one foot hot and the other cold. And, like Nux, Phosphorus, and Sulphur, the Pulsatilla patient may sweat only on one side of the body.

Pulse: The patient may experience a racing pulse in the evening. The patient's heartbeat may be audible. The pulse slows in the morning. The patient may feel a sensation of heaviness or pressure, or a sensation of fullness in the chest every evening.

The patient may experience palpitations, caused by strong emotions like fright, anger, or joy. Palpitations are accompanied by trembling of the limbs. Palpitations start after dinner, usually while the patient is talking.

Modalities: Worse: in a warm, closed room; on first motion; from rest; while lying down; after eating (a good while afterward), especially pork, pastry, or fruit; at sunset; during thunderstorms.

Better: from cool, fresh air; from gentle motion; from cold applications; after crying.

Common Cause of Illness

Poor diet; getting chilly and/or wet; from thunderstorms; abuse of tea; pregnancy; menopause; puberty.

Common Uses

Colds, cough, bronchitis, otitis media (ear infection), sinusitis; asthma; seasonal and food allergies; pregnancy and labor; menopause; puberty; premenstrual syndrome (PMS); headaches; anxiety.

RHUS TOXICODENDRON

Source: Poison Ivy.

It may come as a surprise that a remedy taken from poison ivy can be such a help, but remember a simple homeopathic axiom: "the stronger the poison, the stronger the cure." While the plant may cause illness, the remedy taken from the plant ends it. And, of course, it is to be considered a chief remedy for those suffering from poison ivy.

Theme: This is the grand old "rusty hinge" remedy. Its theme, both emotionally and physically, is that it is the start up, the initial motion that is hard and painful. Gentle progress, however, yields a positive result.

The core of the remedy has to do with motion. Most often you will consider this remedy for cases involving overdoing: over-lifting with strain on the back, too much speaking or screaming the night before. The patient's body is worse from motion, especial-ly from first motion, and yet it will be impos-sible for him to stay still. He has to move to find comfort. Like a rusty hinge, the patient has great pain and stiffness upon first mo-tion, but begins to feel better as he moves in a gentle manner. However, the pain will return once he moves too much or too roughly.

About Rhus Tox

Hahnemann wrote, "There are a great number of characteristic peculiarities in its action. To mention one only: we observe this curious action (which is found in very few other remedies, and in these never to such a great degree), viz. the severest symptoms and sufferings are excited when the body or the limb is at rest and kept as much as pos-sible without movement."

The Rhus Tox Face

Eyes: The eyes are red, swollen, and puffy, as if the swelling were fluid-filled. The eyelids will be swollen and inflamed, and the eye itself may be inflamed. Look for a profuse flow of tears, mucus, and yellow pus. Look for the patient's eyes to water when he yawns.

The patient is photophobic. Light causes his eyes to tear.

Look for the patient to be unable to move his eyes about without a great deal of pain, especially in damp and cold weather.

Ears: The earlobes will be red and swollen. Also look for the glands behind the ears to be swollen. Look for a discharge of thick, yellow pus and blood.

Nose: The tip of the patient's nose will be red, sore, and possibly ulcerated. The whole nose may be swollen. The air coming from the nose will be very hot. This patient sneezes a great deal, especially after getting wet. He may have spasmodic sneezing.

Consider this remedy for those who suddenly have a nosebleed that may be quite difficult to stop, or who suddenly have a great discharge of mucus, apparently without cause.

The patient will experience a loss of the sense of smell.

Mouth: Look for bloody saliva in the mouth when the patient sleeps. The patient sleeps with his mouth open. Look for a great deal of mucous in the patient's mouth and throat.

Tongue: The Rhus patient's tongue is red and cracked. It may be coated, except on the tip. The tip is the keynote: it will have a very red triangular patch on the tip. The whole tongue may be clean and quite red, or the tongue may have a yellowish-white coating, especially at the root. The tongue may be quite swollen, and show teeth marks at the sides.

Throat: There will be swollen glands everywhere. The throat is red and swollen, or may be covered by with a thick, yellow coating.

The patient will feel that his throat is very dry. He will have trouble swallowing solids, and will be very thirsty for liquids, especially warm liquids that soothe the throat and relieve pains. Patients will often feel that they must continually swallow. Swallowing—especially empty swallowing—is very painful.

Countenance: The jaw is an indicator of the type. The Rhus jaw is given to dislocation. It cracks when the patient tries to chew. The patient may hold his jaw very rigid. Yawning may be very painful.

This is a patient with a red face. The face may be very swollen and bloated, and it may also seem a bit stiff, as if the patient cannot move it easily. Look for red and shiny rash on the patient's face, especially on the left check. Consider this remedy for cases of acne rosacea.

The cheek bones are very painful and sensitive to touch. The face, as a whole, may be very cold to the touch. The eyes will be ringed in blue and seem sunken. The lips are brown in color. This is a patient with a sickly look on his face.

The Rhus Tox Patient

Behavior: The Rhus patient is better in dry, warm surroundings, and worse from getting cold or wet.

These patients are likely to be a bit depressed, and a little dark in their humor. They are likely to think that things can never get better. They are given to apprehensions, especially at night, of bad things about to happen. When you ask them questions, they are likely to ramble a bit when they talk, or to move off the subject at hand. They will be slow to answer even if they answer directly.

The patient's voice sounds weak, exhausted, and raw. This is the remedy for "preacher's throat," for those who have stressed their voices into exhaustion by speaking or singing.

In general, this is a very restless patient. He seeks comfort and safety, and yet he cannot rest, cannot relax—he must keep moving.

Characteristics: The action of this remedy is especially felt in joints and tendons, so this is one of our greatest remedies for rheumatic pains in any part of the body. And it should come as no surprise that a remedy taken from poison ivy also affects the skin, especially the scalp and face.

The pain sensation is one of bruising, tearing, and shooting. Joints feel dislocated. Pains feel as if the skin were being torn from the bones.

This is a very restless patient who must change positions more or less constantly in order to find relief from pain.

Pulse: The pulse is small, sharp, and vibrating in nature. It is often weak, faint, and soft, and sometimes imperceptible. The pulse is often irregular. It may be strongly affected by use of alcohol or coffee. The patient may experience a weakness in the area of the heart.

The patient may feel pain in the chest and the left shoulder and arm with coldness and numbness. The pain is worse when the patient raises his left arm, takes a deep breath, or ascends stairs.

Modalities: Worse: in wet weather, especially in wet, cold weather; from cold air, any draft; before a storm; from northeastern winds; on first motion; from over-lifting or straining; from jarring motions, sudden movements; when rising up out of a seat.

Better: from continued gentle motions; from heat, especially from wet heat, such as a hot bath; from being rubbed; from changing positions; from lying on something hard; in warm, dry weather.

Common Causes of Illness

Getting wet when overheated; getting the head wet; over-lifting or straining; from physical overexertion; from drinking ice water or beer when overheated; from anger, even the slightest anger.

Common Uses

Strains, sprains, backache; whiplash; tendonitis; rheumatism; sciatica; rheumatic fever; colds, flu, sore throats, laryngitis, bronchitis; chicken pox; herpes; asthma.

RUMEX CRISPUS

Source: Yellowdock

This is a small remedy, but one that is very useful in the home, especially in the treatment of coughs. Tickling—a sensation of tickling that leads to coughing—is the key here. Cough occurs when the patient laughs or talks. The patient may feel that he will suffocate from coughing. The cough may take on a barking sound. It is worse in open air or when the patient lies down.

Theme: It's all about controlling that cough, and all that the patient will do to stop coughing.

About Rumex

Boericke wrote, "Rumex is characterized by pains, numerous and varied, neither fixed nor constant anywhere. Cough caused by an incessant tickling in the throat-pit, which tickling runs down to the bifurcation of the bronchial tubes. Worse from the least cold air; so that all coughing ceases by covering up all the body and head with bedclothes ... Its action upon the skin is marked, producing an intense itching."

The Rumex Face

Eyes: Look for the eyes to be swollen in the morning. The eyelids are inflamed, especially at night. The eyes themselves may be sore, even without inflammation.

Ears: There are no guiding objective symptoms for this remedy, although the patient may experience ringing and/or itching in his ears.

Nose: There will be a great deal of mucus discharge from the nose (and coughed up from the throat as well). Discharge is watery, and will be worse at night. Discharge is caused by sneezing, which occurs in attacks. Violent sneezing attacks start at night. Nosebleeds may result from sneezing fits as well.

Mouth: For patients with toothache, look for the pain to be less when the patient is eating, or holding cold water in the mouth.

Tongue: The tongue is most commonly colored yellow, although it may be brown or reddish-brown. The tongue is dry. The patient reports that his tongue feels burnt.

Throat: The patient hawks and hawks, and coughs up a great deal of mucus. The hawking is worse in the evening. The patient also coughs and coughs; coughs are shallow and dry, and may be brought on by touching the pit of the throat.

Countenance: The patient has a stoic expression on his face, as if he is holding something back or putting a great deal of concentration into something. (He is: it is taking all his willpower to keep from coughing.) The patient's face is pale when he stands up, and flushed and hot when he is at rest.

The Rumex Patient

Behavior: This is a patient with a very serious expression. He is withdrawn and indifferent to everything in his environment.

Characteristics: The pain sensation associated with Rumex is a bit odd, in that the pains—and there may be many of them—tend to change and move around the body without any consistency. The patient's voice changes in the same way. Tone and pitch may shift at different times, or may change at the same time every day. The voice is pitched higher than usual, and is nasal and hoarse, especially in the evening.

Rumex acts primarily upon the skin—and the Rumex patient may experience maddening itching of the skin—and on the chest, larynx, and trachea. It also acts upon the joints, especially the ankles.

Pulse: The pulse is irregular and throbbing. It races when the patient ascends stairs. The patient reports that he feels as if his heart suddenly stops beating, which is followed by a throbbing sensation in his chest.

Modalities: Worse: from breathing in, especially from breathing in cold air; from any change in temperature; from uncovering; from talking, and, especially, laughing; from motion; from eating, especially after meals.

Better: from staying covered; from covering the nose and mouth when breathing.

Common Causes of Illness

Changes in weather, especially from warm to cold; when the weather pattern is in constant change; seasonally, spring and autumn.

Common Uses

Cough; laryngitis; croup; measles; morning diarrhea.

RUTA GRAVEOLENS

Source: Rue

Rue has for centuries been grown in gardens of Southern Europe and used as an herbal remedy for ailments like epilepsy and hysteria, even rabies. Homeopathically, it is used for more common household ailments.

Theme: Stiffness is the theme of this remedy: stiffness of muscles and tendons, as well as a sensation of stiffness in the eyes. On a constitutional level, you will see a sort of emotional stiffness as well. The eyes and the profuse watering from them are the best clues. This is a patient whose eyes will water for one reason or another. The patient may be given to weeping, or he may complain of eyestrain, but the eyes will water and water and water.

The other visible indications of the remedy type have to do with the body. This is a major remedy for those with strains and sprains and dislocations, especially when they concern the area of the hips. The is a remedy that combines restlessness with paralysis, so it can resemble Arnica and Rhus Tox in that the patient is always trying to find a comfortable position, and tosses and turns in the attempt.

The Ruta Face

Eyes: This is a major remedy for those with eyestrain, so there will be important symptoms related to the eye, although they may not be visible. Look for the eyes to water, especially after the patient has done any form of close work such as reading, sewing, or other similar activities.

The eyes will also itch and the patient will want to scratch them. Look for the eyes to be filled with water after the patient rubs them. The patient will have a sensation of heat, of fire in the eyes.

An interesting keynote of the remedy is that the patient will not be photophobic, but instead will seek and crave light.

Ears: Physical pain in ear, as from a blow or a fall. The patient may report a sensation as if a piece of wood were being pushed into his ear.

Nose: Look for sweat on the nose. Nose-bleeds are common.

Mouth: The gums bleed easily. The mouth and tongue are dry. There is a taste of wood in the mouth.

Tongue: There is a cramp or spasm in the tongue that makes speech very difficult.

The patient is very embarrassed by his difficulty in speaking. The tongue is swollen.

Throat: The patient experiences a sensation of a lump in his throat.

Countenance: This is a grave patient; look for a very serious expression on his face.

The face is tender, painful, as if the patient had been struck. His lips are dry and sticky.

The Ruta Patient

Behavior: This is a fussy patient who is dissatisfied with himself and with all others. Look for him to constantly complain and fuss. Look for the patient to stretch, yawn, and reach out with his hands.

Characteristics: I have always found it a bit odd that Ruta combines symptoms of the muscles, tendons, and joints with eye symptoms, but I have seen this peculiar combination again and again. Ruta is perhaps our best remedy for eyestrain.

The patient will feel bruised in the rest of the body as well as the eyes. Pains are aching in nature, and soreness runs throughout the whole being. The patient feels heavy, sore, and bruised, and yet is restless. This is a remedy to remember for those who have become lame after a strain. This is also a very important remedy for hip pain, especially when the movement of rising up from a chair is most painful. Think of this remedy for cases of low back and hip injury and/or pain.

Pulse: This is a patient with a steady pulse. Look for the pulse to accelerate only during fever, or from anxious emotions.

Modalities: Worse: from reading, sewing, and other "close work"; from overexertion; from cold; from cold, damp wind and weather; when sitting, or, especially, when rising from a sitting position.

Better: when lying still; from gentle motion; from rubbing and scratching.

Common Causes of Illness

Mechanical injury, especially to bones; sprains; over-lifting; overexertion of eyes.

Common Uses

Muscle strains; sprains, especially to wrists and ankles; low back and hip pain; bursitis; sciatica; eyestrain; headache; panic attacks.

SABADILLA

Source: Cevadilla Seed

Sneezing is the key here, as simple as it sounds, but these are sneezing attacks that go on and on in repeated explosions. Sabadilla incorporates all the symptoms traditionally thought of in association with seasonal allergies. In addition, the patient is chilly and very sensitive to cold.

Theme: This remedy, taken from a plant native to the Americas, tends to be acute in nature and lacks a "theme" as such. But the patient who can't stop sneezing may well benefit from a dose of Sabadilla.

About Sabadilla

Morrison writes, "Sabadilla is primarily a remedy for hay fever and coryza. The main keynote symptom is the tremendous sneezing and paroxysmal nature of the sneezing."

The Sabadilla Face

Eyes: Since this is a remedy for those with hay fever, the eye symptoms are exactly what you would expect. The eyelids are red and inflamed. The eyes water, and the watering becomes worse if the patient sneezes, coughs, yawns, or walks in the open air. Look for the watering to most often accompany fits of sneezing. Look for blue rings under the eyes.

Ears: The patient has a very difficult time hearing. Everything is muffled, distant.

Look for the patient to complain of itching or tickling in the ears. This is a remedy (along with Cina) for those with worms, so internally itching ears are also a major symptom for Sabadilla.

Nose: The patient is overly sensitive to odors of all sorts. Smells bring on fits of sneezing. The scent of flowers and the odor of garlic are especially difficult.

There is copious discharge, which is clear and watery. Discharge starts after fits of sneezing. The eyes tear and the nose waters at the same time. Discharge may become thick and clear over time, and may also become yellow-gray. The nose alternates between dry and running, or alternates with one side dry the other running.

The patient cannot leave his nose alone. They rub it, scratch it, blow it, pick it. (Again, this is a remedy for those with worms.)

Mouth: The patient cannot bear to have anything that is either too hot or too cold in his mouth. The patient may have a good deal of saliva in his mouth, may be almost constantly spitting out saliva.

Consider this remedy for cases of toothache, in which pain extends throughout the whole side of his mouth.

Tongue: The tongue is coated with a whitish-yellow in the middle and/or at the back. There may be blisters on the tongue. When the throat is sore, look for the patient to be unable to stick out his tongue.

Throat: The patient has postnasal drip in the back of the throat. This is thicker than the nasal discharge. Dry swallowing is very painful, but the patient feels he must swallow constantly. Cold drinks increase pain, while warm drinks soothe pain.

Countenance: The patient's face is flushed, hot, and red. The lips feel very hot to the touch. The heat in the face increases if the patient drinks wine. Listen for the cracking that the patient's jaw does every time he opens his mouth wide.

The Sabadilla Patient

Behavior: This patient is a bit nervous, and very frightened. He will fixate on some strange notion—usually that he is a victim of a fatal disease—and will not be comforted on that subject. Therefore, he may seem demanding in that he will want comfort.

It is best to try to get the patient's mind off his symptoms, as the symptoms will actually increase if he stops and thinks about them.

Characteristics: The action of the remedy centers on the nose and eyes, specifically on the mucous membrane of the nose and the tear ducts. The patient sneezes in fits and his eyes run with water while he sneezes. The patient is chilly and very sensitive to cold.

The pain sensation is bruising, with cutting pains in the bones.

Pulse: The pulse is small and spasmodic. The patient feels blood pulsing throughout the body, although he fears that his circulation may be stopped.

Modalities: Worse: from specific smells; from cold in any form, especially cold air and cold drinks; at the new and full moon; at the same time every day.

Better: from heat; in open air; from eating, or from swallowing anything (the motion of swallowing soothes); from being wrapped up.

Common Causes of Illness

Seasonal, late summer and autumn; from worms; from fright; from sexual excess.

Common Uses

Colds, cough; asthma; allergies; worms.

SEPIA

Source: Cuttlefish Ink

This remedy was created by Hahnemann for a patient who worked tinting art work with squid ink (sepia-toning). Hahnemann suspected that the ink was poisoning the man, so he created the homeopathic remedy Sepia to cure him. Little did he know that day what an important remedy he had made.

Theme: A sensation of weight is key here. The patient feels as if he were holding the weight of the world upon him, both physically and emotionally. The indications in the physical body have to do with a sensation of heavy gravity, of increased weight, and the limbs feel numb and heavy. And yet, this is also a restless remedy. The patient will suddenly feel restless after sitting in one position for a while. His symptoms grow worse if he sits quietly for too long. Finally, it is keynote for the patient to experience the sensation of a lump or a ball in the throat or any other affected part of the body.

Sepia is one of our great polycrest remedies, and its indications can be for every aspect of the body. It is most often associated with female patients at times of great hormonal shift in their lives: puberty, pregnancy, and menopause. But, Sepia has much to offer as an acute remedy. In acute situations, gender is not an issue in the selection of this remedy.

About Sepia

Hahnemann wrote, "This brown-black juice, which, before me, had only been used for drawing, is contained in the abdomen of the sea-insect, ink-fish (*Sepia octopoda*), and is sometimes jerked forth by the insect to darken the water around, either for the purpose of securing a prey or opposing an attack."

The Sepia Face

Eyes: Keynote here is that the whites of the eyes become yellow. All eye symptoms are worse in the morning and evening. Look for the eyes to tear at these times. There may be agglutination of the eyelids every evening.

This is another eyestrain remedy. Look for the patient to close his eyes and either rub them or pinch the sides of the eyes or the root of the nose. The patient is intolerant to glare and to reflected bright lights.

Ears: Look for eruptions behind the ears, on the lobes of the ears, and on the nape of the neck. Look for subcutaneous ulcers or herpes eruptions. Look for a discharge of yellow pus, which has an offensive odor.

The patient will be very sensitive and intolerant to noises, especially music. The patient may have sudden deafness, as if a plug were placed in his ears.

Nose: Look for a thick, greenish discharge and for thick plugs and crusts of mucus inside the nose. Consider this remedy if there is a chronic flow of thick and greenish discharge, especially a heavy and lumpy postnasal drip. Discharge may come from the nose or be hawked out of the mouth. It is keynote that the patient will have a yellowish discoloration of the skin across the nose. Look for the tip of the nose to be both swollen and inflamed. Look for an eruption on the tip of the nose. The nose bleeds when it is touched, even lightly, or hit. Consider this remedy for nosebleeds that occur during a woman's period or during pregnancy.

This is a patient who is very sensitive to smells, especially to cooking odors, which cause pronounced nausea.

Mouth: The lower lip is swollen and cracked.

Tongue: Generally, the tongue will be covered in a white coating or with mucus, although the sides of the tongue will be red. The tongue is clean during a woman's period.

The Sepia tongue is often stiff, so the patient speaks with stammering.

Throat: The patient hawks up quantities of green, thick, and lumpy mucus. The throat is dry and sore at night.

The patient complains of the sensation of a lump in his throat. During first sleep, the patient dreams that he has swallowed something, which causes him to awaken with a start.

Countenance: The face is yellow or sallow, and is especially yellow around the mouth and/or across the nose. The area of the nose may also be brown, or there may be patches of brown discoloration on the face. Also look for dark brown circles under the eyes, herpes outbreaks on the lips, and warts on the face.

It is common for the Sepia woman to have acne breakouts before her period.

The Sepia Patient

Behavior: This patient usually will present as either indifferent to the illness at hand, or as very sad. Either way, the patient will most often cry when telling you his symptoms. His face may stay stony and calm, but tears stream from the eyes.

Characteristics: The Sepia patient's pain tends to run down the back. Like almost every other symptom in the portrait, it will move in a downward motion only.

The Sepia patient is known for the sensation of sudden exhaustion and for the sensation of having a ball or lump in his inner parts. These patients feel cold, even when they are in a warm place, and they require physical motion and effort to be warm.

Pains are jerking in character, with burning sensations running through the body.

Pulse: The pulse is irregular with an occasional thump.

Palpitations are common, as are sudden flushes. Patient awakens from the hard pounding of his heart. Stitching pains in the left side may accompany the palpitations.

Modalities: Worse: from cold, from anything that chills; from snow, from snowy air, especially a wet snow; on falling asleep; from sitting and standing; from noon until 1:00P.M. and from 4:00P.M. until 6:00P.M. after eating.

Better: from physical exertion; from warmth; from pressure; from crossing legs; after sleeping; from open air.

Common Causes of Illness

Pregnancy and childbirth, menopause; mechanical injuries, especially falls; physical strains and sprains; over-lifting; eating fatty foods; anger and irritation.

Common Uses

Sciatica, backache, strains; premenstrual syndrome (PMS), pregnancy and childbirth, miscarriage, menopause; headache and migraine; constipation; cough, bronchitis, sinusitis; seasonal allergies; chronic fatigue; depression.

SILICEA (SILICA)

Source: Flint

Like Carbo Veg and Calcarea Carbonica, this is another remedy that has a great deal to do with slow and poor digestion and poor assimilation of food. The Silicea patient is also very slow to heal. Therefore, sluggishness is the key to this remedy. This is also a remedy for those with chronic colds and allergies.

Consider that those needing this remedy are often children, as well as businessmen, lawyers, preachers, and students; who work with their minds and neglect their bodies. Note that it is keynote of this remedy that Silicea patients cannot handle alcohol at all; they are very sensitive to it. The key to this remedy is imperfect digestion and/or defective nutrition. The whole body begins to break down, either due to mental stress or an imperfect diet.

Theme: The Silicea patient tends to be weak not only physically, but emotionally as well. These patients are timid, and may lack the power to fight their way back to health.

About Silicea

Tyler writes, "Silica, they say, lacks grit—needs sand. And doses of Silica stimulate mightily these weaklings who are going under, to put up a fight, mental and physical.

"You look up, as poor little Silica is dragged reluctantly in. He is listless; not interested; not frightened.

"You see a pale, sickly, suffering face; and you realize at once that there is something deeply wrong here; no mere ailment—Disease."

The Silicea Face

Eyes: This patient is extremely photophobic, especially to daylight. Also look for the patient's eyes to tear when he is in open air. There is an agglutination of the lids at night.

Ears: Look for swelling of the mastoid with discharge from the ears. The discharge has a fetid smell. Look for crusts in the ears.

The patient has trouble hearing or understanding the human voice.

Nose: Look for dry, hard crusts inside the patient's nose. These crusts bleed when they are removed. Look for the patient to bring food out of the nose when he eats or drinks; milk comes out of the patient's nose when he drinks. The discharge of either mucus or blood will be frothy. The nose is cold to the touch. This patient sneezes in the morning. Look for cracks in the nostrils, especially for cases of chronic and obstinate colds (these are usually accompanied by ear symptoms).

Mouth: This remedy is filled with eruptions in the mouth, especially boils, which can appear on the gums, or abscesses on the gum at the root of a tooth. This is a major remedy for decayed and abscessed teeth. The teeth are very sensitive to cold water. The mouth is dry, with an offensive odor every morning.

Tongue: Typically, the tongue is brown. But it may be covered with yellow or white, the other colors associated with digestive disorders. Tongue may be swollen to the extent that you will see teeth marks lining the sides. The patient complains of the taste of blood in the morning, or of a bitter or soapy taste. The patient complains of a sensation of hair on the tongue.

Throat: The tonsils and glands are chronically swollen. The patient hawks up lumps of old mucus. The patient complains of a pricking sensation in his throat, or of soreness on the left side when swallowing.

Countenance: Look for cracked skin on the margin of the lips. Look for eruptions of the skin on the chin. The lower lip may be swollen. The face is red and swollen, especially in damp, cold weather.

The Silicea Patient

Behavior: This is a timid, nervous, and excitable patient. He is overly sensitive to all parts of his environment, especially to noise, light, and cold. This is a remedy given to violent pains that are of a sticking sensation.

As Tyler noted, however, this may be a timid patient, but it is not a frightened one. He may be disinterested and withdrawn, but he is not frightened. The Silicea patient is far stronger emotionally than he lets on. This is our most passive-aggressive remedy type.

Characteristics: Like the Mercurius patient, every little wound the Silicea patient has tends to become infected. There may be a long-term low-level infection present. The Silicea patient is slow to heal, and slow to react to most stimuli (except to alcohol, which all but overwhelms him).

The Silicea patient is very sensitive by nature. He is sensitive to noise, cold (his hands and feet tend to always be cold) and pain. The pains are sticking in nature, and tend to cluster in specific areas of the body, especially the throat and ears. The pains may be quite overwhelming and violent.

The old texts say that the Silicea patient has a "want of grit." By this they mean that the Silicea seems lacking in vital force, in the ability to stand up and be strong, on both the physical and emotional levels.

Pulse: The pulse is throbbing, but is often imperceptible. In general, the pulse is small, hard, and rapid.

Palpitations are accompanied by a trembling of the hands. Palpitations awaken the patient in the night. He feels throbbing of blood throughout his whole body. Palpitations are caused by nervous exhaustion.

Modalities: Worse: from cold, especially when cold is combined with damp; from getting feet wet; from bathing; from light, noise or touch; from alcohol; during the new moon or during changes in the phases of the moon; from lying on the left side or the painful side.

Better: from warmth; from being wrapped up tight, especially the head; in summer; when lying down and resting; from urinating.

Common Causes of Illness

Mechanical injury; wounds; vaccinations; splinters; poor diet.

Common Uses

Colds, otitis media (ear infection), sinusitis; asthma; night sweats; headache; skin conditions: acne, eczema, keloids, fibroids; abscesses; ingrown nails; constipation.

SPIGELIA

Source: Indian Pink

While this is a remedy often used by homeopaths for those with heart disease (consider it, along with Aconite, for cases in which the heart palpitations are so strong as to be visible in the chest), it is most often needed in home use by those with sciatic pains, especially on the left side of the body. The pains are violent and burning in nature, like hot needles in the body.

Note a general weakness in the patient after he has been moving about in open air.

Theme: The theme for this remedy is a combination of things. First, Spigelia is almost totally a left-sided remedy, meaning that the symptoms are only on the left side of the body. Second, it is a powerful pain remedy, when the pains are severe and piercing in nature.

About Spigelia

Morrison writes, "Spigelia is recognized by its nearly exclusively left-sided focus (left-sided headache and neuralgia, cardiac disorders, left colon infestations, etc.) Most frequently used for headaches of either sinus or migraine types, the remedy is also useful for neuralgia, cardiac disorders and parasitic infections. The pains of Spigelia are of most severe character—piercing and sharp."

The Spigelia Face

Eyes: This patient may have some trouble opening his eyes and raising his eyelids. Look for yellow rings around the eyes. The eyes are red and hot. There is profuse tearing from affected side (usually the left). The patient is inclined to wink and blink. The patient squints, and has difficulty moving the eyes. This patient may have to slowly move his whole head in order to see things to the side. Also note that the right eye itches. The patient rubs just the right eye.

Ears: Consider this remedy for the patient who alternates between deafness and an increased ability to hear.

Nose: While the patient's nose is dry, there is a good deal of postnasal drip. The mucus is either white or yellow and thick. This is also a remedy of violent flow from the nose, either a mucus flow or nosebleed. The eyes water with any nasal discharge.

Mouth: The patient's saliva is white and frothy. The lips are dry, pale, and cracked.

Tongue: The tongue is coated either yellow or white, and it may have fissures and cracks on it.

The patient may complain of burning pains on his tongue.

Throat: The patient is continually coughing and hawking mucus from his throat. The mucus is white or yellow. The patient complains of the sensation of a worm climbing inside his throat.

Countenance: The face is pale and bloated, especially when the patient first awakens in the morning. Look for either blue or yellow rings around the eyes.

The Spigelia Patient

Behavior: The patient will exhibit an inordinate fear of sharp things such as knives, needles, and similar objects. He is also worse from cold, and becomes very afraid if he becomes chilled. He is worse from cold, damp weather, and especially bad in stormy weather.

Characteristics: Spigelia's action centers in two parts of the body, the heart, and the nervous system. In the home, it will most commonly be used for nerve pain, for rheumatism. This pain is usually located in the upper part of the body, in the neck and shoulders. As an unlikely adjunct, it is also often used for the treatment of children with worms (the child typically points to the area of his navel as the most painful part of the body). The patient will be very sensitive to touch. He will feel chilly, may actually shudder from the sensation of cold.

As with most nerve pain, the pain begins at one specific spot and radiates out from there. These are shooting pains. After the pain attack, the whole area will feel sore for a good while.

Pulse: The pulse is irregular. At most times it is fairly slow, but it may race until it seems to be faster than the heartbeat. It tends to stay strong, but slow. There may be a trembling quality to the pulse.

This remedy is known for its unusually strong palpitations. These can be audible palpitations, with the beats visible through clothing.

As this is a major heart remedy, it presents the picture of sudden and severe chest pain that extends from the area of the heart around the whole body. The pain travels from left to right. Pains are accompanied by nausea and vomiting. Chest pains extend into all the limbs. The hands become so stiff that the patient cannot move them. There are cutting pains that extend down to the abdomen, and up to the head, shoulders, and arms. A sensation of suffocation accompanies the attack.

Modalities: Worse: from wet or, especially, stormy weather; from the combination of cold and damp; from any touch or motion; after eating; from any contact with tobacco; from thinking about the pain.

Better: from steady pressure; from dry weather and dry, warm air; while eating.

Common Causes of Illness

Taking a chill; tobacco.

Common Uses

Neck and shoulder pain; headaches, especially sinus headaches and migraines; toothache; sinusitis; angina; worms.

SPONGIA TOSTA

Source: Burnt Sponge

As the Latinized name implies, this remedy is taken from toasted sponge. Since the sponge is a sea creature, it contains substances that make this remedy somewhat related in action to a number of other fine remedies, among them Natrum Mur. Like Natrum Mur, which is, of course, made from salt, Spongia relates to the thyroid, and to cough, asthma, and other breathing issues.

Theme: This is the central theme of Spongia Tosta in home use. It might be said that it seems as if those needing this remedy are trying to breathe under water. They struggle to breathe.

In the same way that the nose is congested, the heart is congested. This remedy is especially for the valves of the heart.

Look for hard swelling of glands throughout the whole body.

About Spongia

Murphy writes, "One of the keynotes of Spongia is dryness of mucous membranes of tongue, pharynx, larynx, trachea. Cough is caused by dryness.

"The dry cough intensely barking, crowing, 'dry as a bone,' or sounding like a saw being driven through a pine board. Dry asthma."

The Spongia Tosta Face

Eyes: The patient will have running eyes, with a gummy discharge that may mix tears with mucus. The eyes are red and tearing. It is keynote of the remedy that the patient will have a yellow, crusted eruption on the left eyebrow. This eruption is painful to the touch.

Nose: The patient's nostrils are held wide open, and may fan in his attempt to draw in air. This is a remedy that most often is needed by patients with a long-lasting, if not chronic, dry stoppage of the nose. It may alternate with drainage.

Mouth: The patient's mouth may have what appears to be a rash running along it, and inside the cheeks. Look for the gums to be swollen and covered in a thin white coating.. They will be painful when the patient chews.

Tongue: The tongue is dry and brown or dry and red. Both the mouth and tongue may be covered in a painful rash. The patient complains of a bitter taste in his mouth.

Throat: Look for swelling of the thyroid, and goiter.

The patient has suffocative attacks at night while sleeping. He awakens with blue lips, and a flushed and hot face. The patient's cough is worse when he lies down in a warm room. The patient is anxious about his breathing, afraid that he will suffocate.

This is most often required as a remedy for patients with cough. A dry, chronic cough is most typical. The cough will have a hollow, barking quality, and may sound as if someone were sawing wood. An asthmatic cough with wheezing is also common. The cough is caused by excitement, cold drinks, and from eating sweets. Cough, and especially asthma are worse during a full moon.

Countenance: Look for an expression of terror on the patient's face. At least, the patient will seem anxious and upset. The face is bloated, and has either a red or blue tint and blue lips. Look for a cold sweat on the chin. Look for swollen glands that are painful to the touch below the left jaw. The whole left jaw is painful, especially when the patient eats.

The Spongia Tosta Patient

Behavior: This is a remedy for anxious and fearful patients inclined to cough with every excitement or disruption. The cough causes anxiety. The patient will fear death through suffocation.

Characteristics: The patient who needs this remedy is having difficulty breathing, and he is very anxiously trying to breathe. This anxiety combines with a sensation of weight and heaviness in the regions of the chest, particularly the heart, and the throat. There is often the sensation of a lump or a plug in the throat.

The Spongia patient coughs and coughs; there is an uncontrollable need to cough that all but suffocates the patient. The cough sounds like a bark, or as if the patient were sawing wood. The patient will throw his head back in order to breathe.

Pulse: This remedy type usually presents one of two pulse pictures. In one the pulse is full and hard, and in the other it is so small as to be almost imperceptible. In either case, the pulse is always rapid.

This irregularity also applies to the heart. Look for irregular action in the area of the heart. Look for a sudden, suffocating palpitation that develops when the patient ascends the stairs. Notice that the patient can bring on the same palpitations if he raises his arms above his head, and that he must lie in bed with his head braced high to have relief. Note that like the patient's cough, the patient's palpitations cause the characteristic wheezing "sawing wood" sound as the patient gasps for breath.

Modalities: Worse: when awakened from sleep; after sleeping; in the morning; from any exertion; from cold, dry weather or wind; lying down with the head low; in a warm room.

Better: from resting with the head lifted; from warm things; from eating and drinking.

Common Causes of Illness

Contact with cold, dry wind.

Common Uses

Cough, whooping cough, croup, bronchitis; asthma; angina.

STAPHYSAGRIA

Source: Stavesacre

This is a remedy often used for acute emotional symptoms, like Ignatia. Like Nux, the key for this remedy is often anger. The Staphysagria patient feels he has been wronged—knows he has been wronged, in fact—but does not know what to do with this anger. Therefore, it stays inside and eats away at him. Some patients needing this remedy will seem to never be angry, while others explode with anger at surprising

moments.

This is a patient with a very low threshold for pain. His whole body seems wracked with pain. The pain is has a knifelike quality.

This is also often a remedy needed by those with a mechanical injury from a sharp instrument, who have been cut and are in pain and shock. For this reason, Staphysagria, along with Arnica and Hypericum, is an important remedy used for recovery after surgery. It is said to be especially helpful when the patient is recovering from cataract surgery.

Note that this remedy is also important for those who have been abused as children. The patient may not have a complete memory of the abuse; only the anger may remain.

Theme: Stabbing is the key. Stabbing pain—even an emotional trauma that "stabs." A knife in the back. Also for literal stab wounds when there is a clean cut.

About Staphysagria

Nash wrote, "Staphysagria, Chamomilla, Nux Vomica, Cina, Colocynth stand very close to each other for cross, ugly, irritable subjects, and there are few cases that one or the other will not fit."

The Staphysagria Face

Eyes: Consider for patients with styes that tend to recur.

The patient's eyes are sunken, with blue rings below them. The eyes are dry, but look for a sudden torrent of hot tears. The eyes will water when the patient is in daylight. The pupils are dilated. The patient may complain of dry eyes in the morning, and of a sensation of pressure in the eyes at night.

Ears: Patient is hard of hearing, and his tonsils are swollen at the same time. The patient may complain of a ringing in his ears when he moves his head.

Nose: The nose is dry, with a great deal of sneezing. Discharge starts suddenly, beginning thick and becoming watery.

Mouth: This is a toothache remedy. The patient's teeth are weak and crumbling. The teeth feel loose. The patient's gums are spongy and bleed easily. The teeth are very sensitive to the touch, especially at night. Tooth pain is worse for cold air or cold drinks. Consider this remedy for tooth decay during pregnancy. Look for increased saliva, which is constantly accumulating in the mouth.

Tongue: There are no objective symptoms of the tongue for this remedy, although the patient may complain of bitter tastes in his mouth. The patient's tongue and mouth may be covered in blisters or ulcers, which will be accompanied by swelling of the glands in the neck.

Throat: The patient swallows constantly when talking. Swallowing and talking are painful. The throat looks dry and rough, with swelling of the tonsils.

Countenance: The patient's whole face will seem sunken, making his nose beaklike. Look for blue margins around his eyes. The patient's face takes on a brown or blue color when he becomes emotional, especially angry. The bones of the patient's face will be tender and perhaps painful if touched. The submaxillary glands are painful, even if they are not swollen. Look for the patient to scratch only his left cheek. The patient's lips are scabby and crusted.

The Staphysagria Patient

Behavior: This is a sad patient, very concerned for his own well-being. The patient may be somewhat forgetful, especially about his injury. He will also have difficulty reading and understanding what he read. He will have even greater difficulty in remembering what he read.

The Staphysagria patient is usually identified by his emotional symptoms. This is a patient who has been hurt or harmed in some way, and knows that he has been treated unfairly and that his experience was not his fault. Usually he is angry and does not know what to do about his anger. He is sullen or sad, and then will erupt into anger and passion. This remedy is often needed by survivors of rape and other forms of physical and emotional abuse, and by those suffering posttraumatic stress. It is keynote of this remedy that the patient will stamp his foot in anger and at feelings of injustice. Also note that the patient has a very strong voice when he is angry and a weak voice thereafter.

Characteristics: The remedy acts on areas of the body where there are many nerves, and on the teeth, urinary organs, and skin.

Pain tends to be squeezing in nature. It may also feel as if the patient has been cut with a knife. Staphysagria is, in general, an excellent pain remedy for situations in which the patient is overwhelmed by pain. Therefore it is to be thought of for cases of terrible toothache and for recovery from surgery, when the patient has been literally cut open.

Pulse: The patient's pulse is weak, frequent, and small. It tends to have a trembling nature. The patient's heart feels weak.

Palpitations are common to this remedy type. Note that listening to music may bring on palpitations. They may also develop after mental exertion or deep emotions.

Modalities: Worse: any negative emotion: anger, embarrassment, confrontation; at the full moon; from sexual excess; from touch of any painful part.

Better: from rest; after a good breakfast; from warmth.

Common Causes of Illness

Mechanical injury, especially a fall; wounds, cuts; recovery from surgery; sexual excess; teething; anger, especially suppressed anger.

Common Uses

Recovery from surgery; wounds, cuts; toothache and teething pains; headache; insomnia; depression.

SULPHUR

Source: Sulphur

The key to seeing the remedy is as simple as red, hot, and damp. This is a hot and sweaty patient, who often seems less ill than he is. Look for glandular swelling throughout the body. Look for a patient who wants to be lazy when ill, who is not interested at all in cleaning or bathing. This is also an itchy patient. Itching will run all through his symptoms. He is scratching his whole body, and is unable to tolerate wool or anything else that itches.

Symptoms are worse from rest, and better from motion. They are worse during any change in weather. All of the symptoms will be worse at night. In general, these patients are better in every way when they breathe open or cool air.

Theme: Combine heat, sweat, itching, and burning sensations, add in a craving for salt and sugar, a gigantic thirst, and an overwhelming desire not to work and you have the acute picture of the Sulphur patient.

About Sulphur

Tyler wrote, "When we were children a precious Riddle Book had it, 'Sulphur comes from volcanoes and is good for eruptions.' And Sulphur is associated in ideas with the Lake of Fire, and Everlasting Burning; and Sulphur indeed causes burning; burning pain in eyes, lips, tongue; in nostrils, face, throat; in fauces and pharynx; in stomach and abdomen; in anus; in hemorrhoids, etc; between scapulae (Lyc, Phos); in fingers, palms (Phos), in skin of the whole body, in parts on which he lies."

The Sulphur Face

Eyes: Typically, the Sulphur patient's eyes will be dry when in a room, and will tear when in the open air. As with every other symptom of this type, the eyes will tend to be hot and itchy. The patient will want to scratch and rub his eyes; to pull them from his head. Look for crusts on the eyelids, for agglutination every night, and conjunctivitis. Consider this remedy for the patient whose every cold goes into the eyes.

Ears: The patient's hearing is very sensitive, and then without warning he is all but deaf. Consider this remedy for sudden deafness in the right ear. The patient may, rather oddly, complain that he feels as if he were not hearing through his ears at all, but through his forehead or brain.

The external ear is very hot and very red. Look for offensive discharge from the ear every eighth day.

Nose: The patient is overly sensitive to odors, and often will smell imaginary odors. And yet, he is immune to his own foul smell. Smells may become trapped in the patient's nose, so that they are the only thing he can smell for days.

The tip of the nose is red, swollen, and shiny. There is frequent sneezing, and discharge can be of almost any sort, but typically it is thick and yellow. There is discharge when the patient is outside, but the nose is stopped when he is inside.

There is chronic blockage of the nose. Look for fanlike motions of the nostrils when the patient attempts to breathe. Look for nosebleeds that start at night, when the patient lies on his right side. Look for redness across the bridge of the nose, and freckles on the nose. In children, look for the patient to pick his nose and eat the result.

Mouth: There is thrush in the mouth, or painful white ulcers. The mouth is dry and sticky every morning. There is a foul smell from the mouth, especially in the morning and after the patient eats. Look for increased saliva in the mouth every time the patient eats.

The patient's gums are red and swollen, and bleed easily. Consider this remedy for cases of toothache that are worse when the patient is in open air, or when air comes in contact with the tooth. The lips are dry, rough and cracked. The lips are bright red.

Tongue: The tongue is white, with red tip and/or borders. In cases of indigestion, look for a white, yellow, or brown fur to cover the tongue every morning. This fur will wear off during the day, leaving the tongue very dry. Consider this remedy when you see a painful blister on the right side of the tongue. The tongue is also swollen, dry, and tends to tremble.

Throat: Throat is red, hot, and dry. The patient hawks and clears his throat constantly. Look for red, swollen tonsils, and swollen and painful submaxillary glands that are hot to the touch. The patient is very thirsty for cold water and cold things.

Countenance: Red is the color of the type. Look for a face that is red and hot, or for very red cheeks. Often the area of the cheeks and across the nose will be a bright red mask. Look for acne on the face. Blackheads on the nose, chin, and forehead are common to the type. Look for swollen veins in the forehead. The lips are bright red. The upper lip is swollen. Lips are dry. There may be herpes on the corner of the lips. The eyes are sunken, with blue rings around them.

The Sulphur patient looks worn out and older than he is.

The Sulphur Patient

Behavior: This is a vague, forgetful patient. He may not give good answers to questions put to him. Do not expect clear or concise symptoms. He very much wants humor, entertainment, and company. He wants games and food; usually salty and greasy foods. He will want to watch television, and play games, especially video games.

Characteristics: The whole idea of the remedy Sulphur is the idea of itch, especially when it is combined with the whole formula described above. The remedy has a special action on the skin. As much as he wants to drink, the patient will not want water on his skin. Look for red, itching rashes of all sorts. Look for the scruffy patient whose skin always looks dirty, no matter how he washes.

This is also a very important remedy for cases involving all sorts of indigestion, for cases of diarrhea that drive the patient out of bed first thing in the morning, and for acid indigestion and acid reflux.

Smell is important in understanding the Sulphur patient. It is characteristic of the type that just like Sulphur, the patient and all of his discharges smells like rotten eggs. Usually, the patient will be unaware of his smell.

Pains are throbbing and, of course, burning in nature. The patient also experiences the discomfort of swelling and congestion in parts of the body. Symptoms seem to ascend, to rush upward, especially hot flushes and rushes of blood to the head.

Pulse: The pulse is rapid, and is more rapid in the morning than in the night.

The patient may complain that he feels as if his heart were enlarged. He may feel a rush of blood to various parts of the body, especially the head, accompanied by itching and burning of his hands.

A fluttering sensation in the area of the heart may give way to palpitations. This may happen while the patient passes a stool, turns in bed, or ascends a stairs or hill.

Modalities: Worse: in a closed room; from weather changes; from bathing; from becoming hot; from touching wool; at 11:00A.M.; at night; from alcohol.

Better: in open air; from motion; from sweating; in warm, dry weather; from walking in open air.

Common Causes of Illness

Junk food diet; vaccination; mechanical injuries, especially falls and sprains; suppressing discharges, especially sweat; alcohol.

Common Uses

Colds, sore throats, coughs, bronchitis, pneumonia, tonsillitis, otitis media (ear infection); asthma; allergies of all sorts; mechanical injury, sprains, backache, bursitis; acid reflux, constipation, diarrhea, irritable bowel syndrome, colitis; skin conditions: rashes, eczema, psoriasis, seborrhea, dandruff, herpes, acne, abscesses; angina, arrhythmia; chronic fatigue; depression.

SYMPHYTUM

Source: Comfrey.

This is a small remedy with very simple uses in the home. It is our best remedy for cases of mechanical injury, especially those that have resulted in fracture. It is also very useful for blunt trauma to the eye and for black eyes. It is also used after amputations for phantom pains and what classically was called "irritable stump." Note: because of the rather specific action of this remedy, its portrait, for a good part, lacks the usual diagnostic guiding symptoms.

Theme: There is no specific theme of behavior. Rather, there is a theme of causation—physical trauma leading to mechanical injury.

About Symphytum

Morrison writes, "Symphytum is a remedy for injury. It has mainly been used for fractures, both acutely and in cases with non-union of fractures. It is also a useful remedy in injuries to periosteum and bone with persisting pains long after the injury. In blunt trauma to the eye, Symphytum is the specific remedy, though Arnica is more useful in injuries to the orbit."

The Symphytum Face

Eyes: As this is a black eye remedy (along with Arnica and Ledum), the first indication is the presence of a black eye. It is also useful for pain in the eyes after a mechanical injury, or for any trauma to the eye. Consider this remedy for all cases of injury in which, upon closing his eye, the patient feels as if the upper lid had passed over an elevation on the bulb of the eye itself. When the patient wakes, he will have great difficulty opening his eye. Look for his eyelids to be spasmodically closed.

Ears: The internal and/or external ears are inflamed. The patient cannot hear well.

Nose: There is pain down both sides of the nose.

Mouth: There are no guiding symptoms for this remedy.

Tongue: There are no guiding symptoms for this remedy.

Throat: There are no guiding symptoms for this remedy.

Countenance: The patient's skin is cold. Consider this remedy for injuries to the face, especially when the face is left swollen, or when the injury impacts upon the maxillary bone.

The Symphytum Patient

Behavior: There are no guiding symptoms for this remedy.

Characteristics: This remedy acts especially when there has been an injury to a bone and the attached tendon has been bruised. It may also be considered for cases in which pain lingers after healing has taken place, and for phantom pains after amputation. Symphytum is also very helpful (as is Arnica) for trauma to the eye, or a black eye.

Pulse: There are no guiding symptoms for this remedy.

Modalities: Worse: touch; motion; sitting or stooping; sexual excess.

Better: warmth.

Common Causes of Illness

Mechanical injury, falls, blows, blunt trauma (especially to the eye); sexual excess.

Common Uses

Mechanical injuries, fractures, bruises to soft tissue, blunt trauma to the eye; phantom pains after amputation; lingering pains after the healing of a mechanical injury.

URTICA URENS

Source: Stinging Nettle

As the remedy is taken from the stinging nettle, the theme of the remedy may be expressed as of being great use to those who suffer stinging or burning pains. This is most often used in the home for cases of burn or chicken pox (consider also Dulcamara). The Skin has itchy blotches on it. The blotches have a burning heat and are violently itchy, driving the patient nearly insane. The skin may also be swollen and fluid filled.

It is keynote of the remedy that the patient's itch disappears when he falls asleep, only to reappear and be even worse when he awakens. The patient will not want to go to sleep because of this effect. The patient is worse from bathing, exercise of any sort, and warmth in any form.

Theme: This is a very small remedy, with a specific action. It is suggested for the home kit because it works so well for those with simple burns. Because of this narrow action, the remedy has very few guiding symptoms other than the burning sensation itself.

About Urtica

Murphy writes, "Urt-U as its common name stinging nettle implies, it produces stinging or stinging-burning pains. Urt-U is one of the best remedies for burns of the first degree, used locally and given internally."

The Urtica Face

Eyes: The eyes are sore, as if they had sand in them, or as if they had been struck by a blow. Listen for the patient to complain of pain and pressure in his eyes and in the bones around them. The patient will rub and press on his eyes and the bones around them.

The patient's vision is weak.

Ears: The patient's external ears will be swollen.

Nose: There may be nosebleeds. It is said that a leaf placed on the tongue will stop this nosebleed. The patient's nose may be swollen. Note that the patient's nose will itch.

Mouth: The patient's lips may be swollen.

Tongue: There are no guiding symptoms for this remedy.

Throat: The patient may complain of pain in his throat. The pain will be accompanied with nausea. The patient may throw up frothy mucus. Nausea will be accompanied by coughing.

Countenance: The patient has an expression of pain. He has a dull aching pain in his head, especially over the eyes.

The Urtica Patient

Behavior: This is a somewhat drowsy patient. He tends to drift off to sleep, especially when he is reading.

Characteristics: In acute use, consider this remedy for two major sorts of pain: First, it is an excellent remedy for those who have been burned. Second, it is a wonderful remedy for those who suffer rheumatic pains of a burning nature. It must also be considered for cases of chicken pox, and for cases where the patient's skin is swollen and fluid filled. This remedy especially affects the skin, nerves, mammary glands, urinary organs, spleen, and liver.

It is a remedy that is given to right-sided symptoms in cases occurring naturally. In burns, of course, it does not matter which side of the body is affected.

Pulse: There are no guiding symptoms for this remedy.

Modalities: Worse: from touch; from cold, damp air, especially snowy air; from cold applications and cold bathing; from eating shellfish.

Better: from lying down, from rubbing.

Common Causes of Illness

Burns; insect stings, especially bee stings; eating shellfish.

Common Uses

Burns; insect bites and stings; fever; chicken pox; rheumatism.

PART THREE

Acute Applications for Homeopathic Remedies

The ear may not be as important in diagnosis as the eye or touch, yet we purpose employing it to its fullest capacity. To the routine physician who asks questions and depends for his knowledge of disease upon what the patient tells him, it is the organ of greatest importance. But we have already seen that we do best when we study disease with our senses, and depend but little upon what the patient says.

—JOHN SCUDDER, *SPECIFIC DIAGNOSIS*

Introduction

I put this guide together to assist readers in understanding homeopathic remedies and their acute uses. It considers various household emergencies, along with the homeopathic remedies most commonly used to treat each of them.

And because this is a guide to "objective" homeopathy, it stresses symptoms that can be objectively witnessed over those that can only be subjectively experienced. This means that I have not included ailments such as headache—an illness for which nearly all the guiding symptoms are subjective in nature. (This may be the reason why headaches are among the most difficult symptoms to treat homeopathically.)

So although this is not an exhaustive guide (see my previous book for that sort of guide), it is targeted toward increasing your understanding of the appropriate uses of homeopathic remedies in common situations, and sharpening your skills in selecting remedies by virtue of objective symptoms.

To make this guide easy to use, the most common household emergencies are divided into three basic categories:

The first category, First Aid, considers the remedies most often called upon to heal cases of physical trauma, ranging from wounds, cuts, and scrapes to blows to soft tissue in the body. First Aid also includes a consideration of injuries to joints and connective tissue under the subcategory of "injuries," and information on dealing with true emergencies, such as fainting and nosebleeds.

The second category of remedies are those needed in the treatment of Acute Ailments. For the most part, illnesses addressed in this category are those that are communicable, such as cold, coughs and flu.

The final category contains information on "homeopathic Band-Aids." As you will remember from past chapters, these are acute treatments of chronic conditions like allergies, indigestion, toothache, and headache. It is not the purpose of this section to suggest that it is possible for an acute treatment to cure a chronic complaint. These remedies are provided to give temporary relief to those suffering from chronic conditions until they can get to a medical professional's office for appropriate treatment.

I also list the remedies most often used for the conditions described in each category, taken from our list of fifty-two in Part Two of this book. These lists will help students who want to start working with homeopathic remedies in a finite and controlled manner. The suggested "first aid" kit of remedies—a much shorter list than the complete Objective Materia Medica in Part Two—gives the reader the option of investing less money in their first purchase of remedies, and the possibility of learning about this aspect of acute treatments before moving on to the others.

In addition to the remedies taken from our Objective Materia Medica, I also suggest some additional remedies that have some importance in treating a particular ailment. Obviously, there are simply too many homeopathic remedies on the market to include them all in the Objective Materia Medica. But since it is important to become familiar with as many remedies as possible, I mention others that you might want to research further in other materia medicas and consider for your home kit.

A quick note about potency and dosage: as I have stated before, the potency 30C is implied as the remedy of choice in all cases, unless another potency is specifically indicated. This is true for all internal remedies, and for all topical remedies created at home by dissolving remedy pellets in pure water. Topical remedies purchased in a prepared state will have their own potency levels. In all cases, remedies are given as needed, and stopped when improvement begins, until needed again.

Finally, it is my hope that the information contained in this section is as clear and concise as it can be so that the reader will have a better understanding of how and why homeopathic remedies are used in the acute sphere. When used correctly, the remedies listed here are all equally effective tools for healing.

First Aid

First Aid treatments are those given in emergency situations before appropriate medical services can be obtained. Therefore, first aid is commonly given at the site of the emergency, and those giving first aid need to be well-versed in their treatment of choice. The wounds, injuries, and emergencies that require first aid also require a calm head and a working knowledge of homeopathy on the part of the caregiver.

Unlike other acute treatments, first aid treatments often do not give the practitioner a chance to run and get his research books. The practitioner must have enough understanding of homeopathy to know the remedies most often used to treat emergencies, and what those remedies look like "on the hoof," in real situations. You, as the practitioner, must learn the remedies well enough to recognize them when they are played out in front of you.

Remedies Highly Recommended for the First Aid Kit

Aconite: Noted for its treatment of ailments that develop quickly, Aconite is also very helpful as an antishock remedy. It is extremely calming to patients who thrash about in fear and shock, and for those who fear death from their injuries. Aconite is often given in alternation with Arnica for cases of physical trauma and shock.

Apis: Since the remedy is taken from bee venom, think of it first for cases of bee stings. It is also useful for other puncture wounds and for injuries to knees. The affected area of the body will be red, swollen, shiny, and hot to the touch. The patient will crave cold applications, and often cold drinks.

Arnica: Perhaps the most important first aid remedy. Consider Arnica in all cases that involve blows to soft tissue and bruises anywhere on the body. Think of Arnica as a remedy that, in general, encourages the healing process throughout the body and assists and supports the body in withstanding pain.

Calendula: While it is most often considered a topical remedy, Calendula may be used topically or internally in the treatment of wounds. It assists the healing of cut, scraped, or ripped skin and acts as a natural antibiotic to keep wounds from becoming infected.

Hypericum: A multipurpose remedy that soothes nerve pain, heals lacerations, and is of great help in recovery after surgery and dental work. Hypericum may be used internally or topically. Hypericum is also an important remedy for those with rheumatic aches and pains associated with injuries, sprains, and strains. The pain will be worse during damp and especially foggy weather. Note that the patient who needs Hypericum often seems vague and foggy.

Ledum: This remedy can be helpful for cases as diverse as insect stings, black eyes, and sprained ankles. Look for the affected area to be black and blue, and cold and squishy to the touch. The patient will want cool applications on the affected area.

Rhus Tox: A superb pain remedy for those who have overworked or over-lifted, for those with creaky joints that sound like rusty hinges, and those with strains and sprains. Rhus Tox is often given after Arnica to complete the healing process for those strained muscles. This is a major remedy for stresses, strains, and sprains anywhere in the body, and for chronic complaints that arise from these injuries. Consider it for cases of rheumatic aches and pains that are worse during wet and damp weather and better from rubbing, heat, gentle motion, and hot baths.

Ruta: Another excellent remedy often used to finish the process that Arnica has begun. Ruta often cures pain in the lower back and hip area, such as that experienced by gardeners. Headache and eyestrain may accompany hip pain. It is also an excellent remedy for cases involving bruising of bone tissue and for shin splints associated with exercise.

Staphysagria: A great remedy for healing clean cuts and stab wounds. Staphysagria is excellent for pain control in patients extremely sensitive to pain. It is also very helpful in recovery from surgery, in which the doctor's incision is the "stab wound."

Symphytum: This is our best remedy for the speedy and complete healing of broken bones. It is often given as a follow-up to Arnica or in alternation with that remedy in cases of injury to both soft and hard tissue. Note that bones should be set in the emergency room before Symphytum is given. Arnica alone should be given until bones are set.

Remedies You May Want to Add to Your First Aid Kit

Bryonia: This remedy is useful for any injury in which the patient cannot move at all because the pain is too great. Bryonia is often considered a specific remedy for cases of broken or cracked ribs. It is also a general remedy for aches and pains, when the patient cannot move the affected area but the pain is improved by gentle pressure. This patient is temperamental and becomes angry in his discomfort, especially when moving or disturbed from rest.

Camphora: This is a good, general remedy for aches and pains associated with stress, sprains, or physical trauma, especially to the upper half of the body. The affected area will have pain that hampers free movement and will also feel cold, as if packed in snow or ice. The patient's feet will also feel icy cold. The patient will crave heat in any form and will be better from heat.

Causticum: This remedy assists those who have fallen and injured their coccyx (tailbone). It is useful for general pain in the lower back and for pain in the forearm. This is also a general rheumatic remedy for those with aches and pains predominately on the left side of the body. This is especially true of the neck. The Causticum patient feels improved during wet weather.

Chamomilla: This is an excellent remedy for cases in which a wound is slow to heal or becomes infected. The emotional symptoms of the patient will often be the indicator of the remedy—the patient is angry, irritable. He tends to rush and thrash about. He will throw things in anger.

China: Consider this remedy for cases in which the wound has bled a great deal. The patient is dealing with the loss of blood as well as the wound. The patient will tend to feel faint, and will be very pale and exhausted. A throbbing headache may accompany the wound. Note: think of this remedy first for cases in which the wound will not stop bleeding and the patient is quickly becoming weaker from blood loss.

Hepar Sulph: This is the remedy of first choice when a wound becomes reinfected, especially if it repeatedly becomes infected as it slowly heals. This is also a remedy for a bruise that fails to heal and becomes pus filled. Think of this remedy for the patient who seems to wound himself again and again, or for the patient whose wounds tend to become infected.

Lachesis: Another remedy for puncture wounds. The affected area will tend to itch, and will turn purple and swell after being scratched. The affected area will also tend to be filled with dark fluid or blood.

Silicea: This is our most important remedy for cases in which the patient is slow to heal, and when every scratch or wound forms scar tissue and unhealthy keloids. Note that the area of the skin involving the wound will look dirty and unhealthy.

Urtica Urens: One of the best homeopathic remedies used in the treatment of burns. This is an important remedy to have in the home at all times.

Remedies Not Contained in the Objective Materia Medica That May Be Useful in First Aid Cases

Bellis Perrennis: Think of this remedy as a deeper-acting Arnica. It often follows Arnica and clears away bruising that Arnica failed to cure. It is another remedy for physical traumas of all sorts.

Berberis: When pain radiates from one spot in either the top half or the bottom half of the body, or radiates throughout the body as a whole, consider the remedy Berberis. It should also be considered (along with Pulsatilla) for pains that shift and move throughout the body. The patient's whole body may feel beaten, stiff, and sore.

Cantharis: A remedy to be considered for wounds, especially puncture wounds that have the sensation of burning to them. This is a deep, powerful burning, as if the affected area had been held to a hot stove. Because of the quality of pain associated with Cantharis, it is also an excellent remedy for burns and scalds when this deep burning sensation defines the case. The patient will be restless in his pain.

Carbolicum Acidum: This remedy is useful for cases of bee stings in which the patient goes into shock. The patient may lapse into a coma.

His life will seem to be slipping away. The patient's face will be very pale, especially around his mouth.

Cimicfuga: This small remedy is very helpful for cases of palpitation or heart attack when the pain moves from the chest to the left shoulder and down the left arm. The patient will not be able to move his left arm at all; it may seem as if it were attached to his chest.

Natrum Sulphuricum: This is one of our most important rheumatic remedies. Those needing Natrum Sulphuricum will be extremely sensitive to damp, even to the dampness present in a basement or a cabin. It is, therefore, helpful to general aches and pains that are worse for damp. It is also to be considered for cases of physical trauma to the head, especially those that also involve long-term headache in the back of the neck.

Opium: Should be considered for cases of stroke (it is one of only three remedies for this purpose that are part of the home kit, along with Aconite and Belladonna), in which the patient is unconscious or semiconscious and in which the patient seems to be asleep. The patient's breathing will be that of a sleeping person, often with wheezing or snoring. The patient's face will be bloated and flushed.

Rhododendron: This is a remedy that mirrors the action of Rhus Tox in many ways. Like

Rhus Tox, it is a rheumatic remedy deeply affected by changes in weather. The Rhododendron patient will feel especially bad just before the onset of a storm. Like Dulcamara, many of the Rhododenron patient's aches and pains will be especially great in spring and autumn, when days are hot and nights are cool. Think of Rhododendron for stiff necks, and for general strains and sprains. Like Rhus Tox, the patient is worse for rest.

First Aid: Wounds

Let me begin by saying that as with other aspects of acute homeopathy, the very fact that homeopathic remedies are being used with wounds does not mean that we can omit the basis of common sense. In other words, wounds still need to be cleaned and examined for the presence of foreign matter before they are dressed and remedies are given.

And it is important that you stop the bleeding when dealing with a wound. This may be done by placing gentle pressure on the wound, or by placing the affected area under running water or applying ice to it.

Once the blood has stopped flowing and the wound is clean, it is important to dress the wound to protect it. In the absence of modern bandages, the wound should be wrapped in clean, dry cloth.

Deep wounds and those to the eyes or ears may require a trip to the emergency room. They may need stitches to heal correctly.

There are different types of wounds, and each requires different treatment:

Contused Wounds

These injuries are caused by the impact of some blunt object to the soft tissues beneath the skin. In some cases contused wounds may cause the skin to split, like those involving blunt trauma to areas of the body where the skin is close to the bone, such as the head. In such a case, the cut as well as the contusion will have to be treated.

Most commonly, contusions will involve damage to the soft tissues and organs beneath the skin. The affected area will tend to be swollen and discolored by bruises. Note that some areas of the body can be more deeply affected by contusions than others. Blows to the head, chest, and stomach may involve internal bleeding and damage that is not visible to the naked eye. In these cases, it is important to note changes such as increased pulse, troubled breathing, a feeling of faintness and/or weakness, and a pale face. These are indications of internal damage, and the patient exhibiting these signs with his contusion should be taken to the emergency room immediately.

For common contusions, the most effective treatment is **Arnica.** This remedy will clear away the bruises as it promotes quick healing to the body. It should be given as soon as possible after the injury, and can be repeated in 30C potency two or three times a day until improvement begins. Then it can be given as needed until the injury clears away. Once symptoms begin to improve, do not repeat the dosage; if symptoms grow worse or reappear, give another dose.

Note that **Arnica** may be dissolved in water and applied topically as well as internally if the skin is unbroken and there are no scratches, cuts, or other open wounds in addition to the contusion. This combination of the remedy—topically and internally in the same potency—will speed the healing of the wound. Never, under any circumstances, treat with **Arnica** if the skin is broken. It will cause the patient great pain. Instead, use **Calendula** to protect the area and keep it from infection when a topical homeopathic is needed for a cut accompanying a contusion.

If you have a case of a contusion that is slow to bruise, and the affected area feels cold and numb, then consider using the remedy **Ledum,** giving it two to three times a day.

When old bruises have failed to be reabsorbed into the body, consider using the remedy

Calcarea. This is an important remedy for cases that involve a failure to absorb or reabsorb.

Bruises

When blood gathers under a contusion, a bruise is the result.

And for most bruises, **Arnica** is the remedy of choice. It will reduce swelling by causing the body to reabsorb the trapped blood. **Arnica** will also relieve the pain associated with the trauma.

Bellis Perennis is called for with cases of deep bruising or bruises that do not heal from the **Arnica** treatment. Consider **Bellis** for cases in which the patient is experiencing deep muscle pain, or cases in which **Arnica** has failed to act after a day or two. (Note that **Bellis** is not a remedy listed in our Objective Materia Medica.)

Think of the remedy **Calcarea** for cases involving bruises that have changed color to blue or even brownish, but have not faded. Think of this remedy first for long-term bruising that fails to fade, as the blood has not been reabsorbed into the body.

Ledum should also be considered as a remedy for those with bruises, most often for bruises of the eye (black eye), ankle, or wrist. As is always the case with **Ledum,**

the patient will feel chilly and his wound will be chilly. He will want his body kept warm, but will want cold applications to his wound.

Ruta is excellent as a remedy for cases in which the bones are bruised. The **Ruta** patient will have great difficulty moving about. Consider this remedy especially for cases of shin splints associated with exercise.

Finally, think of **Hepar Sulph** when a bruise refuses to heal, or when the bruised area becomes infected and the affected area is pus filled. The bruised area will feel as though there were a splinter under the skin.

Incised Wounds

These are wounds in which the skin has been cut by a sharp object, like a knife. The damage is not only to the skin itself, but also to tissue beneath the skin to the extent that the foreign object has entered.

The difficulty with an incised wound is that it may be very difficult to stop the bleeding. And depending upon the depth of the wound, the incised wound may require stitches to heal correctly.

Staphysagria and **Hypericum** are our two most important remedies in dealing with incisions. If the pain associated with the wound is in the wound itself, or if the pain is so great that it seems to overwhelm the patient's life force, consider **Staphysagria.**

However, if the pain associated with the wound seems to travel on nerves throughout the body, especially along an arm or leg, then the remedy of choice is **Hypericum.**

If the wound is shallow and no internal remedy is required, then either **Hypericum** or **Calendula** should be considered. Again **Hypericum** is excellent for the pain associated with the remedy. It will also encourage healing and assist the skin in gathering the two cut parts together (this will especially be true with lacerations). **Calendula,** as always, will protect the area from infection and speed healing.

There are those who would say that the two remedies, **Hypericum** and **Calendula,** could be used concurrently to speed healing, with **Hypericum** taken internally and **Calendula** applied topically. This treatment could certainly be considered for cases of severe incision.

If the incision is deep and bleeding cannot be contained, consider the remedy **China.** In the portrait of this remedy, the patient is weak from blood loss and may pass out. He is weak, pale, and growing weaker as more blood is lost.

If the wound is becoming infected, consider the remedy **Chamomilla.** In the portrait of this remedy, the wound is slow to heal, or is becoming infected. The patient's actions will often indicate the need for this remedy, as the patient will be very angry in his pain and may throw things at those who attempt to help him.

And if the incision is slow to heal, or seems not to be healing correctly, consider **Silicea.** Those needing this remedy will find that their wound is not healing at all, or is healing very slowly. The wound appears to be in danger of infection, and is forming keloids or scars instead of healing cleanly.

Finally, think of **Hepar Sulph** if the wound tends to become reinfected, or in the case of the patient who tends to wound himself again and again.

Note that surgical incisions are to be considered incised wounds for the purposes of homeopathic treatment. Therefore, **Staphysagria** and **Hypericum** will be the most important remedies for surgical recovery. **Arnica** may also be an important remedy to encourage the body's ability to heal after surgery. Dental treatments should also be considered incisions. They are often best treated by dissolving **Hypericum** in water and using the **Aqua Hypericum** as a mouth-wash.

Lacerated Wounds

These are wounds in which the skin is not only broken, but quite often is also ripped. And although lacerations tend to bleed less than do incisions, they may be much slower to heal and can be harder to treat. In lacerated wounds the damage is not only to the skin, but also to the muscles, nerves, and blood vessels that lie below the skin. These injuries can be caused by human-machine contact, such as putting your hand in a garbage disposal. It is important to note that lacerations often are complicated by contamination from contact with the machine or weapon that caused them.

It is also important to note that gunshots should be considered lacerated wounds, because of the ripping damage they cause.

Hypericum is the most important remedy for lacerations of all sorts. Where **Staphysagria** may be the remedy of choice for a nice clean cut to the skin, **Hypericum** is always the first choice remedy for a ragged wound. It will help the skin to heal cleanly and easily. It may be used both internally and topically to enhance its actions. It may be used concurrently with **Arnica;** this is especially true of deep lacerations. In these cases, give

Arnica internally and **Hypericum** externally. The **Arnica** may be given two to three times a day, and the **Hypericum** should be repeated hourly until relief is attained.

If, over time, the wound is slow to heal, the two most important remedies are **Silicea** and **Chamomilla.** The patient's actions will help you decide which to use. If the patient is weakened by his wound, and seems unable to heal and to be fading away, consider **Silicea.** This patient will be chilly and weak. If, however, the patient is angry in his illness or his wound seems to be becoming infected, consider **Chamomilla.**

Finally, if there is a pattern in the patient's health in that every little wound he receives becomes infected, consider the remedy **Hepar Sulph.** This is also the remedy of choice for cases in which a wound tends to become reinfected.

Animal bites. Note that animal bites may be considered to be lacerated wounds, in that the bite rips the skin and damages the tissue beneath it. In acute homeopathic treatment, they are to be considered for treatment just as any other lacerations. But make no mistake about it, animal bites can be dangerous. They may be a cause for a trip to an emergency room or to a medical professional's office, and the practitioner must be told the cause of the wound.

Note also that a particular form of laceration, a scratch to the eye's cornea, will often require the remedy **Hypericum** in order to heal properly. Although the eye heals quickly, **Hypericum** may be given even after scar tissue has formed. For best results, it should be given in the high potency of 1M for one or two doses.

Puncture Wounds

Whether caused by a needle, a nail, a thorn, an insect's stinger, or a splinter, puncture wounds are all considered and treated in the same manner in acute homeopathy. A long, sharp object has cut into the body, and while the injury to the skin is usually insignificant, the damage to soft tissue deeper in the body may be very significant. Also, puncture wounds often become infected. In the worst cases they may cause concern regarding tetanus.

The two most common remedies for use in treating punctures are **Ledum** and **Apis.** **Ledum** is called for if the wound is blue, or black and blue (bruised looking). The skin will feel numb and cold around the wound, and yet the patient may want cool applications on the wound. **Apis** is called for if the wound and the area around it are swollen and shiny red in color and the wound is hot to the touch. The patient will want cold applications on the wound, and he also may be very thirsty for cold water. Further, **Apis** is one of our angry remedies, so the patient needing it may be very impatient with you for your inability to instantly heal his wound.

Lachesis may also be called for in puncture wounds. The area surrounding the wound may itch, and it will swell when it is scratched or touched. The swelling will be filled with dark fluid or blood. The wound will be purple or bluish in color.

Hypericum should also be considered for cases of puncture wounds. As always, the indicator of the remedy is that the wound will hurt not only at the site of the injury: the pain will also travel along a nerve in the body, usually in the arm or the leg.

If a puncture wound has the sensation of burning (as if the skin had been burned on a stove and not punctured), **Cantharis** or **Urtica Urens** may be the remedy. **Cantharis** is useful for general punctures with a burning sensation; **Urtica Urens** is useful for a bee sting with a burning sensation.

Insect stings and snake bites. As noted above, insect stings and snake bites are to be considered punctures because of the quality of these wounds. But, because they may contain poisonous venom in addition to the wound itself, they may require other treatments.

For bee stings, **Apis, Ledum,** and **Urtica Urens** are common treatments. Note the descriptions of the **Apis** and **Ledum** wounds above. **Urtica Urens** will be helpful for bee stings in which the patient's major sensation of pain is burning.

For wasp stings, **Apis, Ledum,** and **Arnica** are the most common remedies. **Arnica** is used when the sting leaves the patient feeling beaten up and bruised. The affected area will be black and blue.

For snake bite, **Hypericum** is considered the best remedy.

Note that some patients will be very sensitive to bee stings. In fact, some may be so sensitive to the sting that their life is in danger. For cases of severe reaction to bee stings, consider either **Apis** or **Carbolicum Acidum.** The **Carbolicum Acidum** patient will be overwhelmed by the impact of the sting. His face will be very pale, especially around the mouth. He may lapse into a coma. The **Apis** patient, on the other hand, will be angry and impatient. Look for the indicative bright red and shiny swelling of the affected area, and for swelling in other parts of the body as well, especially in the throat. The patient will be very thirsty for cold water, and may be unable to swallow anything but water.

Note that, whatever remedy is used, the patient who is allergic to bee stings should get to a hospital immediately for treatment.

Splinters

Finally, while splinters are to be considered puncture wounds, they do have their differences. In the case of a splinter, a foreign object has become trapped in or below the skin.

The treatment of a splinter usually involves the external use of either **Hypericum** or **Calendula**. **Hypericum** is useful for cases in which the patient experiences nerve pain radiating from the splinter. **Hypericum** is also thought to be preventative for tetanus. **Calendula** is most useful if the possibility exists that the splinter may become infected.

Internally, the remedy of first choice is **Silicea**. **Silicea** will actually help the body to expel the foreign object. It will also help heal the wound if any infection is present.

Another common remedy for splinters is **Ledum.** This remedy is especially useful for deeply set splinters and for splinters that have become infected. Look for the area around the splinter to be swollen, red, and pus filled. The patient will tend to be chilly, and the affected area will also feel cold, both to the patient and to the touch. While the patient will want his body to be warm, he will want cool applications to the affected area.

Scrapes and Scratches

These are any wounds in which a break to the skin allows blood to flow out and, quite possibly, infection to flow in. Deep abrasions may also be contaminated with dirt and stone. It is important that the wound be cleansed under running water and the bleeding stopped. Do not touch the wound.

Calendula lotion is the remedy of first choice in dealing with scrapes and scratches. It will heal the wound and protect it from infection. It is especially helpful in scrapes and scratches on the patient's face. **Calendula** may be applied as often as needed. It may also be taken internally as well as used externally.

Arnica is also often used in case of scrapes and scratches. But remember that **Arnica** is only to be used internally, and never externally when the skin is broken. If **Arnica** is applied to broken skin it will cause the patient a great deal of discomfort.

Hypericum is also helpful for cases of scrapes in which the patient feels nerve pain as a result of his wound.

And, finally, **Staphysagria** can be very helpful if the wound seems to be very painful or if the patient seems to be feeling much more pain from the wound than he should (from the appearance of the injury). **Staphysagria** is always a remedy of choice when the experience of pain outstrips the injury itself.

First Aid: Injuries

The category of injuries is both broad and general. In it, we consider strains and sprains, in which the affected areas are muscles, tendons, and/or ligaments. In these injuries, the muscles and the connective tissue around the bone have either been stretched too far, or violently twisted. In minor cases, the tissue has merely been stretched and will pull back to its previous condition in time. In more serious cases, the tissue itself has been ruptured or torn away from its regular position.

In this category we also consider injuries to individual parts of the body, from the head down to the ankles and feet. These injuries may be cause by blows or by strains and sprains. Whatever the cause, this category considers the treatment of the body's inner tissue for cases where the skin is not broken and there is no visible wound.

Note that while we consider injuries to be acute ailments, they may have chronic phases as well. Often parts of the body (especially the joints) that were injured in the past are left weakened, and they are liable to be injured again easily. The chronic complaints based upon acute injuries are often rheumatic in nature, which is to say they are greatly affected by changes in the weather. Some remedy suggestions for the chronic phases of acute injuries are provided below.

Sprains and Strains in General

While sprains and strains may differ in specific cause and in degree of severity, they basically involve the same situation—a muscle, or a part of the connective tissue that joins muscle to bone, has been stretched and/or twisted out of its usual position.

In all cases of strains or sprains, **Arnica** is considered the remedy of first choice. **Arnica** may be used topically by dissolving it in water. A cloth is moistened in the **Aqua Arnica** and placed gently over the affected area. **Arnica** may also be given internally at the same time to increase its healing power.

Note that the affected limb or body part should, if possible, be elevated and kept perfectly still after the topical **Arnica** treatment is in place.

Other than **Arnica,** which may well act as a curative remedy in and of itself, there are a handful of other remedies to consider for strain and sprains. The chief among them are **Rhus Tox** and **Bryonia.** These two remedies will be very easy to tell apart, because the **Rhus Tox** patient will want to keep moving. He will feel that the affected area of his body will tighten up if he doesn't keep it moving. The **Bryonia** patient, on the other hand, will not want to move at all. He will find it too painful to move the affected area, and will keep it frozen from any motion if he can.

Note that even though the **Rhus Tox** patient wants to keep moving the injured part, it still hurts him. But if he doesn't keep it moving it will lock in place, and will hurt all the more on first motion. For this reason, it is called the "rusty gate" remedy; the first motion is the hardest, just like forcing open a gate that has rusted in place. If the **Rhus Tox** moves with continued, gentle motion, the affected part will actually feel better. But if he overdoes his movements, the initial improvement will cease, and the part will be all the more painful with motion.

You may find that **Arnica** is very helpful in starting the healing process in some cases, but that it does not seem capable of completing it by itself. After a while the patient seems to stop getting better. In these cases, you may need another remedy to complete the cure that **Arnica** has begun.

Rhus Tox is the most common remedy used to complete **Arnica's** cure. It is especially helpful for cases of back injury or strain, either acting on its own or following **Arnica.** Consider it as your second remedy, but only if the patient follows the general portrait of the remedy's symptoms. **Ruta** is another remedy that can finish what **Arnica** has begun. This is especially true when the injury has occurred to tendons or ligaments. It also completes cases of lower back injury or hip pain.

Used on its own, **Ruta** is an excellent remedy to consider for cases of shin splints after too much exercise, or runner's knee, which also is caused by overwork. In fact, **Ruta** should be considered (along with **Apis**) for any knee injury. It is characteristic of the **Ruta** condition that the patient will have particular problems going upstairs because of knee pain.

Apis, as mentioned earlier, is another major remedy for strains and sprains. When **Apis** is called for, the injured area of the body will be red, swollen, shiny, and hot to the touch. The patient will want cold applications placed on the injury.

Note that **Apis** and **Rhus Tox** work with special affinity in treating sprains and strains.

Either remedy may follow the other in completing the case. Make sure to follow the total pattern of the patient's symptoms in selecting which to use first.

In some cases, **Rhus Tox** will be seem to be perfectly called for as the remedy of choice, but will fail to work. In those cases, consider the remedy **Anacardium** (which is not included in the Objective Materia Medica).

For old sprains and strains that refuse to heal, consider the remedy **Zinc,** (also not included in the Objective Materia Medica) which is also excellent for nightly muscle cramps in the legs that wake the patient from his sleep.

If a joint, especially the knee or ankle, has been injured repeatedly until it is permanently weakened, consider **Natrum Mur.** If soft tissue has been permanently weakened, consider **Calcarea.**

For rheumatic complaints originating from injuries or repeated injuries to a specific set of muscles or joints, there are several remedies to consider, based generally upon the symptoms and their reaction to weather changes.

For pains that begin suddenly when there is a cold wind, consider the remedy **Aconite.** If the aches and pains are worse in wet or damp weather, consider **Rhus Tox.** If the aches and pains are worse in damp, and, especially, foggy weather, consider **Hypericum.** If the aches and pains are worse just as wet weather—especially a thunderstorm—is coming on, consider **Rhododendron** (a remedy not listed in the Objective Materia Medica). If the aches and pains are better in damp weather, consider **Causticum.** If the aches and pains are worse in the spring or, especially, the fall, when days are hot and nights are cold, consider **Dulcamara.**

Injuries to the Head

Head injuries, especially those caused by car accidents or other mechanical means, are nothing to fool around with. An ambulance should be called immediately, and any first aid remedy given should be given to keep the patient in the best shape possible until he can get to the hospital.

After a serious head injury, the patient may vomit, and frequently his mouth will be filled with blood. It is, therefore, very important that the patient not be allowed to lie on his back, because he risks the possibility of choking on his own blood or vomit. So, gently turn the patient to his side, and make sure his mouth is open to prevent the inhalation of blood or vomit.

The danger of a blow to the head is, of course, a concussion. The important symptoms of concussion include headache, disrupted sense of sight, trembling throughout the body, and rapid pulse. The patient will tend to be nauseated and to want nothing more than to sleep. The situation may be even worse if the patient's pulse begins to slow and if he becomes semiconscious or unconscious, and if his skin becomes cold and pale.

Even if the patient is coherent and insists that nothing is wrong with him, make sure to take the blow to the head seriously. Try to get the patient to rest, even if he is sure that he is fine. And, if you suspect that anything is out of order in his behavior or symptoms, call that ambulance.

Note that **Arnica** patients will often insist that they are fine when they are not. They do this because they are in shock and because the **Arnica** patient fears being touched. They equate touch with pain, and will therefore lie and tell you they are fine to get you to leave them alone. So the patient with a blow to the head who insists he is fine is virtually crying out for **Arnica.** In any case, whether the patient cooperates or not, and whether he is conscious after the blow or not, **Arnica** is the remedy of first choice for those with head injuries.

If after **Arnica** has been given (and, in severe cases, remember that it can be repeated until improvement begins), you notice that the patient has half-open eyes, as if he lacked the strength to keep them open, and he complains of pain in the back of the head, then you may want to follow the **Arnica** with **Gelsemium.**

If the patient does not seem to fully recover after the treatment with **Arnica,** and especially if his symptoms primarily include a headache that never seems to go away, then give the patient a dose or two of **Natrum Sulphuricum.** This remedy is known for its excellence in curing concussions and head injuries after which the patient does not seem like his old self.

Finally, for the patient who, after a trauma to the head, experiences a throbbing headache and sees sparks before his eyes, consider the remedy **Belladonna.** The **Belladonna** patient will not be able to bear any sort of light or noise. He will want to be in a quiet place. He will tend to be sleepy in his pain, but will be unable to sleep.

Eye Injuries

Again, these are not to be fooled around with, as nearly any injury to the eye can have serious repercussions.

The most general treatment for any injury to the eye involves giving **Arnica** (either in the usual 30C or the high potency of 200C or 1M, depending upon the seriousness of the injury) internally, while dissolving **Hypericum** in cool to just-warm water (whichever the patient desires). This solution is used to moisten a cloth, which is then gently placed over the eye.

Some texts call the remedy **Aconite** the "Arnica of the eye," and strongly suggest that you use this remedy internally instead of **Arnica.** I suggest that you use the portraits

of the two remedies to decide which to use. The **Arnica** patient will tend to say that he is fine and will refuse to let you examine his eye. The **Aconite** patient, on the other hand, will tend to be nearly hysterical in his pain and will fear the worst from his injury.

A blow to the eye, or a black eye, may call for the usual remedy, **Arnica.** But, if the area of the injury is black-and-blue and cold to the touch, and the patient reports that the affected area is numb and desires cold applications on his eye, give the patient **Ledum** to cure the injury. Note that **Ledum** also often acts as a secondary remedy given after **Arnica** to complete the cure.

Another remedy for blunt trauma to the eye is **Symphytum.** In this case the injury will take on a purplish color.

For cases of foreign objects in the eye, consider using **Aqua Hypericum** to wash the object away. If the object resists the actions of **Hypericum,** or if pain persists after the object is gone, consider using **Aqua Euphrasia** in just the same way. Usually, the eye that needs **Euphrasia** will be watering profusely because of the discomfort caused by the foreign object. Note that, if you discover that any foreign object has become embedded in the eye, you must get the patient to an emergency room or medical professional's office as soon as possible.

For cuts in or around the eye, dissolve **Calendula** in water and then moisten a cloth with **Aqua Calendula.** Apply this cloth to the wound, and then apply gentle pressure until the bleeding stops. Continue to apply **Calendula** to the injury to complete the healing process and keep the cut from becoming infected. The remedy **Aconite** may be given internally, while **Calendula** is used externally for cases of cuts in or around the eye.

If the cornea of the eye is scratched, consider one of a handful of remedies. The first remedy to consider is again **Hypericum,** which may be taken internally or used directly as **Aqua Hypericum** on a clean cloth. Another remedy is **Belladonna.** It may be used either for a blow to the eye or a scratch on the eye if the eye becomes bright red, bloodshot, and very hot. The eye itself will tear profusely, and becomes very sensitive to light. The patient will complain of a throbbing in the eye. He will usually be is such great pain from his injury that he cannot sleep or sit still; he will pace in pain.

Another remedy to consider is **Apis.** In cases that call for **Apis,** the eye again will be red and swollen. Look for the patient's eyelids to swell. The eye itself may swell so that the iris of the eye will look as if it were sitting in a shallow depression. Note the characteristic shiny redness of the affected part. The eye will be hot, and the patient's tears will also be hot. The patient will want cold applications on the eye.

Now, sometimes injuries to the eye will take on two different and distinct stages. The first is from the moment of injury to the flow of clear tears. As the tears take on color and become thicker, the second stage has begun.

Mercurius is often the remedy needed to clear away the second stage of an eye injury. When **Mercurius** is called for, the discharge from the eye is yellow or yellow/green and thick. The eye will be incredibly sensitive to light, and any glare will cause great pain. The discomfort will be worse at night.

The patient who needs **Pulsatilla** for the second stage of an injury will also have yellow or yellow/green discharge, but he will become worse by being in a warm room. Both the patient and his eye will be better for sitting by an open window or going outside. Cold applications will also make the patient feel better. Note that, in general, the **Pulsatilla** is a gentle, yet demanding patient. He tends to feel very sorry for himself in his plight, and will play upon your feelings of guilt and pity to keep you doing what he wants.

Ear Injuries

Injuries to the ear, especially the internal ear, can be just as serious as eye injuries. The most common injury to the ear happens when a foreign object—anything from a stick to an insect—is stuck into the ear. In this case the ear canal may be damaged, or worse, the eardrum punctured.

In this case, it is important to seek medical attention immediately. This is especially true if the patient has a history of ear infections and/or chronic discharges, or if you have reason to believe that the eardrum has been punctured.

If the situation does not seem so serious, you may choose to remove the object yourself. Make sure to look into the ear and see if you can locate and identify the object. Gently remove it. After doing so, you may wish to put a drop or two of either **Aqua Hypericum** or **Aqua Calendula** into the ear with a dropper. Make sure that the water is warm beforehand.

Now, make sure that you treat the patient as a whole, and not just the ear. If the ear pain or injury has started suddenly, or if the patient seems in a good deal of pain and is overly anxious or fearful as a result, give **Aconite.** This remedy may be repeated as necessary until the patient begins his improvement.

Neck Injuries

Neck injuries can, of course, be very serious things. If a patient has had a severe neck injury—for example, from a car accident or a fall from a horse—call 911 immediately. **Arnica** should be given until help arrives.

But most injuries to the neck, or neck pains in general, are far more benign. Most are caused by sleeping badly or by everyday stress. Sometimes, like back pain, the neck can be stressed by over-lifting. The problem that challenges us is that general, acute neck pain can become a chronic condition so easily. At this point it is often affected by the weather.

If the neck pain is caused by whiplash because the neck has been sharply shaken in an accident, the remedy of first choice is **Bryonia.** The **Bryonia** patient will not want to move his neck at all, as every slight motion brings on great pain. Further, he will not want his neck touched by anyone, but gentle pressure on his neck will actually make it feel better.

Hypericum may also be considered for whiplash. Here the pain will be accompanied by a sensation of numbness or tingling. The pain will extend from the neck to the patient's shoulder and into his back.

Natrum Sulphuricum is a remedy for neck pain, just as it is for head injury. Think of this remedy for cases involving neck injury or pain as a result of physical trauma. Note that **Natrum Sulphuricum** may be considered as a secondary remedy to **Arnica,** which would often be the remedy of first choice for cases of neck injury due to blunt trauma.

There are several remedies to consider for the patient who is suffering from the condition torticollis, or "wry neck," in which neck pain and stiffness combine to restrict the motion of the neck. For instance, if the neck is more painful on the left than on the right, and if the stiffness extends to the area between the shoulder blades, the usual remedy is **Causticum.**

Chelidonium will also have the neck frozen and more painful on the left. But in this case, the pain in the neck travels to the right scapula. In addition, the patient will say that his head feels heavy. The head particularly and the whole patient in general will also feel cold, and the patient will crave heat in any form. Note that **Chelidonium** is not in the Objective Materia Medica.

If the neck is stiff and fixed in a raised position (as if the patient is looking up at the ceiling), then the remedy to consider is **Cimicifuga,** which is also not in the Objective Materia Medica. The patient needing **Cimicfuga** will experience tenderness in the whole of the upper spine.

A good general remedy to have on hand for pain or stiffness in the neck is **Berberis,** which is also not in the Objective Materia Medica. Berberis is a rheumatic remedy that is an excellent choice for pains that extend from the neck into the shoulders, the arms, the hands and the fingers. The **Berberis** patient is worse from standing, and better from resting.

Other remedies for rheumatic pains in the neck include **Rhododendron,** which is excellent if the pain and stiffness are dominant on the right side and if the pain is worse in wet weather. The pain extends into the shoulder and arm, and down even into the wrist and hand.

Rhus Tox is an excellent general remedy for aches and pains in the neck brought on by damp and/or wet weather. The pain will be improved by gentle rubbing or pressure. It will also be better if the patient continually and gently moves the pained area. A hot shower or a warm application will generally improve the pain as well.

Finally, **Dulcamara** is the remedy to consider if you feel that your neck pain started because you "slept funny." The **Dulcamara** patient is improved by heat and is worse from getting chilled. Often the neck pain will recur annually, especially in the autumn, when the days are warm and the nights cool.

Shoulder Injuries

Shoulder pain is more often associated with chronic stress than it is with a specific physical trauma. If may be caused by carrying an unbalanced load, like the student who carries a too-heavy backpack to school, especially if he carries it only over one shoulder.

Most of the time, what is called shoulder pain is not really exclusive to that part of the body. Most shoulder pain will begin in the neck, and extend down through the shoulders. It may extend through the entire upper half of the body.

Therefore, in considering a remedy for shoulder pain, make sure to also find out about other closely associated areas of the body. Make sure your answer is not hidden away under "neck pain," and you are missing it by insisting that there are solid lines limiting pains to certain parts of the body. There are not.

If the pain in question extends pretty much through the whole upper half of the body, the remedy **Berberis,** noted above, may often be the answer although it is not in the Objective Materia Medica. The **Berberis** pain extends from the neck to the shoulder, arm, wrist, and hand.

If the patient complains that his neck feels as if it were grinding down on his shoulder every time it moves, or if the interior of the shoulder feels dry and as if it were grinding on itself when moving, then the remedy may be **Bryonia.** As usual with this remedy, the patient will not want to move in general and will be all but unable to move his shoulders.

The patient needing the remedy **Camphora** will also have difficulty moving because of pain. Here the pain tends to center in between the shoulder blades and radiate from there. The affected area is cold as well as painful. And the patient's feet may be cold as well during periods of pain. The patient will crave heat in any form.

As usual, **Rhus Tox** will be useful here as well. The patient needing this remedy will feel tightness and a burning sensation in the shoulders as well as general pain. The patient will feel that he needs to constantly move his shoulders to keep the muscles from shrinking and locking in place. Think of this remedy first for cases in which the pain is caused by overwork or over-lifting.

Finally, consider **Sulphur** for cases in which the patient has pain only in his left shoulder. This pain may be chronic and rheumatic in nature. Look for the patient to bend his shoulder forward to relieve the pain. This is a pain that tends to develop slowly and build over time. Look for the patient's hands, and possibly feet, to be hot and sweaty during times of pain.

Injuries to the Spine

The spine may be jarred or injured in an accident, such as a car accident, or by an accidental fall. If you suspect that the injury may be at all serious, call 911 immediately.

For less serious injuries, **Arnica** is the remedy of first choice. Let the severity of the situation and the patient's degree of pain determine whether you use the lower 30C or higher 1M potency. You may need to follow the **Arnica** with **Hypericum,** which may be given if pain continues after healing has begun. Give **Hypericum** in the regular 30C dose, as needed, for two or three days or until improvement has begun.

Note that **Ignatia** is sometimes considered to be a remedy that is specific to the spine and injuries of the spine. Consider this remedy if the patient displays the usual emotional pattern of Ignatia.

Back Injuries

As with the other parts of the body in this category, the back is usually injured either by over-lifting, stressing or straining, or by physical trauma, like a fall or car accident. And like those other injuries, back injuries are to be considered acute situations, although they may have chronic implications if they are not properly treated.

In most cases, pain in the upper back will be associated with shoulder pain. Therefore, pains that begin in the neck or shoulders and travel downward, or pains centered between the shoulder blades should be treated with remedies listed under "shoulder injuries." The back remedies listed here tend to be those associated with either lumbago, or lower back pain, or with sciatica, which is back pain that involves the sciatic nerve and travels downward into the leg.

When the patient has lower back pain caused by an injury or a strain or sprain, the remedy of first choice is **Arnica.** It will be all but impossible for this patient to find a comfortable position. Every surface will seem too hard. This patient will be like the princess with a pea placed under her mattress: sleep will be all but impossible. Yet the patient may insist that nothing is wrong with him, and certainly will not want to be touched or examined.

Sudden, sharp pains in the lower back suggest either **Aconite** or **Belladonna.**

Cases that respond to **Aconite** will occur after the patient has become overheated while out of doors or when he is in contact with cold wind. This patient will be restless and even frantic in his pain.

The **Belladonna** case, on the other hand, will involve a sudden, severe, cramping pain in the lower back. The patient in this case cannot thrash about, but must stay very still because his pain is so great. The patient will feel as if his back will break from the pain. Look for the patient to have a bright red face and a hot head while in pain.

Another patient who cannot move because of his pain is the **Bryonia,** but the **Bryonia** patient will want to rest against a hard object or lie on the floor to get relief.

If the patient is totally and completely paralyzed by his pain, think of **Causticum.** The pain will tend to be worse on the left or to begin on the left side of the body, and will experience a sensation of weight as well as pain. This is a rheumatic remedy in which the patient will feel better in wet or damp weather.

If the pain becomes so great that the patient is actually nauseated because of his back pain, consider **Antimonium Tartaricum.** In this case the pain continues without ceasing. The patient will be worse from cold and will be covered in a cold sweat. He will try to stand and will feel better when standing.

For general backaches and lower back pain, especially chronic lower back pain, think of **Natrum Mur** and **Rhus Tox.** The **Natrum Mur** patient will experience pain from stress or emotional upset, the **Rhus Tox** from overwork or over-lifting. Both will want to rest because of their pain, but only the **Natrum Mur** patient will be able to do so. This patient will take to his bed in pain. The **Rhus Tox** patient will want to rest, but will feel that he has to keep moving to keep his back muscles from freezing up.

And don't forget **Rhododendron** as an alternative or a follow-up remedy to **Rhus Tox.** As is often the case, the symptoms can look a great deal alike, but the **Rhododendron** patient's pain is worse on the right side of the body. Further, the **Rhododendron** patient is worse as a thunderstorm approaches. His pain may also be worse during cold, wet weather and may improve and grow worse with each little change in the weather.

Sepia is another good general remedy for those with lower back pain. The patient will desire firm support for his back and will feel that his lower back is heavy with pain. There is also a sensation of stiffness associated with the pain. The **Sepia's** lower back is often chronically weakened by his pain. Look for a sensation of coldness between the shoulder blades to accompany the pain.

Chronic lower back pain associated with constipation often calls for **Nux.** Here the patient will be very much worse from any contact with cold, especially cold wind. The pain will have a bruising nature. This is an impatient, angry, demanding patient. The pain will often be caused by overwork and working hard to meet deadlines.

If the lower back pain has become truly chronic and seems hopeless, consider **Calcarea.** The **Calcarea** patient has usually surrendered to the situation and will tell you that he has a "weak back." Most often, the weakened lower back will be associated with overweight and with weak, underdeveloped abdominal muscles.

If lower back pain is associated with specific motions or body positions, we have some other remedies to consider:

Backaches that become worse when the patient stoops may require either **Dulcamara** or **Sulphur.** The **Dulcamara** patient will be worse from exertion and worse from damp or cold. The **Sulphur** patient will be hot and sweaty in his pain. The **Sulphur** pain will dominate on the left side of the body.

For true lumbago, the best remedy may be **Ruta.** The patient will often feel that his lower back pain extends into his hips and legs. Often the pain will be terrible in the mornings before the patient can get out of bed. In fact, getting out of bed or out of a chair may be the most painful thing you can ask a **Ruta** to do. The backache will be better from gentle pressure and from lying down on the back.

If the patient with lower back pain cannot bear to be in a sitting position, consider **Ammonium Muriaticum,** which is not in our Objective Materia Medica. The pain in this case will extend into the patient's coccyx (tailbone) when he is sitting.

Finally, again, consider **Berberis** for lower back pain that extends throughout the entire body and into the extremities, and when the pain is centered in the region of the kidneys and extends from there. It is also useful for cases in which the pains shift and wander throughout the body. The back pain will be worse from any movement, and from standing up.

For cases of Sciatica, in which pressure on the sciatic nerve causes pain and numbness in the buttocks and legs, we have some other remedies to consider.

For cases of sciatic pain that are worse on first motion, consider **Rhus Tox** or **Gelsemium.** The difference is that the **Gelsemium** patient will stay still or will move only very slowly because of the initial pain. The **Rhus Tox** patient, on the other hand, will move through the pain, and will continue to move the affected area to keep stiffness from setting in.

For sciatica in the left leg, consider **Causticum, Colocynthis,** or **Kali Bi.** The **Causticum** pain is accompanied by numbness and the patient will walk unsteadily, as if his legs were about to give out from under him. His ankles will feel weak. The **Colocynthis** patient's pain will shoot all the way down the left leg to the foot. Numbness will accompany pain. Pain will be worse from motion, although this is a restless patient who may want to keep moving in spite of pain. The **Kali Bi** patient has left-sided pain that occurs only in one specific spot. The patient will be able to point to the exact spot that is painful.

Right-sided sciatica suggests **Lycopodium** or **Magnesia Phosphorica.** The **Lycopodium** patient will have pain in the right leg that is worse from pressure, and, especially, from lying on his right side. The leg feels numb and heavy. The pain is worse at 4:00P.M. The **Mag Phos** patient, on the other hand, has pain that is lightning-like in nature. The pain is sudden and electrical, and worse from any sudden motion, like the jerking that comes from sneezing. The affected areas feel numb and still.

Sepia patients will experience sciatica in both lower limbs. The legs will feel heavy, lame, and stiff. The patient will have difficulty moving. A pain in the heels will accompany sciatic pains. The patient will often turn to exercise to relieve pain. He may experience chronic sciatica.

Another remedy for chronic sciatica is **Arsenicum.** The **Arsenicum** patient is weary from chronic rheumatic pains. This is a patient who likely will suffer from long-term periodic attacks of sciatica that are worse at night, and better from heat and gentle motion. The sciatica will have a stinging sensation.

Finally, consider **Natrum Sulphuricum,** which is not in our Objective Materia Medica. This is an excellent general rheumatic remedy to consider in general cases of sciatica that tend to be worse on the left side. The patient will have a pattern of pain that moves from the left hip down to the knee. The **Natrum Sulph** patient is sensitive to changes in weather and to damp weather. He is sensitive to any form of damp.

Hip Injuries

Again, injuries to the hip tend to involve either physical injury or stress and strain. And, again, it can be difficult to discern exactly when a condition is lumbago and when it becomes hip pain. It is wise, therefore, to consider the remedies listed under both conditions.

Arnica is, of course, the remedy of first choice for hip pain after a physical trauma or from a fall. If the pain from the injury extends along the nerves in the body, **Hypericum** may be called for as a second remedy to complete the case. Or an **Arnica** rub may be used externally while **Hypericum** is given orally. If **Arnica** fails to complete the healing process or if bruising persists, consider the remedy **Bellis Perennis.**

But perhaps the best remedy for use in treating those with hip pain is **Ruta. Ruta** is especially called for when the patient's spine feels bruised, and when the patient feels as if his legs will fly out from under him if he tries to rise out of a chair. In fact, no other motion is as difficult for the **Ruta** as rising out of a chair. In addition to this pain, the **Ruta** patient's hips feel weak. Note that **Ruta** may be used as a second remedy with **Arnica** instead of **Hypericum,** and will complete its action in healing the pain.

Chelidonium may also be considered for patients who experience rheumatic pains in the hips and thighs. The muscles surrounding the entire hip joint will feel rigid and shrunken. The pain is worse on the right side. The affected area will feel cold, as if rubbed with ice. The patient will crave heat in all forms.

For women's hip pains during pregnancy, consider the remedy **Kali Carbonica.** For women's hip pains that occur during the onset of menopause, consider **Cimicfuga.** Neither of these remedies is listed in the Objective Materia Medica.

Injuries to the Coccyx

Injuries to the coccyx, or the very end of the spine, almost always occur as a result of a fall. The pain associated with this injury may be severe and long lasting.

As always, in the case of a fall or a blow to a particular part of the body, **Arnica** should be considered the remedy of first choice. However, be aware that I have often found that **Arnica** alone will not completely clear this condition.

Perhaps our most important remedy for injuries to the coccyx is **Causticum.** Just as the remedy relates to the neck, it also relates to the coccyx. The **Causticum** patient, like the **Arnica** patient, will feel bruised. He will have difficulty in walking, and will feel numbness in his lower limbs as well as coldness along with the pain of the injury. The patient's whole body will feel achy and bruised.

As always, **Rhus Tox** and **Bryonia** may be considered for cases of injury associated with a fall. And again, the difference between the two is that **Rhus Tox** patients will want to continually move the affected part of the body, while the Bryonia patient will want to stay still. Both will like gentle pressure on their injured area, which will soothe the pain.

Bellis Perennis should also be considered for cases in which **Arnica** seems called for, but fails to heal. If bruising persists in the affected area, consider Bellis.

Hypericum may be called for if the injury seems to extent from the area of impact and radiate along the nerves. **Hypericum** should especially be thought of as a secondary remedy to **Arnica,** and may be given as a follow-up to **Arnica.**

Kali Bi is a remedy to consider for cases of coccyx pain that are worse from sitting and from walking. Look for a sensation of jerking or twitching to accompany the pain.

If the coccyx injury becomes chronic, think of **Silicea.** This is often the remedy for elderly patients who suffer from long-term bouts of coccyx pain. This is a timid patient who longs to be taken care of. Constipation may accompany the discomfort in chronic coccyx pain.

Knee Injury

Injuries to the knee are perhaps most often sports injuries. They are caused either by a blow to the knee, a fall, or straining the joint.

Unless the injury is caused by a blow to the knee, in which case we will consider **Arnica** the remedy of first choice, the most commonly used remedy for knee injury and pain is **Ruta. Ruta** is, in general, consider *the* knee pain remedy. And, most commonly, the pain associated with **Ruta** will travel from the knees to the hips. The patient will have great difficulty getting up from a chair or out of a car.

Apis is the other important remedy associated with the knee. When **Apis** is called for, look for the knee to be red, swollen, and shiny looking, and hot to the touch. The patient will be crying out for cold things—especially ice—to be put on the knee. The knee pain may have a stinging sensation or a burning sensation.

If the knee condition becomes chronic, it is likely to call for **Rhus Tox** in treatment. As always with this remedy, the **Rhus** patient will want to gently move his knee to keep it from locking up. The knee will be most painful on first motion, and will actually feel better from gentle motion. It will also feel better from warm applications.

Finally, don't forget that little remedy called **Berberis. Berberis** may be the answer if the pain seems to radiate out from the knee to the whole body, and, especially, up into the hip. The patient will complain that he feels as if he has been beaten, that his whole body radiates pain. His whole body will feel stiff and sore. The patient will have trouble supporting his body weight on his knee.

Ankle Injury

When you twist your ankle, you might just reach for the **Arnica.** The simple fact is that it seems to be the remedy of choice for all the other strains and sprains, but this time you'd be wrong. For ankle pain, no remedy is as important as is **Ledum.** Consider this remedy if the joint feels numb and sort of "mushy," as if there is no way that ankle is going to support body weight. The ankle will be swollen and purple or bluish in color, or a bruised black and blue. It will have a sensation of coldness, and yet the patient will want cold applications on the injury, as heat makes the pain even worse.

As with insect stings, the remedy other than **Ledum** that is most often called for is **Apis.** The ankle will be red, swollen, shiny, and hot if **Apis** in needed. The patient will call out for ice to be put on his injury. As with **Ledum,** the patient will be unable to walk on the ankle.

If the ankle can support the body weight, even if the patient does not believe it, then you should consider the remedy **Causticum.** In these cases the ankle will feel torn and will crack and pop when the patient moves it, but the joint will actually be able to support the patient. **Causticum** is sometimes the remedy if the ankle injury is becoming chronic and rheumatic. Look for the pain to be better during wet weather in these cases.

Two other remedies associated with chronic ankle pain are **Natrum Mur** and **Rhus Tox.** As always, **Rhus Tox** injuries will be worse when the weather is damp, cold, and wet. The pain will be worse on first motion and better for slow, gentle motion. The patient will continue to work the ankle gently to keep it from locking up. The pain will be relieved from heat, especially wet heat, like a hot bath.

Natrum Mur, however, is usually associated with ankle pains in middle-aged persons who have injured the same ankle repeatedly until it seems permanently weakened. Use **Natrum Mur** if the patient seems to be very careful with his ankle, and yet continues to injure it again and again.

First Aid: Fractures

Like injuries, fractures are caused by falls, blows, or accidents, but in this case the affected areas are bones. If physical trauma causes a break to a bone but the skin is left intact, the injury is referred to as a "simple fracture." If the bone is not completely broken, the injury is called a "greenstick fracture." But if the injury extends from the bone to the tendons, ligaments, and/or skin, the injury is called a "compound fracture." The compound fracture is obviously the most complex condition, and the hardest to treat.

In the case of any fracture, do not move the patient; make him as comfortable as possible as you call for an ambulance. If the skin is broken, clean and cover the wound.

Whether the skin is broken or not, nearly all fractures involve bruising and swelling of the affected area, so **Arnica** should always be considered a remedy of first choice. In simple fractures, **Arnica** may be given topically as well as internally, but in compound fractures, **Arnica** must never be used topically.

In all compound fractures, **Calendula** should be applied topically to guard against infection and to speed the healing of the wound.

As always, **Hypericum** may be given either externally or internally for fractures that involve nerve pain. This will most often only be the case with compound fractures.

For cases involving shock, like car accidents resulting in fractures, **Aconite** may be given in alternation with **Arnica** to soothe the shock and stabilize the patient until help arrives.

Ledum is also an important remedy for cases of fractures of all sorts, but it should not be the first remedy used. Instead, **Ledum** is an excellent remedy to follow up **Arnica** and to clear away the bruises that **Arnica** has begun to heal.

Another excellent follow-up to **Arnica** is **Symphytum.** This remedy will greatly heal the bone itself once the initial trauma has been cleared by **Arnica.** Be sure never to give **Symphytum** before the bone has been set, as it may cause the bone to set prematurely and incorrectly.

Bryonia is a remedy that may follow **Arnica** or be used alone as a treatment for cracked or broken ribs. **Bryonia** may also be considered for any fracture causing pain so intense that the patient dare not move at all.

The remedy **Calcarea Phosphorica** may be used as a follow-up to **Bryonia** in healing fractured ribs. It also will be very helpful in treating fractures that are very slow to heal, or are not healing at all.

Another remedy used for those breaks that are slow to heal is **Silicea. Silicea** is very important in that it will help the body to reabsorb splintered bone chips that can damage nerves or blood vessels.

In concluding this section on treating fractures, it is important that I point out that homeopathic remedies will not replace the need for allopathic treatments such as x-rays to assess the damage, and a cast to hold and protect the injured bone while it heals.

First Aid: Emergencies

The emergencies covered in this text include issues involving the heart—from palpitations to heart attack and stroke—as well as shock, sudden nosebleed, and burns and scalds. Objective symptoms are of the utmost importance in all of these cases, since the patient may not be in any condition to answer questions.

With the occasional exception of nosebleeds, all these emergencies require professional medical attention. Any homeopathic remedy administered should be given as a stopgap to medical treatment.

Palpitations

Palpitations are wild beatings of the heart that are accompanied by a sensation of weight in the area of the heart. Some may be very painful, and nearly all will interfere with the patient's breathing. Palpitations may be caused by emotional upset, stress and overwork, blood loss, or pregnancy.

Palpitations may be difficult to differentiate from heart attacks, so be sure to take this symptom picture very seriously. Call for emergency medical help immediately.

Sudden powerful palpitations suggest two major remedies, **Aconite** and **Belladonna.** Both of these remedies commonly have symptoms that start suddenly and can, in **Belladonna's** case, leave just as suddenly. The **Aconite** patient will have a fever accompanying his palpitations. Look for his skin to be hot and dry in his fever. An important keynote symptom of **Aconite** is that the patient's pulse will be slow, while the palpitations are rapid. The **Aconite** patient will be in a terror from his palpitations, and will often feel that they will kill him. He will be hard to control and get to rest, and will thrash about. He may actually attack those who are trying to help him.

The **Belladonna** patient, on the other hand, will not strike out, although he is in anguish over his sudden condition. Instead, he will be overwhelmed by his pain. He will not be able to tolerate light or noise. He will be *willing* to rest but is unable to.

The **Aconite** patient's face will be bright red in color, while the **Belladonna's** face will be a darker red, flushed the color of deep sunburn. The **Belladonna** patient's face will also be very hot, as it is characteristic that a rush of blood to the face and head will accompany the palpitations. The **Belladonna** patient will be nauseated and may vomit. He also will have trouble breathing and may faint.

Note that, where the **Aconite's** skin is hot and dry, the **Belladonna's** head and face stays hot and dry, while the skin on the rest of his body is usually covered in a cold sweat.

If the patient with palpitations cannot sit still but must keep moving for relief of his symptoms, then consider **Rhus Tox** as the remedy. The patient will report numbness in the left arm in **Rhus** palpitations. He will also experience pain and trembling in the area around his heart. Note that as long as the **Rhus Tox** patient is allowed to keep moving he can obtain relief from his palpitations. If he is forced to stop, the palpitations begin once more. (Note that cases of palpitations in which the left arm is involved to the point that it seems attached to the side of the body, and cannot be moved at all during the attack, may call for the little remedy **Cimicfuga,** which is not a part of our Objective Materia Medica.)

On the other hand, the patient who cannot move at all during the palpitations may require **Bryonia.** A great difficulty in breathing is keynote here, as it is for the remedy **Spigelia.** Like the **Rhus** patient, the **Bryonia** patient will likely experience numbness and pain in his left arm. This patient will only take the shallowest of breaths. He will be unable to move, and most important, he will be unable to talk or answer questions.

The **Spigelia** patient may look a good deal like the **Bryonia** patient. He, too, seems to be suffocating during the attack, and his pain will grow worse if he moves, especially if he tries to sit up or move his chest or head forward. The **Spigelia** patient may want his head held high in order to achieve relief. Note that in most cases a bad mouth odor will accompany palpitations in **Spigelia.** The pulse will be intermittent during palpitations.

The palpitations themselves are intermittent in cases calling for **Lachesis.** Both the heart-beat *and* the palpitations will be intermittent and spasmodic. The patient will feel very weak. Although he very much wants to rest, he will be unable to lie down because it makes him feel as if he is suffocating. He is worse from resting in general, and especially worse from sleeping. The patient will actually feel worse when he wakes up than he did when he fell asleep. The **Lachesis** patient will also feel worse from moving his hands. It is important to note that the **Lachesis** patient will keep talking through all this, even if he merely mumbles or raves and makes no sense.

Another patient who cannot move is the **Digitalis** patient. In this case, however, the patient is *afraid* to move; afraid that any motion will actually cause his heart to stop beating. These palpitations tend to begin suddenly, and are accompanied by severe pains in the region of the heart. It is said that the **Digitalis** palpitations are so severe that you can actually see the motion in the patient's chest through his skin. This patient cannot talk, in that talking increases the palpitations, as does any motion or attempt to lie down. The patient will have a cold sweat all over his body. Note that **Digitalis** is not a part of the Objective Materia Medica.

The patient who needs **Phosphorus** will likely feel as if there is a steel band around his chest, pulling tighter and tighter. It is important to note that the symptoms in this case will move from the chest up into the throat. This is a very weak patient, and an emotional one.

The **Mercurius** patient may be one who is already very ill before the onset of the palpitations, but whatever their cause, they keep him from taking a deep breath. If he does attempt to do so, he will have a fit of coughing, which further weakens him. The patient may even cough up blood. This is a very weak, sweaty patient who is worse at night. He will often have a very bad body odor, and may have a bad mouth odor as well.

Another very weak patient is the **Arsenicum,** but where **Mercurius** patient is totally weakened and fairly still, the **Arsenicum** patient is weak and fussy, as if he is wrestling Death itself. He may often struggle to get up during the palpitations, although a very sick **Arsenicum** will lie very still, as if he has given up. This is a fearful patient, and he does not want to be left alone, even for a moment. This is a remedy for those who chronically suffer from palpitations, especially elderly patients. They will be worse at night, especially right around midnight.

The **Nux** patient may also experience chronic palpitations. These are usually brought on through overwork (in its constitutional presentation, **Nux** is the archetypal "Type A" driven personality, who is given to heart conditions of all sorts) or through poor diet, including alcohol, tobacco, caffeine, and red meat consumption on a daily basis. Bouts of anger may also trigger the palpitations. These palpitations are usually worse at night. They usually begin with the patient feeling his clothing is too tight across his chest. The palpitations themselves are slow to come on, and involve a sensation of heat and throbbing in the region of the heart. Note that the **Nux** patient will feel cold, and will need to be kept warm throughout the attack.

The **Pulsatilla** patient's palpitations are also often emotionally triggered, and may be caused by sorrow or bad news. The attack will usually begin with the patient's sensation that he cannot breathe. Then there will be a burning sensation around the heart. The **Pulsatilla** patient will want to sit by an open window and breathe cool, fresh air to attain relief. This is a highly emotional patient who will want comfort and company.

Heart Attack

It is often hard to differentiate between symptoms for different conditions, for example, lower back pain and hip pain. In the same way, the exact line separating palpitations from heart attacks may be difficult to discover. Therefore, it is important to take the situation very seriously in either case, and call for an ambulance before you consider any homeopathic remedy.

The symptoms associated with heart attack are very similar to those of palpitations: shortness of breath; pain in the chest that sometimes spreads into the arms, neck, or back; nausea; a feeling of faintness; irregular pulse. The patient's lips may even turn blue when breathing is difficult. In severe cases, the patient's breathing or heartbeat may stop altogether.

If the patient is conscious, prop him into a half-sitting, half-lying position to ease circulation. Keep him warm and loosen any tight clothing. If the patient is unconscious, monitor his breathing and heartbeat.

The group of remedies used here are basically the same as those used for palpitations, with **Aconite, Belladonna, Rhus Tox, Phosphorus, Lachesis,** and **Arsenicum** chief among them. Check the listing under palpitations for the indicators of these remedies. Do not hesitate to use the other remedies listed under palpitations if they seem called for. In addition to these remedies, consider:

Spongia is a remedy whose symptoms are linked with motion. The patient is worse for any kind of movement. If he moves, he feels as if he cannot breathe. Movement also gives the patient the feeling that he will faint. The pain in the area of the heart is throbbing in nature. The heart pounds so that it feels as if it would burst through the chest. This is an anxious, exhausted patient, covered in sweat.

Also consider **Cimicfuga,** a remedy not contained in the Objective Materia Medica, for cases involving intense pain in the area of the heart. The pain will extend into the left arm. The pain in that arm will be so great that the patient will not be able to move it at all. The left arm will be frozen in place.

Finally, remember the remedy **Cactus** for cases of heart attack. As with **Phosphorus,** the patient will feel as if he has a steel band around his chest that it is tightening. But instead of moving up into the throat, the symptoms will travel into the left arm. The patient will have terrible trouble breathing. Note that **Cactus** is not contained in the Objective Materia Medica.

Stroke

In cases of stroke, blood flow has been cut off to the brain, usually by a blood clot. The other cause of a stroke is when a blood vessel in the brain bursts, and a cerebral hemorrhage brings on the event.

As with any other condition, a stroke may be minor or devastating in nature. Minor strokes may involve only somewhat lesser symptoms, such as general weakness, a slight loss of muscular control over speech, and a general confusion. These symptoms may be common in elderly patients.

In a more serious event, however, the patient's major objective symptoms include a sudden confusion on the part of the patient, along with a sudden inability to speak. Also check for a pounding pulse, another important symptom. Finally, check the patient's eyes, as unequal dilation—one eye being fully dilated and the other not—is a sign of stroke. The patient may or may not lose consciousness. If fully conscious, he may complain of a terrible headache.

If you suspect a stroke, call for an ambulance immediately. Keep checking the patient's pulse and breathing. Do not move the patient into another room or to his bed. If possible, gather the patient gently into a half-sitting, half-lying, fully relaxed position. Loosen any tight fitting clothing and keep the patient comfortable and warm.

There are only three important remedies to consider for cases of stroke. Two are important remedies both for palpitation and for heart attack, and are important here because they speak to the suddenness of the attack. These remedies are **Aconite** and **Belladonna.** Be sure to check the listing under palpitation for each of these remedies in addition to the information given here.

The suddenness and the severity of the attack may lead you to **Aconite.** This patient, although severely stricken, will still thrash about and refuse to be still or comforted. He will talk of death and predict that he will die from his illness. In fact, the patient in need of **Aconite** might really be in danger of death, and might appear to be struggling to hang on and stay alive. Although he wants to keep moving, the **Aconite** patient may have to sit down or rest because he feels as if he cannot breathe when he stands or walks. He can only breathe when he is resting. He may also be very thirsty. As always, fear, anxiety and a fevered heat accompany the illness. The patient's face will be bright red and very hot, and his skin will be very dry as well.

The Belladonna patient will resemble the **Aconite** patient in many ways. The attack will be just as sudden and as severe for the **Belladonna** patient, but it may end just as suddenly, unlike **Aconite's.** The patient's face will be red, but it is usually a darker shade of red than in the **Aconite** case. Think of the color of very bad sunburn for the **Belladonna** patient. (In fact, **Belladonna** is an excellent remedy for severe sunburns, especially to the face and head.) And, while his face will be hot and dry like **Aconite's,** his body will be covered by a cold sweat. The Aconite patient's skin is dry over the whole body. Finally, the **Belladonna** patient usually will not thrash about, he will, instead, want to lie down in a dark and cool place, away from noise and light. He wants to rest, even if his attack will not let him.

Finally, consider the remedy **Opium,** which is not a part of our Objective Materia Medica. The patient needing **Opium** for symptoms of stroke is in a state of total collapse. He may be either semi-or totally unconscious. Often, he will be unable to answer any questions at all. If he can move or communicate at all, he may seem to be drunk and very out of it. Listen to this patient's breathing. It will sound deep and slow, like that of a sleeping person. His breathing may also have a wheezing to snoring sound attached to it, again like a person asleep. Look at the patient's face for indicators. The **Opium** patient will have a flushed, bloated face. His eyes will be half open, and half closed. Touch the patient's hands for indicators. The **Opium** patient will have damp palms, and will often have limbs that twitch through the whole attack. If the patient is able to communicate, he may complain of a burning sensation in his chest and of feelings of weakness and vertigo.

Note that, when dealing with a stroke patient, no matter what remedy is called for in the terrible moment of the attack, **Arnica** is considered to be the most important long-term remedy for bringing the patient back to his former self. The **Arnica** should be given in a 30C dose two or three times a day for several days after the stroke to help the patient heal.

Fainting

Simply put, fainting is caused by a temporary depletion of the blood flow to the brain, which causes a lack of oxygen to the part of the brain that controls human consciousness. Left to itself, the body very quickly puts things to right and consciousness returns.

However, fainting often seems like a melodramatic thing, and it causes a good deal of manic behavior by those who witness it. Many things, from bad news to stuffy rooms, can bring on an attack of fainting. It should be considered a minor emergency unless it is concurrent with a great physical trauma and accompanied by a pale face and an inability to breathe (which, together, could indicate internal bleeding).

If fainting is caused by a physical trauma, then the first remedy considered is **Arnica.** And if it is caused or accompanied by great pain, consider **Aconite, Chamomilla,** and **Cocculus.**

In the case of **Aconite,** the suddenness of the faint is the key to the treatment. In **Chamomilla,** the intensity of the pain builds more slowly. In **Cocculus,** the patient will demonstrate the keynote symptom of doubling over in pain, and trying to soothe the pain by pushing his fist into the painful area.

If the patient's pain is not severe, consider **Hepar Sulph.** And if the patient faints after losing a good deal of blood or after fighting a long-term illness, consider **China.**

If the patient faints because a room is too warm and airless, consider **Pulsatilla.** And if a patient faints from deep emotion, especially grief, consider **Ignatia.**

Finally, if a patient faints from a specific fear, consider these remedies: for a fear of needles, give **Silicea;** and for a fear of the sight of blood, give **Nux.**

Burns and Scalds

In homeopathic terms, these two injuries are treated in the same manner. But before any treatment is given, it is important that the severity of the injury be determined so that proper first aid is given.

Most burns and/or scalds in the home are usually of a minor sort, caused by the hot stove or boiling water involved in food preparation. When a superficial burn or scald does not involve broken skin, the best thing to do is to plunge the whole affected area into cold water and to hold it there for a good ten minutes. Either **Hypericum** or **Calendula** may be added to the water to cut the pain of the injury.

After the initial plunge into water, the minor burn or scald may be treated topically. You may dissolve any of the remedies listed below in water and apply a clean cloth saturated in the liquid remedy, or you may use any of the many homeopathic salves on the market. Be sure not to use any remedy based in petroleum jelly in the treatment of a burn or scald, however, because it will seal the burn into the skin and make matters worse. In addition to topical treatment, the same remedy may be taken internally to enhance its actions. And make sure that the patient under treatment for a burn or scald drinks plenty of water.

Burns and scalds can be very serious things. In the case of severe injury, it is important to call for emergency medical assistance immediately, and to give initial shock remedies until help arrives.

For the shock that accompanies serious burns or scalds and that often precedes the patient's awareness of pain, the same two major remedies are suggested here as elsewhere, **Arnica** and **Aconite.** Consider **Arnica** for cases of shock in which the patient seems a little slow and a bit removed from the situation at hand. On the other hand, **Aconite** is the better choice if the patient is very fearful in his shock, or if he says that he is dying and thrashes about in pain. In some cases the two remedies may be alternated until improvement begins.

In an emergency like a burn or scald, usually **Arnica** and/or **Aconite** will be given in a single dose, before the burn remedy itself is given.

When dealing specifically with a burn, it is important to remember not to remove any clothing that has been burned next to the skin, as it could bring the skin along with it. The same is true for jewelry. Remove jewelry only if it will not remove skin and increase the injury. Instead, lightly drape the area with a clean cloth. If possible, the cloth should be saturated with the remedy **Urtica Urens** dissolved in clean water. The **Aqua Urtica Urens** will help reduce the pain associated with the injury and will promote healing. Finally, if blisters or boils appear as a result of the injury, make sure that you do not burst them.

In the case of scalding, it is important to gently and slowly remove any clothing from the patient's body that was saturated with the hot liquid, because the saturated cloth will hold in the heat and increase the scald. As with burns, the affected area of the body can be covered in a clean cloth saturated in **Aqua Urtica Urens** to soothe the injury.

Urtica Urens is, in fact, perhaps the best remedy for use for simple burns and scalds. It may be taken internally as well as used topically. Think especially of **Urtica Urens** if the patient complains that his injury has a stinging sensation associated with it.

Cantharis, a remedy not listed in the Objective Materia Medica, is another excellent burn and scald remedy, and one that you may want in your first aid kit. Instead of a stinging sensation, the wound that needs **Cantharis** will have a deep burning sensation and will be improved by cold applications. The patient needing **Cantharis** will also be restless in his pain.

A third major remedy for burns and scalds is **Arsenicum.** Consider this remedy when the patient seems overwhelmed by his injury; cases in which the patient seems to be losing his life force in his attempt to overcome his injury. The patient will be very thirsty for cold water, but will only take small sips. Look for nausea and diarrhea to accompany the injury.

For more serious burns or scalds consider the remedies **Chamomilla** and **Kali Bi.** The **Chamomilla** patient will be furious in pain, and impatient for the pain to end. His face and head will be covered in sweat. If the injury is severe, the patient may go into convulsions.

The **Kali Bi** patient will also have more severe burns, but the remedy is usually called for when the injury itself covers only a small part of the body. In these cases the patient can point to the exact spot of his pain.

Should a burn become infected, consider the remedy **Hepar Sulph.** The remedy should be taken internally while **Calendula** is used topically.

In the final stage of a burn, consider the remedy **Causticum** for use on the scar tissue if it is still painful. And if the wound is slow to heal or does not heal at all, use the remedy **Silicea** to promote healing.

Nosebleeds

Nosebleeds may begin in several different ways. They may be the result of blunt trauma or mechanical injury, or they may occur at the end of an acute respiratory ailment, such as a cold, in which the nose has been blown and blown. Or they may, in some cases, be something that a patient is vulnerable to, especially a child.

Nosebleeds are seldom dangerous. Only if the blood flow cannot be stopped should emergency help be sought. In most cases, the bleeding can be stopped by pinching the end of the patient's nose together for a few minutes. You should start out for the emergency room if bleeding persists after fifteen minutes of pinching the nose.

Fortunately, there are a handful of remedies that should help you in your attempt to stop the bleeding.

The first one to consider will only help if the cause of the nosebleed is known to be a mechanical injury. In this case, **Arnica** is, as usual, the remedy of first choice. So if the bleeding was caused by a punch in the nose, **Arnica's** your choice.

Perhaps the best all-around remedy for the patient with a nosebleed is **Vipera,** which is not listed in our Objective Materia Medica. If you can discover no specific cause for the nosebleed, and have no particular guiding symptoms to go on, a dose or two of this remedy at 30C usually sets things right.

If the nosebleed starts very suddenly in a patient not given to nosebleeds, then the first remedies to consider are **Aconite** and **Belladonna.** The Aconite nosebleed often will start after the patient has become chilled outdoors and then comes inside the warm house. The **Belladonna** nosebleed, on the other hand, often will occur after the patient has become overheated. The **Belladonna** nosebleed will also be accompanied by a sensation of headache and congestion in the patient's head. The patient may see lights or sparks in front of his eyes during the headache. He will be exhausted by the nosebleed and will want to lie down in a cool, dark place.

The **Aconite** patient, on the other hand, will be fearful and anxious concerning his nosebleed. He will not lie down, will not rest. Instead, he thrashes about in his discomfort. Note that the blood will be bright red, and the patient's face will also be bright red and hot to the touch.

Other remedies involving bright red blood are **Ipecac, Ferrum Phos,** and **Phosphorus.** For the **Ipecac** patient, the bright red blood flowing from the nose will be accompanied by nausea. The patient may vomit during the nosebleed.

The **Ferrum Phos** patient will be dizzy during his nosebleed, and will have very pale skin. The patient will complain of a sensation of throbbing throughout his whole head and, especially, in his nose during the nosebleed.

The patient who has a weakness toward getting nosebleeds, whose Kleenex always seems to have a little blood on it, and whose nosebleeds are typified by a flow of bright red blood most often need the remedy **Phosphorus** to set things right. **Phosphorus** is also a remedy for those who get nosebleeds during colds.

Another remedy for those given to nosebleeds is **Rhus Tox.** In this case, the nosebleeds tend to happen at night. Also, in acute circumstances, consider this remedy for nosebleeds that occur after the patient has been over-lifting or straining. Look for the patient's nose to be swollen during the nosebleed.

Finally, if the blood from the nose is dark rather than bright the first remedy to consider is **Lachesis. Lachesis** is an excellent general remedy for any nosebleed in which the blood is dark red. The patient's face may also take on a dark red coloring.

Note that, since **Vipera** and **Lachesis** are taken from specific snake venom, whose action in the human body is to keep blood from clotting, it makes sense that in homeopathic form they would be such excellent medicines for stopping a nosebleed.

Acute Ailments

For our purposes, the acute ailments responding to homeopathic remedies will be acute respiratory ailments like colds and flu, and their related ailments, coughs and sore throats. These are quite likely the most common communicable illnesses that are dealt with on an annual basis in the American household, so you will be able to do a great deal of good for your loved ones if you can grasp the appropriate use of just a handful of homeopathic remedies.

As always, unless otherwise advised, all remedies are discussed in the 30C potency, and all are to be given as needed until improvement begins.

Remedies Strongly Suggested for the Acute Ailments Kit

Aconite: As is always the case, the speediness of the onset of symptoms is of the greatest import to this remedy. It is perhaps our best remedy for the first stage of a cold. Aconite will quickly cure or greatly lessen the impact of a cold if it is given soon enough after its onset.

Allium Cepa: Our great homeopathic remedy taken from the humble onion. Think of what happens to your eyes when you slice an onion, and you have a perfect picture of the patient needing the remedy. The eyes flow with bland tears, the nose flows with acrid mucus.

Apis: This is an important remedy for sore throats when they follow the general formula of the remedy's symptoms—the interior throat will be bright red, shiny looking, and swollen. It is also a remedy for those with fever, whose faces are bright red and hot to the touch.

Arsenicum: An important remedy for all acute ailments, from colds and flu to sore throats. This patient has been weakened by his illness, but unless he is very, very ill, he is also unwilling to just get into bed and rest. This is a restless, fussy patient who is thirsty, especially for warm tea with lemon, but who is able to take only the smallest sips of liquid when he receives it. This is a fearful patient, who is always chilly and does not want to be alone. Consider this remedy for respiratory ailments in which digestive symptoms accompany respiratory distress. Note that Arsenicum is a right-sided remedy, and that the patient's symptoms will begin on the right side of his body or will be worse on that side.

Bryonia: Consider this remedy for acute ailments in which the patient doest not want to move at all, when discomfort keeps the patient from moving. This patient is sometimes called the "Bryonia Bear;" he is a cranky patient who most often wants to be alone. He will be a very thirsty patient, but will drink little. Consider this remedy if, as with Nux, constipation accompanies the acute ailment.

Euphrasia: Euphrasia is often thought of as the homeopathic remedy whose symptoms are in opposition to Allium Cepa's. The eyes and nose both flow in both remedy portraits, but in Allium Cepa, the eyes flow with bland tears, the nose flows with acrid mucus. The opposite is true in Euphrasia—the eyes flow with acrid tears, the nose flows bland.

Ferrum Phos: Keep Ferrum Phos on hand for general cases of fever in which there is no specific guiding symptom that will lead you to another remedy.

Gelsemium: Gelsemium is the remedy for "malaise." There is a general weakness about the patient, often a weak voice.

Hepar Sulph: In acute ailments, Hepar Sulph, like Mercurius, nearly always suggests that an infection is present. It is keynote that the patient needing this remedy will feel as if he has a stick of some sort caught in his throat.

Kali Bi: Kali Bi is an important remedy in the third and final stage of a cold. It will clear away coughs and colds that just drag on and on. It is an excellent sinus remedy and helpful even for cases of sinus headache if the patient's pain appears in specific spots, so that that patient can point to the exact spot of sinus pain. It is also an excellent remedy for those with postnasal drip.

Mercurius: This remedy is most often called for in acute ailments that have become deeper issues in which an inflammation or infection is present. The Mercurius patient is most often sweaty in fever, and almost incapable of dealing with changes in room temperature. He is worse at night. He is a patient who smells ill, who especially exudes a foul odor from his mouth.

Natrum Mur: No home kit is complete without Natrum Muriaticum. It is perhaps the leading remedy for colds in the nose, and a remedy that is helpful in both the first and second stages of a cold. The patient will want to take to his bed and rest. He will be very thirsty. Always consider this remedy for colds that begin with a great deal of sneezing.

Phosphorus: One of our most important remedies in acute ailments. It is a major remedy for weakened or lost voices, and for colds and flu that move from the head into the chest. This is a remedy for those with loose coughs that may bring up mucus or blood. This is a sensitive patient who needs encouragement in order to get well. The Phosphorus patient will be improved by cold drinks.

Pulsatilla: This is an excellent remedy to have on hand at all times for cases of sore throat, fever, or colds in which the patient is thirstless, even in the heat of fever, emotional—Pulsatilla patients can be quite demanding and even tearful during illness—and almost totally incapable of being in a warm, closed room. The Pulsatilla will want a window open in order to breathe, or better still, will want to go for a walk in the open air. Pulsatilla is an excellent remedy for the third stage of a cold.

Rhus Tox: Like Phosphorus, this is an excellent remedy for those who have lost their voice, particularly from overuse. The Rhus Tox patient will be better from warm liquids, whereas the Phosphorus patient will be improved by cold drinks. Note that the Rhus Tox patient with a cold will likely have a nosebleed accompanying the cold.

Sulphur: One of our most important remedies for those with colds and flu. As always, the Sulphur formula of being hot, sweaty, and itchy will be present, along with a desire for happy company, and salty or sweet foods. The patient will be very thirsty and will drink just about anything. Consider this remedy for cases of respiratory ailments accompanied by digestive distress, especially by diarrhea that drives the patient out of bed in the morning. Note that Sulphur is one of our great left-sided remedies. Symptoms will be worse on the left side of the patient's body, or will begin on the left side and move right.

Remedies That You May Want to Add to Your Acute Ailments Kit

Camphora: The key to understanding the Camphora patient is knowing that, like the substance camphor from which it is taken, the Camphora is "minty fresh." This is one of our chilliest patients. the patient sneezes and sneezes and sneezes as his cold begins. Think of Camphora for patients with colds that involve very little mucus flow.

Carbo Veg: This is an important remedy for cases of sore throat and cough, especially when these are accompanied by long-term hoarseness. This is a good general remedy for cough that interferes with the patient's breathing. It is, therefore, one of our most important remedies for cases of whooping cough.

Chamomilla: Think of this remedy first for cases of sore throats in young children, particularly if the child is angry in his pain. Look for one side of the patient's face to look pale, the other to be reddened. The common sensations of pain are burning and/or stinging.

Dulcamara: Think of this remedy first for cases of cold and sore throat (and, especially, of hay fever) that occur in spring or fall, when days are warm and nights are cold. Think of this remedy especially for cases in which the patient becomes ill annually at this time of year, either with an acute ailment or an allergy.

Eupatorium: Think of Eupatorium as "deeper Bryonia" for cases of flu in which a sensation of aching bones is even deeper than it appears in Bryonia. The pain is so great the patient may feel as if his bones were actually breaking.

Ipecac: Think of this for any acute ailment in which the patient feels nauseated and in which that patient may vomit as part of his symptom portrait. It is important as a bronchitis remedy, for instance, in which a simple cold has moved deep into the patient's chest and the patient is having a terrible time breathing. The cough, which is intended to bring up mucus, may also trigger vomiting.

Lachesis: Think of this remedy for cases of sore throat—especially severe sore throat—if the patient is unable to swallow liquids but is able to swallow solids. Look for the interior throat to be the characteristic purple-red that indicates this remedy. It is also an excellent remedy for colds in which the patient's eyes and nose tear a great deal, but his mouth is very dry. This is also a suffocative patient, who will easily feel as if he cannot breathe. This is especially true just as the patient is drifting off to sleep. He will suddenly become fully awake, convinced that he will suffocate if he sleeps. Lachesis is a left-sided remedy. Symptoms will begin on the left side of the body and move toward the right.

Lycopodium: Lycopodium is, along with Arsenicum, one of our great right-sided remedies. So look for the patient's symptoms, especially sore throat, to begin on the right side of his body and move left, or to be worse on that side of the body. Lycopodium patients will generally be improved by warmth and warm applications. He will be better from warm drinks. He is also worse at 4:00P.M.

Nux: Think of this remedy for acute ailments that are very slow in developing. The patient feels sicker and sicker each day until an ailment fully forms. The first symptom of illness is usually a sensation of chilliness throughout the patient's whole body. The patient is even cold during fever. This is a remedy of dryness—the patient's nose is often stopped up, without flow. In the same way, the cough is dry. And look for constipation to accompany acute ailments.

Rumex: This is an excellent remedy that will help with coughs that develop with colds or hay fever. The cough is shallow and dry, but maddening. This is a patient who labors not to cough and whose cough is generally triggered by a "tickle in the throat." Talking, breaking deeply, and laughing will all trigger the patient's cough, as will touching the patient's throat.

Spongia: This cough is usually identified and treated on the basis of sound alone. It is a ringing, distinctive cough that has been described as sounding like "sawing wood" and "a dog barking." Either way, the Spongia patient's cough has a jarring sound that always surprises and startles when heard. The Spongia patient is, like the Lachesis patient, easily made to feel as if he is suffocating. The patient may awaken in the night because he feels as if he will stop breathing in his sleep.

Remedies Not in the Objective Materia Medica That You May Want to Have On Hand

Baptisia: This remedy may be an important addition to your home kit if you find that you are often treating patients with fever. Like Aconite and Belladonna, the Baptisia patient will have a sudden high fever and a bright or dark red complexion, but the Baptisia patient will often seem sicker from his fever—he may seem to be slipping away. Often he will fall into a sudden, deep sleep that can be most frightening. Like the Arnica patient, the Baptisia patient will report that he feels bruised and beaten up in his pain. And, like the Arnica patient, he can be slow to answer and vague in his answers.

Baryta Carbonica: An important remedy for those with the sore throat that is associated with chronic conditions like bronchitis and tonsillitis. These are sore throats that are slow to develop but become very serious. Both the tonsils and the lymph glands behind the neck will be swollen and sensitive.

Drosera: This is an excellent remedy for those with coughs that share the characteristic symptom of a violent tickle in the throat causing a spasm of coughing. The cough can all but overwhelm the patient. Look for him to have to support this chest or stomach as he struggles to stop coughing. The patient may retch or gag during his spasms of coughing.

Kali Iodatum: Think of this remedy for patients with colds who, while their body feels hot and cold in alternation, are always better from warmth and applications of heat.

This is a remedy type with a great many discharges, from the nose and from the eyes. All discharges are acrid, and the eyes and nose are swollen and pained. Note that some of the patients needing this remedy are those who seem to catch cold all the time, after every exposure to weather changes, and especially during damp weather.

Phytolacca: Although it is not commonly needed, you may want to have this remedy on hand, because the pain of the sore throat is so great that no patient will want to wait while you order it. Look for the interior of the throat to be swollen and very dark red in color. The root of the tongue, the soft palate, and the tonsils will also be swollen. The patient will be unable to speak due to his pain, and will not be able to swallow anything hot.

Stramonium: Stramonium is a remedy you may want to have on hand, because it is used to treat high fever: fevers that are accompanied by hallucinations. The patient will stare without blinking. He will want to escape, as if he could run away from his fever. The patient will also be worse and even more terrified in the dark, although he will not be able to bear too bright a light either.

Colds

The common cold may be said to come in three stages. The first stage is from the onset of the cold—however it begins, whether with sneezing, sore throat, body chills, or other beginning symptoms—to the first flow of mucus. The second stage of the cold is the stage of clear mucus. The third and final stage is the stage of colored mucus.

There are homeopathic remedies that will work to clear each individual stage of a cold, and there are some remedies that will take you through more than one stage. Therefore, when you treat a cold, you should be prepared to closely watch the patient's symptoms and how they shift during its course. Shifts in symptoms may or may not imply that a shift is needed in the remedy. That is determined only on the basis of the individual patient, and his experience of the cold. But be aware that you may have to use one, two, or even three different remedies to clear the cold away. The remedies will depend, of course, upon the vital force of the patient, and his ability to throw off the ailment on his own. So stay aware when treating a cold, and you should be able to clear it away quite nicely, based solely on the information you can gather with your eyes, ears, and fingertips.

Remedies for the First Stage of a Cold

When you consider remedies for the first stage of a cold, first determine whether the cold came on quickly or slowly. For the cold that develops very quickly, the first remedy to consider is **Aconite.** Often, the **Aconite** cold will develop as the result of the patient having been in contact with a cold, dry wind, or from having become deeply chilled. The cold will begin with a great deal of sneezing and with a quick, high fever. The patient's face will suddenly be very hot, and he will be flushed bright red. Another early symptom of the cold will be a tickle in the throat that very quickly becomes a sore throat. Note that the **Aconite** patient, although exhausted by his cold, will be very restless. It will be very difficult for you to get him to just lie in bed and rest. Also note that, as **Aconite** is a quick remedy, it will do little or nothing for the cold unless it is given in the first hours.

The **Belladonna** cold will develop very quickly, just like the **Aconite.** And, like **Aconite,** the **Belladonna** cold will usually begin with a sore throat and a fever. A dry cough is likely to appear soon after. The first symptom is usually that **Belladonna** fever: a sudden, high fever that leaves the patient's face dark red, like bad sunburn, and very hot and dry. The rest of his body, however, will be covered in a cold sweat. Bouts of fever will leave the patient alternating between hot and cold. Unlike the **Aconite** patient, the **Belladonna** patient will be unable to bear noise or fuss or any form of bright light. He will be sluggish, especially in fever, and will want to rest in a cool, dark place. He will want to go to bed and sleep, but try though he might, he usually will be unable to sleep.

Remedies for the First and Second Stage of a Cold

Some remedies straddle the bridge between the stage one and stage two cold. Two important ones are **Camphora** and **Natrum Mur.**

Camphora is an excellent remedy for the first stage of a cold, and it also may help support healing in the second stage. The patient needing **Camphora** will first feel the onset of the illness with chilliness throughout his body. He will become very, very cold. Next, he will begin sneezing, and it is the sneezing that will confirm the onset of the cold. Although the patient sneezes a great deal, it is keynote of the remedy that the patient's nose will never produce much of a flow of mucus. Instead, the patient's nose will feel very, very stopped up and pressured. A headache located either in the forehead or the front sinuses and a sore throat are likely to complete the picture of this cold.

Natrum Muriaticum is one of our most important remedies, not just for colds and allergies, but for many, many different types of ailments.

In the case of colds, the first symptom in the usual **Natrum Mur** cold is sneezing. The patient's nose will close up and sneezing will begin. The patient will lose his sense of smell and taste because of his blocked nose. Listen for the patient to speak with a nasal voice. Think of **Natrum Mur** as the best general remedy we have for colds. The symptoms of this remedy are those that we usually equate with what we consider to be the most typical cold.

In addition to that blocked nose, the **Natrum Mur** patient has fits of sneezing. When it begins to run, the patient's nose will have a clear and somewhat thick flow of mucus like raw egg whites. There may be a fever, but it will not be a major feature of the ailment. The patient may also have a sore throat, for which he will want cold drinks, like ginger ale. He may also want salty foods that will make his throat feel better. The patient feels just rotten, and will tend to just want to go to bed and be left alone. He does not want to be fussed over. Note that other symptoms of the Natrum Mur cold include postnasal drip, cold sores, and lips that become so dry that they tend to crack.

Nux is another remedy that straddles between stage one and two of a cold, and it may be given for either or both, as long as the symptom portrait matches the remedy. The **Nux** cold is very slow to come on. Over a period of days or more, the patient will feel that he is slowly getting sick, and that something is wrong. He may have a bit of a sore throat for a day or two and then it goes away again. Then another symptom may appear and fade. Finally, the patient begins to get cold. He will feel as if he cannot get warm, whatever he does. This is commonly the first real symptom of the illness. Early symptoms will include fever, which makes the patient feel all the colder, and a frontal headache, which may last for days. The patient soon develops a cough, which irritates the headache. And the nasal flow begins. It is keynote of this remedy that the patient's nose will flow during the day, and be stopped up without any flow at night. What flow there is in the daytime will be watery and clear. The **Nux** will wake up feeling terrible, after having had a terrible night's sleep. All of his symptoms seem to gather and to grow worse in the morning. This is an irritable and impatient patient. He may seem impossible to please.

Sulphur is another remedy that straddles the first and second stages of a cold, and in many ways it will display a picture that is opposite of **Nux.** For one thing, while the **Sulphur** cold can be as slow to develop as is the **Nux** patient's, the **Sulphur** patient is pretty often cheerful throughout the whole process. He tends to want to have happy company, even when he is at his sickest. He wants to play cards and watch movies with his friends and loved ones. He loves to get magazines and presents. In fact, the **Sulphur** may often seem to be less ill than he really is, so parents and friends will feel as if he is tricking them by saying that he is ill.

The mucus flow begins quickly with the **Sulphur** cold, and will flow in great amounts, so the **Sulphur** patient's bed and surroundings will be littered with used tissues. The mucus will be clear and watery in nature. And the **Sulphur** patient will be hot, sweaty, and itchy. He will usually crave salty things like potato chips, and will also tend to want greasy things like pizza, even when sick, as the cold will seldom interfere with his hunger. While the **Sulphur** patient is hot, his feet may become cold, so he puts his feet under the covers. But he also cannot bear to have his feet covered, so he will take them out again, only to place them there once more soon after. The **Sulphur** cold may often be accompanied by stomach distress. In the case of the **Sulphur** cold, the patient may be driven from his bed in the morning by a sudden case of diarrhea. Note that the **Sulphur** cold may start on the left side of the patient's body, or the patient's symptoms will be worse on the left side of his body.

Lycopodium is another remedy that is used for both stage one and stage two of a cold. And it is the opposite of **Sulphur** in that the symptoms will be worse on the right side of the patient's body, or will begin on the right and move left. Most often the **Lycopodium** cold will begin with a sore throat, often a very mild sore throat on the right side. The cold will spread from there to a full-fledged head cold. The throat will be dry, and the patient typically will not be thirsty for anything, although warm drinks will soothe the sore throat. In more severe colds, look for the patient to complain of a headache that begins over the right eye and moves over the left eye as well.

The **Lycopodium** patient's nose will be stopped up, and he will have to breathe through his mouth. Although there will be little mucus flow, the patient will feel that he has to blow his nose very often. The **Lycopodium** patient will tend to be a little chilly and will seek warmth. He will tend to lose his appetite altogether or, if he continues to eat, will have digestive problems along with the symptoms of the cold. The **Lycopodium** patient tends to belch and feel bloated. If anything, he will tend to want to eat sweets.

Some remedies, while they may certainly be called upon in the treatment of acute colds, are very useful for those who tend to have a weakness for colds and have them more often than the average person.

One of these remedies is **Arsenicum,** which is often the cold remedy needed by elderly people with a tendency to catch cold with every change in the weather. These colds tend to appear first with the sensation of chilliness throughout the whole body. The patient will say that he feels as if he has ice water running in his veins. Another common first symptom is a tickle in the nose located in one specific place which then spreads throughout the whole nose, and sneezing begins.

The chilly **Arsenicum** patient yearns to go to bed and to get "cozy." Unlike the chilly **Nux** who cannot get warm, the **Arsenicum** patient can become quite warm and comfortable if put to bed and covered well. There is one exception to the **Arsenicum** patient's chilliness, and that is his head. If he gets a headache with his cold (and these patients often do), he will want cool air on his face and the rest of his body kept warm.)

Once it begins, the **Arsenicum** patient's nasal discharge will be thin and watery, and quite often painful and acrid. The discharge will cause a burning sensation to the nose. The patient's eyes may also tear a good deal, and that may have the same burning sensation. The patient's eyes may be reddened from the discharge.

This is a fussy patient who may not be willing to just stay in bed unless he is very ill. He may constantly get up and fuss about in the house. Unlike the messy **Sulphur** patient, who leaves a wake of tissues wherever he goes, the fussy **Arsenicum** patient may refuse to leave a used teacup on the dresser and will get up to take it to the kitchen to wash. He may tell the doctors what to do, and he does not want to be alone, as his symptoms and fears about his illness will greatly magnify when he is alone.

Phosphorus is another remedy to consider for those who tend to catch cold easily and often; this is especially appropriate for children with a weakness for colds. The **Phosphorus** cold will usually begin with a sore throat that feels much improved from eating and drinking cold things. Cold drinks and ice cream may upset the patient's stomach, however. The patient may become nauseated or even vomit once they warm up in the stomach.

The key to understanding the **Phosphorus** cold is that, at some point, it will end up in the patient's chest. It may start there, or, more commonly, it will begin in the throat and move into the head and especially the ears. (The constitutional **Phosphorus** has two weak links, his ears and his chest. The ears act as a steam valve to relieve pressure and protect the constitutional type's underdeveloped lungs. Therefore, you will find a pattern of earaches, deep chest colds with bronchitis, and so on throughout the childhood of a typical **Phosphorus** patient.)

You do not need to be constitutionally a **Phosphorus** type or a young child for this remedy to work in an acute situation. You only need to match the remedy's pattern with your own pattern of illness. So any acute cold that moves into the ears and chest may be greatly improved by **Phosphorus.**

As the cold takes hold and discharge begins, look for the **Phosphorus** patient to have discharge from one side of the nose, while the other side is blocked. These discharges will alternate throughout the cold. Note that the patient's tissues may often be blood-streaked.

The patient will also suffer from ear pressure and a loose or dry cough. The patient may cough up a good deal of mucus, and that mucus may contain some blood. This cough may become the driving force of the illness in this case. The patient may be wracked with pain from the cough, and may complain that he feels as if he has a steel band around his chest. The cough will be worse if the patient comes into contact with cool air, or from laughing or talking.

This patient never wants to be alone; his physical symptoms will actually grow worse if he is left alone. This is a sweet patient who appreciates all that is done for him.

Remedies for the Second Stage of a Cold

Let's consider some remedies for the common cold that has moved from stage one to stage two.

Two of the most common and helpful remedies for colds are **Allium Cepa** and **Eu-**

phrasia. You can tell which cold fits each of these remedies easily enough, because their symptoms are opposite of each other.

Allium Cepa is made from an onion, and you only have to picture your reaction when you cut an onion to get the idea of this remedy's symptoms. The patient needing this remedy is already in stage two. He is dealing with nasal flow as well as a great deal of discharge from the eyes. The tears are thin, watery, and bland, and their flow does not harm the eyes or face, just as when you cut that onion. The discharge from the nose is also thin and watery, but unlike the tears, it is acrid and leaves a sensation of rawness behind. You have seen the **Allium Cepa** patient before. He's the one whose nose is crusted, red, and sore-looking around the bottom of each nostril. He has to wince a little every time he has to touch a tissue to his sore nose, yet he continues to sneeze and sneeze and sneeze, and his eyes and nose continue to flow.

In addition to this, the **Allium Cepa** patient also feels hot, raw, and headachy. This rawness may flow into the patient's throat and chest. This patient is very thirsty, and feels better in fresh air and worse in a warm room.

The **Euphrasia** patient's symptoms are the opposite. His eyes and nose will also flow and flow, but in this case the tears are acrid, while the nasal flow is bland. The patient's eyes are reddened and burn from the tears. In opposition to **Allium Cepa,** the patient will feel worse in open air and better in a warm, closed room. The **Euphrasia** patient is worse in the daytime and when he lies down, but his symptoms, especially his cough, will feel better when he eats. This cough will tend to be a later symptom of the cold. It will be loose in nature and will bring up mucus.

If the discharge from the eyes and ears are both acrid, consider the remedy **Kali Iodatum.** Both discharges are watery and irritating, so the patient will have red eyes and a swollen, red nose. He also has a red face. A helpful symptom in identifying this patient is the fact that he will swing between being too hot and too cold, but he is worse from heat in any form. This is a very thirsty patient who may be among those vulnerable to colds in general. He may catch cold with every change in the weather.

The remedy **Lachesis** may also be considered at this stage in the cold. The **Lachesis** patient will experience a great deal of discharge from both the eyes and the nose, but this flow is accompanied by a dry mouth. Look for the patient's tongue to be dark about and from the dry mouth.

In addition, the **Lachesis** patient will have a sore throat, sometimes a severe sore throat. He may have trouble swallowing liquids, and may only be able to swallow solid food. The Lachesis patient will be very protective of his throat; he may not be able to bear anyone or anything to touch his throat. A cough will usually accompany the cold. Note that, if his throat is touched, the patient will experience a spasm of coughing.

Sleep will be an issue for the Lachesis patient. He may be unable to sleep, because he will feel as if he is suffocating just as he falls asleep. And he will often sleep into aggravation, and feel worse after sleeping than he did before.

Consider **Carbo Veg** for colds that strongly feature headache, and for second stages of colds in which the patient's head feels pressurized, to the point that the pulse of every heartbeat pounds throughout the head. The patient's nose will be totally blocked and pressurized during the night, but mucus will flow during the day.

Because of the blockage and sinus pressure, the patient will feel as if he cannot breathe, and will have great difficulty breathing. He will need moving air or he will feel as if he is suffocating, and he may want a window open or a fan to help him breathe.

Another patient who has difficulty breathing is the **Ipecac** patient. This patient will have labored breathing, as if he is having an asthma attack. He will also have a great deal of discharge from the nose and the eyes. The flow does not lessen symptoms, however, as the patient will lose his senses of taste and smell.

The **Ipecac** patient will also have a loose cough, and there will typically be a rattling of mucus in the chest. But no matter how much the patient coughs, the coughs fail to bring up the mucus. The coughing may be so bad that the patient becomes nauseated, and may then gag and vomit up mucus.

Note that it is the severity of the nausea and vomiting that most clearly indicates the need for Ipecac, not the symptoms of the cold itself. **Ipecac,** like **Phosphorus,** is a remedy to consider in stage two of a cold when that cold is moving into the chest and the chest is filling with mucus.

Remedies for the Third Stage of a Cold

In stage three of a cold, the mucus begins to change color, usually to green or yellow. The color of the mucus, as well as its specific quality, will help you to determine the needed remedy. Normally, for cases of colds that are moving along nicely to a satisfactory end, the two most common remedies are **Pulsatilla** and **Kali Bi.**

When **Pulsatilla** is called for, the mucus will have changed to a yellow or yellow-green color, and will have a fluffy quality. It will be somewhat thicker than the clear mucus, and will gather into a large blob or cloud in the patient's tissue when he blows his nose. The patient will crave fresh air, which will improve his symptoms. He will be unable to bear being in a closed, warm room, even if he feels chilly. He may need to go outside for a walk to feel better. His symptoms will be worse in the evening, and better in the day. He will not be thirsty, even during fever, and he will have lost his senses of taste and smell. The **Pulsatilla** patient may be needy, keeping you running as he lists his needs and wants, but what he wants, more than anything else, is attention.

The **Kali Bi** patient, on the other hand, will tend to have discharges that are more green than yellow. This discharge will be tougher than the **Pulsatilla** patient's, and will be ropy in nature. The **Kali Bi** patient may pick his nose, trying to get the mucus out, as it is very difficult to get out by blowing the nose. The patient's nose may be filled by dried crusts or mucus plugs. The cold may be accompanied by a sinus headache, typically located in the forehead or the frontal sinuses. It will impact only a small area, and the patient will be able to point to the exact location of the pain. The patient may also suffer from postnasal drip during the last stage of the cold, and may have to constantly clear his throat to remove the mucus flow.

Two other remedies indicate that the cold is not clearing away, but that it is moving deeper into the body in stage three, and may lead to a much more serious ailment. The need for either of these remedies suggests that an infection is already present in the body. These remedies are **Mercurius** and **Hepar Sulph.**

The patient who needs **Mercurius** will, in addition to any number of cold symptoms, have swollen glands in his neck. He will also have tenderness, pain, and sensitivity in the region of those glands, in his jaw, and in his teeth.

It is keynote of the remedy that the patient's tongue will be swollen so that you will be able to see the shape of the patient's teeth running down the sides of his tongue. In addition to a swollen tongue, the patient will have increased saliva and often will drool on his pillow each night. The patient's mouth will have a foul smell. He will tend to have a hoarse voice. He will also have a sore throat, inflamed tonsils, and a dry cough that is worse at night. (In fact, all the **Mercurius** symptoms will be worse at night.) This patient cannot bear changes in temperature, which affect him much as weather changes affect rheumatic patients. But he is also a chilly patient, so is most comfortable in a warm room. He sneezes a great deal. His nose will tend to drip mucus, and will be red, swollen, and very sore. The **Mercurius** patient will have mucus that is thick and white or yellow, like pus.

The **Hepar Sulph** patient will also have a sore throat in addition to the other symptoms of his cold. The throat will be very sore, and will tend to have the sensation of a stick caught in the throat. The **Hepar Sulph** patient will have mucus that is either clear or green in color.

Note that **Hepar Sulph** is often a follow-up to **Aconite,** as both are remedies for colds that are brought on from exposure to cold, dry wind. The patient will be worse from any contact with cold, which will make him sneeze and sneeze. This patient will have to stay completely covered up because of his sensitivity to cold. Even exposing his hands or feet in a cold room may worsen symptoms.

Flu

When a patient is ill, it is sometimes hard to get an exact diagnosis. This is very true when it comes to colds and flu. It may be very difficult in a given case to determine the exact line that separates a cold virus and its actions in the human system from an influenza virus and its impact. So it is strongly suggested that you read all the remedies listed in both categories, whether you determine that the patient has a cold or the flu.

And remember, while colds are mostly an irritant, influenza can be serious. Every year, many thousands of people are still killed by flu. So don't hesitate to get professional help for the patient who is very ill.

Flu may include all the symptoms of a cold. Further, it usually will involve body aches and pain. For this reason, perhaps our most commonly used flu remedy is **Bryonia.** Following the general pattern of the remedy, the **Bryonia** patient will be in a great deal of discomfort. And he will not want to move, due to that discomfort. Motion, no matter how slight, increases his symptoms.

The **Bryonia** patient will tend to be slow to develop his full symptoms, and the flu will be very slow in developing. He will tend to sneeze a great deal, and the spasmodic movement caused by the sneeze will greatly irritate him. In fact, this patient is sometimes referred to as the "Bryonia Bear." This is a highly irritated patient and many caregivers will choose to leave him pretty much on his own.

The patient's eyes will tear a great deal, and there will be a great deal of nasal flow as well. Both eyes and nose will be watery, but the mouth will be dry. However, no matter how thirsty the patient is, he will drink infrequently, because he does not want to move. He will drink a great deal when he does drink.

Body aches will tend to be centered in the chest, and will feel as if the ribs were breaking. The cold symptoms will tend to move into the chest as well, bringing along a painful, deep cough. A severe headache will usually be a major part of the picture. The headache will tend to be frontal, in the forehead and/or frontal sinuses. The **Bryonia** with this headache will not even want to move his eyes because of the pain.

If body aches are a more important part of the illness, with the patient in so much pain that he feels as if the bones in his body were breaking, then consider the remedy **Eupatorium.** Think of it as a secondary remedy to **Bryonia,** only to be given if the first remedy fails to work.

Both **Bryonia** and **Eupatorium** will be chilly patients, and in both cases, chill may be the first sign of illness. But the **Eupatorium** patient will be extremely cold, and the chill will tend to be centralized in the area of the patient's spine. He may feel shivers running up and down his spine. As with **Bryonia**, the **Eupatorium** will not want to move, as any motion makes his pain that much worse.

Rhus Tox is another remedy to consider for those with flu who are experiencing body aches and pain. The pains will especially be located in the patient's limbs, and the patient will have to keep moving them to keep his body warm and reduce the pain.

Look for the **Rhus Tox** to have a red, very swollen face. Look for his tongue to be dry and smooth and have a red triangle on its tip, and for his lips to have a brownish color.

The **Rhus Tox** fever will be worse at night, especially around midnight. At that time, it may be high enough that the patient mutters to himself. The fever will be accompanied by a dry cough, which will be worse when the fever is in its chill stage.

The **Rhus Tox** flu may involve the digestive tract—the patient's fever may be accompanied by diarrhea. The patient will be greatly exhausted by diarrhea.

Gelsemium is another remedy to consider for flu that, as with both **Bryonia** and **Eupatorium,** develops with a change in the weather. The **Gelsemium** patient will not be as ill as either the **Bryonia** or the **Eupatorium** patient. He will tend to feel dizzy and too tired; in fact, this tired feeling is most often the sign of the onset, as the patient feels more and more exhausted over a period of days leading up to his illness. His cold-like symptoms will tend to begin with a sore throat. The patient will experience a pain in swallowing that extends into his ears. Mild fevers are also common, as are slight body aches. The patient will want to rest, will often lie about in somewhat of a stupor, with his eyes partially closed.

The patient will tend to suffer from a sensation of heaviness throughout his body, and like the **Eupatorium** patient, will experience a chilliness running up and down his spine. The **Gelsemium** patient will also suffer from a headache, during which his eyes will take on that characteristic symptom of being half-closed. This patient is sometimes too hot, sometimes too cold, and never just right.

The **Arsenicum** flu patient will never be too warm. He is always chilly, and seeks warmth of any sort. He likes to be in bed heavily wrapped up, and he likes the warmth of a fire. He is refreshed and improved by sipping warm liquids, especially tea with lemon. The flu that **Arsenicum** speaks to is the stomach flu, and it is also an important remedy for food poisoning. **Arsenicum** is the remedy of first choice in flu that involves both vomiting and diarrhea. The patient with the flu needing Arsenicum will be greatly debilitated by his illness. Each bout of diarrhea or vomiting leaves him weaker but he may be too nauseated to eat or drink anything. He may also begin to look older than his years in his illness.

In addition to these symptoms, the **Arsenicum** patient may have many of the symptoms usually associated with a cold. To get a more complete picture of the remedy read the listing for **Arsenicum** under that category.

When the flu involves nausea, diarrhea, and perhaps vomiting, another remedy to consider is **Sulphur.** This patient will be very different from the **Arsenicum** patient. In this case, the patient is hot and sweaty. Diarrhea will drive him out of bed in the morning. The flow will be hot and will cause the patient to itch. This will be a thirsty patient who will drink a great deal of cool and cold liquids.

The cold remedy **Camphora** may also be used to treat those with flu. When **Camphora** is called for, the patient will be greatly chilled, and covered with an icy sweat along with bouts of diarrhea. He will complain of an icy burning throughout his abdomen. And, although cold, he may refuse to be covered.

Finally, you should always consider **Mercurius** to be an excellent remedy for those with flu and who have become very ill. Look for this patient to have swollen glands in his neck and a swollen tongue. You will be able to see the indentations of the patient's teeth on the sides of his tongue. The patient will have a great deal of saliva in his mouth at all times.

This is a patient who is extremely sensitive to changes in temperature. Being too hot or too cold will greatly increase his symptoms.

Fever

The presence of a fever is always a sign of the body's immune system being on alert and attempting to cleanse the body. In this sense, fevers are a good thing, in that they are signs that the body is working as it should. Therefore, when a patient exhibits a mild fever that in no way threatens his health, you may want to decide for yourself whether to treat the symptom or not. If the fever persists or grows higher, however, then you will want to treat homeopathically, since the homeopathic remedies will not suppress either the fever or its root cause in any way. Instead, the remedy called for by the fever and its associated symptoms will help clear away the infection or other cause of those symptoms.

Most fevers, it should be noted, include three distinct symptoms, each of which flows into the next. The first symptom, cold, usually begins with a sensation of exhaustion, as the chill begins in the extremities and moves to the body as a whole. This symptom may remain for minutes or hours before moving on to the second symptom.

The next symptom is heat. The heat of fever is usually associated with a dry tongue, a desire for liquids, and a racing pulse. This second symptom can stay in place for several hours.

Finally, the third major symptom associated with fever is sweat. As the increased body temperature burns away the toxins or infectious agents, the fever breaks and the patient's body becomes covered with sweat. This may mark the end of the fever, or the beginning of the next cycle of symptoms.

Remember that this description is of a general pattern, and does not describe every fever. Some patients will only experience heat, others only cold, and some may have sweat throughout or not at all.

Consider the remedies listed below when fever stands alone as a symptom, or when it is the most prominent feature among many.

And since fever often is associated with colds and flu, you may want to read about other remedies listed under those categories to help you in your remedy selection.

There are two major remedies that you may have to choose between for high fevers that start suddenly and frighteningly: **Aconite** and **Belladonna.** In both cases, the fever will be high—so high, in fact, that the patient may hallucinate or cry out. In both cases the patient will also have a face and head that are bright or dark red, and very hot and dry.

In the case of **Aconite,** however, the patient's whole body will stay dry and the patient will experience heat throughout his whole being. The patient's face may turn pale during the fever if the patient sits up. This is a very anxious and worried patient, and he will be very restless as well. This patient may insist that he is dying during the heat of the fever. Look for the patient's fever to be worse in the evening and to build toward midnight.

The patient needing **Belladonna** will often feel chilled during the high fever, and may be covered with cold sweat on every part of the body except the head. His tongue will be red and cracked. His abdomen will be very tender to the touch. As with **Bryonia,** the **Belladonna** patient may experience discomfort with every movement.

The **Belladonna** patient may be belligerent and delirious during his fever. He will feel a sensation of pounding throughout his head and body. The **Belladonna** patient will be very sensitive to noise and to light, and will want to lie down in a cool, dark place. Often he will want to sleep but will be unable to.

Stramonium, a remedy not listed in the Objective Materia Medica, is another remedy for cases of high fever that are often accompanied by hallucinations and delirium. This is a very high fever. The patient has a very red face. And, like **Belladonna,** the **Stramonium** patient cannot bear bright light. But, unlike **Belladonna,** he will be unable to stand dark places as well.

Baptisia is another remedy you may want to have in your home kit that is not included in the Objective Materia Medica. The patient with a **Baptisia** fever will become very ill very quickly. He will seem to be slipping away due to his fever. In this case, the fever will be very irregular; it will go up and down, although it will tend to be at its highest in the late morning. As with **Belladonna** and **Aconite,** the patient will have a dark red complexion. And, as with the remedy **Arnica,** the patient will feel as if he had been beaten up and was bruised from head to toe. And, as with **Arnica,** he will seem vague and will be slow to answer questions, as if his thinking was clouded or delayed. Further, the **Baptisia** patient may drop suddenly into a deep sleep during the heat of fever.

Note that the patient's sweat, urine, and stool are all offensive, and that this patient may have very bad breath as well. Diarrhea may accompany fever.

Apis is a good remedy to have on hand for cases of fever. The patient needing **Apis** will not be thirsty during his fever, no matter how high it may go. Because of this, look for the **Apis** to have a very dry mouth and throat, and to have great difficulty swallowing.

The Apis fever will typically spike at four in the afternoon (this is also true for **Lycopodium**). While the **Apis** patient does not sweat a great deal, his skin may alternate between dry and moist. He will not want heat or warm applications of any sort.

This is another patient who may experience delirium during his high fever. The patient may mutter or cry out in his unconscious or semiconscious state. He will also tend to move his head from side to side in his pain.

Mercurius may be needed for cases of fever accompanied by chills, or when the patient alternates between heat and chills. The **Mercurius** patient will be covered in chilly sweat during fever. He will be extremely sensitive to changes in temperature, and will experience a spike in his symptoms if he becomes too warm or too cold.

Not all fevers are as high or as frightening as those listed above. For cases of fevers that are not too high and do not have any specific guiding symptoms associated with them, **Ferrum Phos** is the remedy of choice. In fact, **Ferrum Phos** is an excellent remedy to have on hand as a first-choice general remedy for those with fever. The **Ferrum Phos** patient will tend to be thirsty, but not in any exaggerated manner. He will also tend to be a bit chilly, and may shiver. He may also experience frequent sweats during fever.

Ferrum Phos may also be of help for cases of colds in which fever is the first symptom. The patient will have a red face. He will also want to keep his face cool, and will want cool applications during fever.

China is another important and rather general remedy to have on hand for cases of fever. The **China** fever best illustrates the general pattern of fevers in that it has three distinct stages. Stage one is chills: the patient will shake and shiver with cold. The second stage is heat, during which the patient will experience the full heat of the fever. Finally, in stage three, the patient will begin to sweat, and this sweating will be accompanied by a huge thirst. The third stage of the fever also includes great exhaustion. Consider the remedy **China** when you see all three stages clearly displayed.

Arnica, which is usually thought of as a remedy for physical trauma, may also be helpful for cases of fever. As in the case of physical trauma, the **Arnica** patient will all but deny that he has a fever. He will not seem to care that he is sick. He will tend to be confused, and may have trouble answering any questions. He may slip into sleep while talking. As is common to the remedy, the fever will leave the **Arnica** feeling bruised and beaten. He will feel that his bed is too hard, and will be unable, like **Rhus Tox,** to find a comfortable position.

The **Arsenicum** patient with a fever will be greatly exhausted, and yet he will remain restless and rather fussy unless he is very ill. He may also become very afraid during a high fever, convinced that he is going to die. Either way, the **Arsenicum** will want you to stay by his side, and will never want to be alone.

The **Arsenicum** patient will want to stay warm—except for his head, on which he wants to feel cool, fresh air. It is not uncommon to find him sitting by an open window, with his entire body, except for his head, completely covered.

The **Arsenicum** will be thirsty for warm liquids, which he will drink one small sip at a time.

In the **Phosphorus** patient, heat and chills will alternate, and the he will be thirsty only during heat. Sweats will occur at night, especially in the early hours of the morning. Sweat will cover the patient's head, hands, and feet. The patient may also sweat up and down his spine.

The **Rhus Tox** patient with fever is another who is restless, despite his exhaustion due to his ailment. The **Rhus Tox** will move about constantly in order to keep comfortable. He will toss and turn seeking a comfortable position. This is a very thirsty patient.

Look for the **Rhus Tox** patient to have a face that is both red and swollen. Look for him (like the **Phosphorus** patient) to have blue rings around his eyes. Note that his tongue is dry and smooth, and has a red triangle on the tip. Note that a red rash may cover the patient's whole body during fever, that body pain and/or diarrhea may accompany fever.

The **Ipecac** patient is also very thirsty, especially during the short chill phase of the fever. When the fever is in its heat stage, look for the patient's extremities to be covered with a clammy sweat. The **Ipecac** patient will be very nauseated; he will tend to vomit, although the vomiting only weakens him further.

Note that **Ipecac,** a remedy so associated with nausea and vomiting, is also one of the few remedies associated with a completely clean tongue. Counterintuitive as it may seem, look for the **Ipecac** tongue to have no coating, no teeth marks, no excess saliva. It will look very clean and pink.

Another remedy with fever and a clean tongue is **Cina.** In cases needing **Cina,** look for the patient to first feel very hungry, and then very nauseated, and then to vomit before the onset of the heat of fever. The patient's face will stay very pale, and he will remain thirsty during both heat and chill. Note that the **Cina** patient will typically have dilated pupils during fever.

Another patient who will be very nauseated during fever is **Antimonium Tartaricum.** This is a very weak patient who is convinced that he will die of his ailment. The patient will experience a profuse cold sweat during fever. Notably, he will be very tired and will want to sleep, but will be afraid that he will die if he sleeps.

Some remedies for "simple" fevers include **Nux, Natrum Mur** and **Phosphorus.**

The first remedy to think of in a simple fever is **Nux,** especially if the patient is angry.

In fact, anger is so much a part of this remedy that **Nux** is contraindicated if the patient is sweet and pleasant. The fever will be slow coming on, and will usually begin with a sensation of chills. Once the patient is chilly, he cannot become warm. The fever is accompanied by a headache, which has the sensation of a nail being driven into the patient's head. It also may be accompanied by constipation.

The **Natrum Mur** simple fever starts in the midmorning. The patient will want to go lie down to combat the fever. He will be very thirsty, especially for cold water. Although this patient drinks very often, his tongue will be very dry.

The **Phosphorus** patient will also be thirsty for cold water, and will want ice cream and other cold things to eat. But he will become nauseated when these things warm in his stomach, and he may then vomit them back up. This is a weak, sweet patient, who does not want to be left alone. He will have a stopped-up nose that forces him to breathe through his mouth.

For the patient who has a fever of unknown origin, or who experiences fevers often, consider **Sulphur. Sulphur** should also always be considered if your best-selected remedies have failed to act. The **Sulphur** patient will most often experience a great heat on the top of his head, accompanied by a sensation of chill in his extremities. This is a patient who is thirsty, especially for cold things, and for sweet things like ginger ale. The fever may be accompanied by diarrhea, which will drive the patient out of the bed first thing in the morning.

If the fevers return chronically without apparent cause, consider **Carbo Veg.** The **Carbo Veg** fever follows three stages: sweat, which leads to shortness of breath (a theme symptom of **Carbo Veg),** which leads to chill. This patient will be thirsty during the chill stage. His extremities will be cold and covered in a cold sweat.

Look for the **Carbo Veg** to have dull eyes that seem to have sunken into his head. He will not be able to bear light in any form. He will need to sit in moving air in order to feel that he can breathe.

If the patient is chronically given to fevers, consider **Calcarea.** These fevers will alternate between stages of chill and stages of heat. The patient may also experience a sensation of external coldness accompanied by internal heat. Palpitations may accompany the fever, as will a rapid pulse. Look for a cough to accompany the fever, as will diarrhea, which is made up of undigested foods. This is an anxious and very weak patient.

Finally, remember the fever symptoms associated with what may otherwise be consider "flu" remedies:

Gelsemium is notable for the patient's complete lack of thirst during his fever. The patient will have the sensation of heaviness throughout his whole body. The fever will be accompanied by a headache, during which the patient's eyes will be half closed. This patient will want to lie still and be quiet. Note that the **Gelsemium** patient will alternate between fever and chills, and that the chills will tend to occur in the evening and originate in the patient's hands and/or feet.

The **Bryonia** patient will be chilly during his fever. He will be very thirsty, and will drink a great deal each time he drinks. The fever will be worse at night, and each time the patient moves.

And the **Eupatorium** patient will experience a fever that is highest in the early morning. He will have chills during his fever, and terrible body aches and pains. He will also experience periods of sweating, but not during the chill phase.

Sore Throat

Since it is hard to separate the sore throat from the other symptoms associated colds and flu, I will be brief here, with the exception of remedies not previously mentioned. See the other listings in this section and refer to the Objective Materia Medica for a more complete picture of the remedies and the symptoms associated with them.

And a final thought: sore throats can be difficult to treat as standalone symptoms, because they rely on so many subjective symptoms, for example, "burning pain" versus "stinging pain." Therefore, to treat objectively it is important to gather information about symptoms other than those relating just to the throat when possible. After all, nearly every sore throat looks red and inflamed.

Many sore throats will have the characteristic pain sensation of burning. **Belladonna, Aconite, Apis** (whose pain may also be "stinging" in character), and **Causticum** are chief among these remedies. Some sore throats involve loss of voice, and **Phosphorus, Gelsemium, Causticum,** and **Rhus Tox** are chief among these. Some, like the sore throats that need **Belladonna** and **Aconite,** develop quickly, while others, like the **Nux** sore throat, develop slowly. Some begin on the left, like **Lachesis** and **Sulphur,** while others begin on the right, like **Arsenicum** and **Lachesis.** Finally, some patients with sore throats crave cold things, like the **Apis** and **Sulphur** patients, while others, like the **Arsenicum** and **Sulphur** patients, want warm drinks to soothe their pain.

The most commonly called for remedies for patients with sore throat are **Apis, Lachesis, Rhus Tox,** and **Phosphorus.** The **Apis** sore throat follows the general theme of the remedy in that the throat feels as if it had been stung by a bee. The sensation of pain is stinging and/or burning. The interior throat will look red and swollen, and may be so swollen that swallowing is difficult. Most important to determining the remedy is that the interior throat will look shiny but is dry. The patient is very thirsty for very cold things, and warm drinks will actually increase the pain. Like the **Lachesis** patient, the **Apis** will not want anything near his throat, and will not want it touched.

The patient needing **Lachesis** will feel as if his throat is the most vulnerable part of his body. He will protect it with all the energy he has, so take care in how you approach him in asking to see his throat. The interior of his throat will be the purple/red hue that is characteristic of the remedy. The pain symptoms will either begin on the left and move right, or be dominant on the left. Note that the patient's pain will be worse from swallowing liquids, most especially from swallowing warm liquids, and better from swallowing solids.

Both **Phosphorus** and **Rhus Tox** sore throats may develop as part of an overall viral attack, or from overuse of the throat and stress of the voice (this used to be called "Preacher's Throat"). Either can be caused by overtalking or oversinging.

The **Phosphorus** patient will feel a sense of exhaustion, tightness in his chest, and voice loss and sore throat. He will want cold water and foods to soothe his throat. (Note that he may become nauseated as those foods warm in his stomach.) This patient will want to talk and laugh, but will be worse from both.

The **Rhus Tox** patient will find that his throat is most painful on first swallowing. Therefore, he may continually swallow to keep his throat lubricated. He will want warm drinks to soothe the pain.

Rhus Tox and **Phosphorus** are often needed as sore throat remedies in children. Two other remedies commonly used in treating young patients with sore throats are **Aconite** and **Chamomilla.**

The young **Aconite** patient often becomes ill after playing outside on a cold, clear day. This is the child who is bundled up and gets overheated while playing and then, when he cools down, takes a chill from a cold, dry wind. He comes in from the exposure, and seemingly within minutes, becomes sick. The sore throat, which is usually accompanied by fever, begins out of nowhere and with no warning, and seemingly without cause. This patient will be chilled, even when he is in the heat stage of his fever. Look for the patient's face to be red, and his skin to be red, dry, and hot. The young patient will be very restless; it will be all but impossible to get him to go to bed and rest.

Where the **Aconite** patient is restless and somewhat anxious, the **Chamomilla** patient is downright mean and very irritable. He may actually even throw things at you as you try to help him. Look at the patient's face: you will likely find that one cheek is red and/or swollen, and the other is pale. (This is a great remedy for the child who is teething that shows this characteristic symptom.)

The **Chamomilla** patient usually will take sick when he goes outside into cold weather after taking a shower in gym class and not bothering to dry his hair. In other words, he tends to follow the pattern of always being overheated and ignoring the cold, until he gets cold, at which point he also gets sick.

Chamomilla is such a common sore throat remedy for children that it is the first one you should think of for cases in which the child is irritable. The most important subjective symptom is that the patient will feel that, if he were just able to cough up some mucus from his chest, he would feel all better. So he coughs and coughs, but nothing comes up.

In some cases, a sore throat, particularly if it is a recurring sore throat, may be related to tonsillitis. This may especially be the case for sore throats that need **Belladonna** or **Ferrum Phos.**

The **Belladonna** sore throat develops quickly, as is keynote to the remedy. Look for the tonsils, as well as the interior throat, to be bright red. Look for the patient to swallow constantly, although swallowing pains him. Note that the throat may be so swollen and painful that the patient will not be able to swallow either food or drink. Often a high fever will accompany the sore throat.

The **Ferrum Phos** sore throat, on the other hand, is far less dramatic. All of the symptoms will be similar to those of **Belladonna,** but not nearly as frightening. Like the **Belladonna** patient, the **Ferrum Phos** patient will have a fever, but one that is not nearly as high. And, in the case of **Ferrum Phos,** the patient will be thirsty for cold things, which will soothe the throat.

Whether or not the cause is specifically tonsillitis or not, the sore throats requiring **Mercurius** or **Hepar Sulph** involve some sort of infection in the patient's system.

The **Mercurius** sore throat will involve swelling of the interior throat and the tonsils, as well as swollen glands under the jaw. Look at the patient's tongue for a major symptom, as the **Mercurius** tongue will be swollen, and you will likely see the indentation for his teeth around its sides. The patient will also have an increased flow of saliva. Because of all the saliva, the patient must keep swallowing, although swallowing is very painful.

The **Hepar Sulph** patient will experience the pain sensation of a bone or a stick being caught in his throat. This patient is also very protective of his throat, as if feels very vulnerable, both inside and out. Note that the interior throat will be very swollen and that there will be a great deal of drainage down the throat. The throat will be very sensitive to anything that is cold, even to cold air. Note that when the patient swallows, the pain extends into his ears.

Remember that in cases calling for **Mercurius** or **Hepar Sulph,** it is unlikely that the sore throat has begun quickly or out of nowhere, as it seems with **Belladonna.** These sore throats are slower to develop, and develop out of some other illness such as inflamed tonsils or a cold that has become something more serious.

Two patients whose symptoms will be similar enough to be confusing are the **Arsenicum** and the **Lycopodium.** Both patients will have sore throats that begin on the right side and move left, or which are dominant on the right side of their throat. Both will be chilly patients who crave warmth and are better from drinking warm liquids. Both will seem shriveled and shrunken by their illness, and rather pitiful. And neither will want to be left alone, although the **Arsenicum** patient will tend to want you to stay in the room with him, while the **Lycopodium** patient will want you to leave his room, but to stay nearby in case he needs you.

One way you can tell them apart is by the time of day in which they are worse. The **Arsenicum** patient is always worse at night, especially as midnight approaches. The **Lycopodium** patient, on the other hand, is worse in late afternoon, especially around 4:00P.M. (Note that, in some cases, the **Lycopodium** patient will be worse at 4:00A.M.)

Another way you will often be able to tell these two apart is by the subjective symptom regarding the quality of the pain. The **Arsenicum** patient's sore throat will be burning in nature, while the **Lycopodium** patient will complain of the sensation of a plug or a ball caught in his throat.

Some sore throats come and go quickly, while others are longer lasting. The remedies most commonly associated with long-term sore throats or with recurring sore throats are **Nux, Carbo Veg, Causticum,** and **Gelsemium.**

The **Nux** sore throat is slow in coming, long lasting, and slow to fade. The patient will experience a scraping sensation in his throat. The **Nux** sore throat seldom involves that single symptom. Most commonly, it is linked to negative emotions, like anger, and to chronic sinus problems that leave the patient's nose blocked and postnasal drip irritating the back of his throat. The **Nux** patient is chilly and may suffer from chronic constipation in addition to his other ills.

The patient needing **Carbo Veg** will experience hoarseness and throat pain that also threatens to become a chronic condition. Both the pain and hoarseness are worse in the morning, and again in the evening. **Carbo Veg** should especially be considered when the throat pain has developed after the patient has failed to fully recover from another more serious condition, like flu or, especially, measles.

The patient needing **Causticum** has, like the **Phosphorus** or the **Rhus Tox** patient, likely stressed his voice and is now hoarse and in pain. But unlike the **Phosphorus** and **Rhus Tox** patient, the **Causticum** case is long lasting. In fact, this remedy may be used as a backup to the other two for cases they fail to cure. The **Causticum** sore throat is obstinate and hard to cure. Often the patient will experience pain in his chest as well as his throat.

Gelsemium is another remedy to think of for cases in which the patient is still suffering the effects of flu or some other disease. The patient is depleted and exhausted, and his voice will be more weak than hoarse. He will have difficulty swallowing.

Finally, there are two important remedies for those with sore throat that are not a part of our Objective Materia Medica. They are **Baryta Carbonica** and **Phytolacca.**

Baryta Carbonica is another excellent remedy to consider for those who are plagued with recurring tonsillitis. In sore throats calling for this remedy, look for the patient's tonsils and the glands behind his throat to be swollen and very tender. Look for these sore throats to start rather slowly, but to get worse and worse until they seem to be sucking all the life's energy away from the patient.

Swallowing will be very painful, especially empty swallowing. The patient will only be able to swallow liquids. Look for the pain and its accompanying cough to get worse as midnight approaches. Look for the patient's pain to increase if his feet get cold. In general this is a chilly patient who is worse for cold in any form.

Note that this remedy is one that usually speaks to conditions that are chronic in nature, especially chronic tonsillitis and bronchitis.

The patient needing **Phytolacca** will have perhaps the most painful sore throat of all. You may want to have it on hand for the rare instances in which it might be needed for this reason. Look for a throat that is sore, swollen, and dark, dark red in color. Look for the root of the tongue, the soft palate, and the tonsils to be swollen as well.

The patient will often be unable to speak because of the pain. He will have trouble swallowing anything, most especially anything hot. He will complain about the sensation of a lump—most especially a red-hot lump—in his throat.

A high fever will accompany the sore throat. The fever will alternate between the stages of high heat and chills.

Note that the patient needing this remedy may also experience muscle pain in his exterior neck.

Consider this remedy for cases of tonsillitis and mumps that follow the pattern of the remedy.

Coughs

You may think of the remedies listed here as a continuation of those listed earlier for the third stage of colds. As cough is usually a symptom associated with the second, or, more often, third stage of a cold, you will seldom find cough as a stand-alone symptom. Therefore, the remedies listed here will often be useful for clearing up the final stages of a cold that has either lingered or grown into something deeper.

Note that you must also refer to the section of this text dedicated to cold remedies to have a complete picture of the kit remedies used to combat coughs. **Phosphorus, Rhus Tox,** and **Lachesis,** among others, may also be considered general "cough" remedies, while **Mercurius** and **Hepar Sulph** may be considered remedies for cases in which the cough is part of a portrait indicating that what started as a simple ailment like a cold has developed into something more serious.

Often, you will be able to tell what remedy a patient with cough needs by the sound of the cough alone. This is particularly the case for those needing **Spongia, Drosera** and **Rumex.**

The **Drosera** cough is perhaps the most distinctive of the three. It has a rat-a-tattat nature. This is a ringing, loud cough, one that resonates throughout the patient's being. Often the cough, like the **Rumex** cough, will begin with a tickling in the throat, although the patient will usually insist that it originates deeper, down in his abdomen. The patient will also complain of a sensation of constriction in his throat. And the cough will occur in spasms, spasms that are, on occasion, violent enough to cause the patient to vomit, and are so violent that the patient will have to support his chest or abdomen during his coughing fit.

Note that Hahnemann considered **Drosera** to be the leading remedy for patients with whooping cough.

The **Spongia** cough is also very distinctive: it has the quality and rhythm of either a barking dog or a saw cutting through wood. This is a raspy, irregular cough that is surprising in both its suddenness and intensity. Often, it will awaken the patient while he sleeps, usually in the early part of the night, before midnight. The **Spongia** patient cannot bear cold in any form and needs to be kept warm and calm. He is worse from talking and for any excitement.

Note that you should look for the **Spongia** patient, like the **Lachesis** patient, to feel as if he is suffocating. Like **Lachesis,** he may awaken suddenly with a feeling that he had stopped breathing in his sleep.

The **Rumex** cough is shallower and gentler, yet more maddening. This is a cough caused by a tickle in the pit of the throat, and it seems to be triggered by everything, especially by the patient taking a deep breath. But it is also triggered by the patient's talking, laughing, or having his throat touched. It is keynote of the remedy that the patient will have to invest all his time and energy in keeping himself from coughing. He will even pull the covers up over his nose and mouth in order to warm the air he breathes before the cool, fresh air can trigger the cough. The cough may also be triggered if the patient lies down, so he may have to go for long, exhausting periods of time trying to sleep propped up. So this patient will be just miserable. He will not eat or drink, talk, or sleep, and will breathe as shallowly as possible, all to avoid that terrible, nagging cough.

Two remedies are commonly used when a cough begins to move into a deeper situation. They are **Ipecac** and **Antimonium Tartaricum.** In cases needing either of these remedies, nausea is as strong a symptom as is the cough itself.

Ipecac is a remedy of first choice for cases of cough that are moving into bronchitis, which often happens with surprising speed. This is a deep and loose cough. You will be able to hear mucus rattling around in the patient's chest, and the patient will cough in an attempt to bring the mucus up. Often coughing will trigger bouts of nausea that may end in vomiting.

Look for the **Ipecac** patient to experience bouts of suffocation with his coughing. The cough is also aggravated by warmth in any form, especially a warm, stuffy room. Nose-bleeds frequently accompany coughing.

The **Ipecac** patient needs rest, and to be kept still, because any motion aggravates the cough. He is thirstless, and nauseated by the very thought of food.

The **Antimonium Tartaricum** patient has been compared to the drowning man going down for the third time. He can seem to be drowning in the mucus in his own system. Listen for the rattling in his chest.

Where the symptoms of **Ipecac** develop very swiftly, those of **Antimonium Tartaricum** develop very slowly. In cases needing this remedy, a simple ailment has slowly developed into something more serious, usually bronchitis. And, where the wild coughing of the **Ipecac** patient fails to bring up mucus, the **Antimonium** patient is, in general, simply too weak to cough up his mucus. Instead, he gasps for air. Look for the patient to alternate coughing and yawning, and note that coughing may end in vomiting for the **Antimonium** patient as well.

The **Antimonium** patient will be very thirsty for cold water, which he will drink in frequent small sips. He will be averse to all forms of food, however.

The **Antimonium** patient will tend to have icy cold limbs and extremities, and a head that is hot and sweaty. Look for the patient's head to tremble when he coughs.

Homeopathic Band-Aids

From time to time, everyone suffers from motion sickness or heartburn, or gets a headache or a toothache. It is easy to think of these as purely acute situations, but often the ailments, especially if they are recurring, are indications of some deeper illness.

So the remedies listed here are included only as a short-term solution until proper treatment can be found.

In many cases, the action of the remedies will indeed be short term. It all depends upon the true cause of the symptoms. For instance, the toothache caused by a rotten tooth cannot be cured by any homeopathic remedy. Ultimately, only a proper filling will cause the pain to stop. But if the tooth itself is sound, and the toothache is caused by sinus pressure on the nerve of the tooth, then the remedy may be curative in its action.

Some things, like a headache or a case of simple indigestion can be simple acutes. But they need to be considered as part of a deeper chronic situation and proper professional care needs to be sought if they recur or link to other symptoms.

So think of these remedies as you did the First Aid remedies: they will get you through the night when symptoms suddenly flare, but they may not ultimately replace the need to find appropriate professional care.

The remedies listed here are to be given in 30C potency unless otherwise noted.

Remedies Strongly Suggested for the Common Complaints Home Kit

Arnica: Think of Arnica first for any case of tooth or mouth pain after dental surgery or after the dentist fills a tooth. Also, think of this remedy first for cases of emotional upset that is the result of the patient hearing bad news. Arnica is as important to emotional healing after emotional trauma as it is to physical healing after physical trauma. Note that Arnica is also a useful remedy to think of for cases of insomnia that follow bad news, or for those who suffer from nightmares.

Arsenicum: This is perhaps our most useful remedy for cases of diarrhea that also involve a great deal of nausea and vomiting, and for cases of chronic diarrhea that have greatly weakened the patient. It is useful for diarrhea in elderly people. The patient will be chilly (except, perhaps, his head, which will be hot and want cool applications or air), weak, and fussy. This is a restless patient who, unless he

630

is very ill, will not want to just get into bed and stay there. This is a thirsty patient, but he will only sip a little liquid at a time. He often will want warm liquids to settle his stomach. All symptoms will be worse as midnight approaches. Consider this remedy for diarrhea caused by fear.

Bryonia: This is another remedy for constipation. This patient will be very thirsty and will drink large quantities of water, although he will drink infrequently, because he will want to rest and not want to move to drink. Think of this remedy for all cases of indigestion that develop in warm weather, especially from eating or drinking cold things in hot summer weather. The Bryonia throws up immediately after eating.

Calcarea: Calcarea often relates to the body's ability to absorb substances, so the patient who requires this remedy for his indigestion is having difficulty properly absorbing his food. Because of this, Calcarea is often needed for patients with chronic indigestion, patients who commonly feel bloated and feel a pressure on their waist. Think of this remedy as well for patients with diarrhea that is caused by stress and overwork. The patient's stool will contain particles of undigested food. When he is feeling sick to his stomach, the Calcarea patient will also be beset with damp, cold feet and a clammy sweat on the top and back of his head.

Carbo Veg: This is our "belchy" patient, the one who is sitting in the corner burping after dinner. Further, this belching is sour and smelly, and it gives scant relief. Heartburn may also leave the patient wracked with discomfort. The patient may feel faint from his indigestion, as if he cannot breathe. He will want moving air, like the air of an electric fan, to be able to breathe. Note that the patient may have an attack of hiccoughs instead of belching. This is an excellent remedy for that problem as well.

Chamomilla: Intense pain is the key to this remedy; intense pain in a very irritable patient. In cases of indigestion, the patient's abdomen will be swollen to the point of being drumlike. The patient will pass gas with no relief. In cases of toothache, the pain is just as severe, and it is made worse by any contact with cold, whether from cold drink or air. The pain from contact with warm drinks is just as great. Nothing satisfies the Chamomilla in his pain. Look for his face, especially in cases of toothache, to have one cheek red and the other pale. Consider this remedy for cases of diarrhea brought on by anger.

China: Think of this remedy first for cases of indigestion that develop after the patient has already suffered from another more serious ailment. This patient will commonly have to lie down after every meal, as it will take all of his body's energy to digest his food. This patient may be disgusted at the sight of any food or drink. His abdomen will be swollen and drum-like. He will pass much gas, but without relief. The patient will experience a cutting pain in the area of the navel that is relieved when the patient bends over. Think of this remedy for cases of abdominal distress that occur after eating fruit. (Note that the two remedies China and Phosphoric Acid have a strong relationship in cases involving indigestion associated with recovery from a deeper illness. Each remedy may follow the other in curing the case.)

Coffea: This is perhaps our most commonly used toothache remedy. It is the remedy for the patient who is manic in his pain, and cannot stop talking, settle down and rest. The tooth itself will be sensitive to heat, and will become much more painful from any contact with heat. The pain will be soothed by cold, however, so look for the patient to hold ice cubes over the tooth or over his jaw to soothe the pain. This is also an important remedy for cases of insomnia in which, like children on Christmas Eve, the patient is too "wound up" to sleep, and for cases in which the patient cannot quiet his mind enough to sleep. Think of this remedy for cases of insomnia that occur after hearing good or exciting news.

Ipecac: This is an excellent remedy to have on hand as it not only is a remedy for nausea that leads to vomiting, but it is an excellent children's remedy. As Chamomilla may be considered a general sore throat remedy for children, Ipecac is the first choice remedy for children with indigestion of any sort. Look for the adult needing this remedy to seem like the Carbo Veg patient: chilly, bloated, belching, and burping, or hiccoughing. Nothing relieves him, and vomiting is the usual result. The patient will experience a sinking sensation in his stomach before vomiting.

Lycopodium: This is perhaps the most gassy of all remedy types. Look for the Lycopodium to loosen his belt and undo his pants while at the dinner table. Gas begins with the first or second bite, and he is fully bloated by the end of the meal. The Lycopodium is chilly, and tends to be crabby. Although he does not want to be left alone, he does not want to be in the same room with others either. So look for the Lycopodium patient to go to his den, where he can pass gas and listen to the sounds of the family from afar. The Lycopodium will be at his worst at 4:00P.M., and sometimes at 4:00A.M.

Nux: This remedy is the king of constipation. Nux is the major remedy for constipation and indigestion that is brought on from a poor or too rich diet. It also is a remedy for those who have had too much alcohol and are suffering from hangover, and for digestive headaches. The Nux patient is very cold, and cannot get warm. He is angry, and cannot bear noise, which makes his head hurt. Like the other symptoms, chronic digestive symptoms may be very slow to develop and may last for a long, long time. Consider this remedy for cases of indigestion or diarrhea brought on by anger.

Petroleum: This is perhaps our most important remedy for travel sickness. Think of this remedy for the patient with persistent nausea while traveling. This nausea will be accompanied by a great amount of saliva accumulated in the patient's mouth. The patient will vomit if he eats or drinks anything. Along with nausea and vomiting, the patient will suffer from pain in the back of his head and from stiffness in his neck muscles.

Podophyllum: As Ferrum Phos is to fever, Podophyllum is to diarrhea. Keep this remedy on hand at all times, as it is an excellent general remedy for those who have acute diarrhea. Most of the time, a dose or two of the remedy will end the problem. It is useful both for cases of painless diarrhea or diarrhea preceded by severe cramping in the abdomen, and for cases of profuse diarrhea.

Pulsatilla: Gentle Pulsatilla is such a sweet and timid patient that it will take you some time to realize that he is driving you crazy. He is also demanding, needy, and among the most self-pitying of patients. He will, therefore, always need you to be doing something for him. This patient does not want to be alone. He is worse in a warm room, and will usually have to open a window or even go for a walk outside to feel better. This is a very common remedy for indigestion and digestive disorders of all sorts, particularly for cases caused by overeating that result in diarrhea, especially diarrhea at night.

Sulphur: The idea of a homeopathic Band-Aid could not exist without the remedy Sulphur. This is the general tonic of remedies. It is commonly used in a single dose to jump start healing when the best-indicated remedy fails to act. It is the supreme remedy for chronic functional complaints when pathology is not present. Look for the common theme of the remedy—a patient who is hot, sweaty, and itchy. This is a talkative patient. Look for the mark of the remedy on his face—a mask of redness flushing across both his cheeks and his nose.

Remedies You May Want to Add to Your Kit

Apis: Apis is not commonly thought of as a remedy for those with constipation, but it should be. It is one of the most helpful remedies for cases of acute constipation. The most important symptom associated with the constipation is that the patient will feel an incredible sensitivity in the region of his waist, and will not be able to bear tight clothing around it. The discomfort will extend through-out his abdomen. The patient who needs Apis doesn't want to go to the bathroom to try to pass a stool. He is fearful that it will be so painful that it will not be worth it, so he will not want to even attempt to pass a stool.

Belladonna: The suddenness of the pain and the suddenness of its departure are key to understanding the use of this remedy. Also important to the remedy is the presence of dry heat. For instance, think of this remedy for cases of toothache in which the pain is sudden and the patient's mouth is dry. The tooth will throb in pain. The same will be true of the patient with diarrhea: the pain comes suddenly, followed by stool. Both will stop suddenly. This patient will be sleepy because of his pain. He will want to sleep, but will be unable to.

Causticum: This is a remedy to consider for cases of acute constipation. The patient will feel sore, especially in the region of his anus. The pain will be especially great when the patient is walking. And the patient's walk will be hurried, with something of a crippled gait. This is an anxious and restless patient whose face is bright red during constipation.

Cocculus: Think of this wonderful acute remedy for colic and diarrhea when the abdomen is swollen, distended, and filled with gas. This is a very gassy patient. This is also an important remedy for those with motion sickness that involves vertigo, dizziness, nausea, and vomiting. The patient will have a sensation of hollowness or emptiness in his head, chest, and abdomen.

Colocynthis: This is a very important remedy for acute cases of diarrhea in which diarrhea will be accompanied by severe spasmodic pains. The patient will say that he feels as if his stomach is being ground between stones. The key to understanding the use of this remedy is that the pain will extend upward into the patient's neck and throat. Cramping may extend into the patient's limbs. Think of this as the remedy of first choice for any case that combines the pain of colic with diarrhea, especially if the patient has to bend over or press hard on his abdomen to relieve pain.

Ignatia: This is an important remedy for cases of indigestion and for diarrhea, either of which may occur after the patient experiences strong emotion, especially grief. The patient's sense of smell will be an important component to the Ignatia patient's indigestion. The patient may become nauseated from smelling cigarette smoke, or at the smell of any food. Note that there is perhaps no better remedy for emotional upsets than Ignatia. This is the remedy for the hysterical patient, for the patient with wild mood swings, and, most especially, for the patient trapped in his grief after the loss of a loved one. It is also helpful for cases of insomnia from grief.

Lachesis: Consider this remedy first for cases of indigestion of any sort, acute or chronic, that are the result of an irregular appetite, as is the case with the patient who does not have regular eating habits and eats heavily in one meal and next to nothing in the next. Like the Nux, the Lachesis patient will crave alcohol, and may have digestive disorders as a result. Look for this patient to be sluggish after every meal, like the snake who supplies the remedy with his venom. The patient will be very sleepy and will want to lie down after every meal.

Mercurius: The Mercurius patient typically has some sort of infection in his system.

Therefore, he usually has swollen glands and a fever. He will be very sensitive to temperature changes, and will tend to be covered in sweat. He will tend to have a swollen tongue and a great amount of saliva. This general picture may extend to or be the result of an infected tooth, or extend into the patient's digestive tract. This is a remedy to consider in the patient who is suffering from pains of colic that are associated with slimy diarrhea. Look for the patient's thighs and legs to be covered in sweat during the bouts of diarrhea. The patient may have dark-colored urine as well, and his urine may also contain blood.

Sepia: On a more chronic level, Sepia relates to grief as much as Ignatia does. The Sepia patient, however, has greatly suppressed his grief, and often experiences it as a sensation of weight in a part of his body. Like Calcarea, Sepia is often required for cases of chronic indigestion that involve a patient's loss of ability to absorb nutrients from his diet. The most telling symptom here is that headache and indigestion will alternate. The aforementioned weight will also be located in the patient's stomach. Consider this remedy for cases of chronic constipation in which the patient feels he must exercise to be able to pass a stool. Often, the patient's face will be yellow during indigestion and constipation.

Silicea: As with Arsenicum, the patient needing this remedy cannot digest any food at all, no matter how simple (Sulphur, in a chronic digestive disorder, may experience this as well.) But the Arsenicum patient tends to be nauseated in the evening, while the Silicea patient is worse in the morning. Both will be chilly, and both will be worse after every meal, but diarrhea follows indigestion in the Arsenicum patient, and constipation accompanies indigestion in the Silicea patient. In severe cases, the patient will not be able to bear even the taste of water and may vomit after drinking it.

Remedies Not in the Objective Materia Medica That You May Want to Have on Hand

Anacardium: This is our true "heartburn" remedy. The discomfort will usually begin two to three hours after the patient has eaten. It will often begin with the sensation of a bad taste in the patient's mouth. Look for the patient to suffer from terrible bad breath as part of his indigestion. The patient will feel acidic and bitter, and may have the sensation of a plug in his stomach. This is a gassy patient who will actually feel better if he passes gas. He will also feel better if he can eat just a little food. He will be worse from drinking cold things.

Borax: Think of this remedy for cases of travel sickness that involve a dread of downward motion. For this reason, this obscure little remedy has taken on special importance in the modern age, in that it is the remedy of first choice for cases of travel sickness on airplanes.

Graphites: Think of Graphites as a remedy of first choice for cases of indigestion that chronically begin two hours after the patient has eaten. This patient suffers from belches that taste of the food he has eaten, or that taste salty. He will also suffer constrictive pains in his stomach, and a weak feeling all over that leaves him trembling. The belches will make him feel a little better for a short time. He will also feel better from sitting in a comfortable chair. He will become worse by eating anything else or by drinking cold things.

Hydrastis: The acute illness associated with this remedy will usually begin with a change in the patient's sense of taste. Suddenly, everything will start to taste funny. Bread will especially taste odd: yeasty and sickening. Then the patient will start to feel nauseated, with a pain in the pit of his stomach. The patient will feel toxic, and totally sick (like Nux). Then he will begin to vomit, and will vomit up whatever

642

he eats. From that point food disagrees with the patient, and he has no appetite.

Phosphoric Acid: This is our third remedy, along with Arsenicum and Silicea, for the patient suffering from indigestion as well as overall exhaustion. And it is another remedy for those, especially the elderly, who suffer from chronic indigestion. Consider it strongly for patients suffering from a loss of vital fluids, whether it is from dehydration due to diarrhea or vomiting, or because they have lost blood due to illness or surgery.

Tabacum: Along with Petroleum, this is our most important remedy for cases of travel or motion sickness. The patient needing this remedy will be icy cold and quite giddy. He will vomit, sweat, and turn pale and icy cold. The major symptom of the remedy is that the patient will feel as if his head were tightly wrapped by a steel band. He will be worse from the smell of cigarette smoke, which will greatly increase his nausea.

Veratrum: Veratrum is such an important remedy in so many cases of indigestion and diarrhea that you may want to add it to your kit. Think of this remedy for any case that combines colic with nausea and vomiting. The colic will be associated with pain that feels as if the patient were being stabbed by knives all over his abdomen. During his pain and during diarrhea—which will be profuse and watery—the patient's forehead will drip with a cold sweat. This patient will crave cold water.

Indigestion

Television commercials have already defined the territory of symptoms that, gathered together, make up our understanding of indigestion. For our purposes we will consider indigestion to be anything other than the normal digestion. In other words, the patient is experiencing bloating, gas, belching, a sensation of suffocation, cold sweats, and perhaps even vomiting instead of digesting his meals easily, extracting nutrients and simply and painlessly disposing of the wastes.

As with some of the illnesses previously mentioned, it is hard to get an exact line as to when a remedy should be considered for constipation alone, and when it should be considered for constipation accompanied by indigestion. So think of this category as the least specific—pertaining to any malfunction of digestion and/or elimination. Three more specific categories follow: heartburn, which involves the acid reflux disease that has replaced ulcers as the American complaint; constipation, which relates to dry, hard-to-pass stools; and diarrhea, which pertains to loose and, perhaps, involuntary stools. You may need to read more than one section at times, to get the full picture of the listed remedies.

I give a good deal more subjective information in this section than in previous sections to be more complete in the symptom pictures. The reason for this is simple: while it is very easy to select a curative remedy objectively when it comes to digestive disorders, doing so often depends upon your willingness to study the nature of the patient's vomit or stool. Since I am assuming that you may not wish to do so, I also give subjective information to help you with your remedy selection.

In my opinion, indigestion is far more often a chronic complaint than a simple acute—unless you've just had dinner at the home of a person who has undercooked the chicken. So the remedies listed here are given with the idea that, at some point, you will look at your diet and not depend upon a pill of any sort to clear up the symptoms.

And speaking of diet, perhaps the best place to start in considering indigestion is with the King of Indigestion, **Sulphur. Sulphur** is, perhaps, our most important remedy for malfunction in any part of the body. In terms of digestion, it speaks to a form of indigestion that is uniquely American, because the indigestion that the **Sulphur** patient suffers from is based upon his cravings. He craves greasy things. He craves salty things. He loves fried things. He loves pizza and hamburgers, and, especially french fries and potato chips. He loves sodas of all sorts. Sugar in all its forms. He loves beer and pretzels and nachos. He craves donuts at 11:00A.M. in the morning, and a candy bar in the mid afternoon. And this is how and what he eats. Because of what he eats, the **Sulphur** patient will, over time, develop indigestion. He will experience this indigestion with bloating, and with a swollen and very tender abdomen. He will have an excess of stomach acid, and a tendency to belch and pass gas. He will have a sensation of heat throughout his body, especially on his head, and will be sweaty. In addition to this, he will tend toward itching.

Think of **Sulphur** for cases of indigestion that evolve into irritable bowel syndrome, in which the patient will alternate between constipation and diarrhea. Also consider **Sulphur** for cases of low blood sugar, in which the patient screams for sugar at 11:00A.M. in the morning.

This is a smelly patient; as sulfur is the smell associated with rotten eggs, you can imagine that the gassy **Sulphur** patient is sort of a rolling, belching odor factory.

This is also a remedy for those who combine indigestion with diarrhea. In this case, the patient will experience painless diarrhea that drives him out of bed first thing in the morning. During bouts of diarrhea, the patient may be covered from head to toe with a hot sweat. The diarrhea may leave the patient with an itching sensation in his anus.

If you were to give **Sulphur** to this patient, you would do him a great deal of good, and he would, for a time, experience a great improvement. But he must ultimately change his habits, especially his diet and exercise program, to be made well.

Another belching machine is the **Carbo Veg** patient. This is another remedy in which the patient will tend to wear his digestion down over time. This patient will be so bloated that his abdomen will become like a drum, with the skin drawn tight. The patient's clothing around his stomach will get too tight. He may even think that his stomach is going to burst from the pressure. So he belches, burps, or hiccoughs (**Carbo Veg** is a good remedy whichever he is doing), but these bring scant temporary relief.

Think of **Carbo Veg** first for cases of simple acute indigestion caused by overeating, so think of it on Thanksgiving Day. Look for the patient needing this remedy to be chilly, to feel as if he is suffocating, and, most important, to need air to be moving to feel that he can breathe.

He may fan himself with a magazine, or he may want to sit in front of an electric fan.

Think of **Nux** if the patient has not been overeating, but has, instead, been eating foods that disagree with him. This is especially true if the patient has been drinking as much as he has been eating, or if the indigestion begins after eating too much dairy (**Lycopodium** will also have this symptom).

Typically the overindulgence may have involved a meal of red meat, potatoes in some form, sour cream, red wine with the meal, some other alcohol before and after, cheesecake, and a cigar. This, the diet of the American businessman of the early 1960s, is the core craving of the constitutional **Nux.** And those who live on this diet, especially with the alcohol and tobacco, often have the chronic indigestion of the remedy type. Others will need the remedy acutely after an occasional night of debauchery. It is perhaps our best remedy for a hangover, after all.

The **Nux** patient with indigestion is belching, and he will have a bitter taste in his mouth. He will not have any hunger in his distress, but he may still crave alcohol as the "hair of the dog that bit him." He will experience cramps in the stomach, accompanied by a headache that has the sensation of a nail being driven through his head. He is irritable, and cannot bear tight clothing, noise, or bright lights. His face will be red when he has indigestion.

Think of this remedy first for cases of indigestion, especially for long-term indigestion accompanied by constipation.

Think of **Hepar Sulph** for cases of indigestion in which the patient has suffered from nausea, belching, and intestinal gas, and has already taken a lot of allopathic drugs to no avail. This is an unusual use of a remedy usually associated with sore throats and flu.

Hepar Sulph and **Nux** can look alike, in that both patients will tend to crave alcohol. The **Hepar Sulph** patient will crave vinegar, spicy foods, and, especially, wine, and will be averse to anything fatty. And both **Hepar Sulph** and **Nux** patients can have indigestion that occurs after eating spicy or acidic foods. Like **Nux,** the **Hepar Sulph** patient will tend to be irritable, and to speak and drink quickly. You may think of **Hepar Sulph** as a good follow-up to **Nux** for cases that **Nux** does not fully cure and in which the patient has taken different allopathic drugs to control his indigestion.

Cases of indigestion that are accompanied by constipation and a headache may also require **Bryonia.** But the circumstances by which the patient gets his symptoms of indigestion are quite different. **Bryonia,** happily, tends to be more of a truly acute remedy for indigestion than **Nux.** Think of this first for cases of indigestion that occur in the hot weather of summer. The patient is overheated on a summer's day, and then drinks ice-cold liquids (especially beer), or eats fruit like watermelon, and then ends up sick.

Bryonia will experience a rolling nausea that will force him to lie down. He will become more nauseated with any movement, so he will want stay very still and quiet. He will become nauseated at the thought of food, and even the smell of food will upset him. He will become worse if he eats and is likely to throw up immediately afterward. His nausea will be accompanied by both headache and constipation. The patient will be very thirsty for cold water throughout his nausea, and will drink large amounts.

If the **Bryonia** patient's indigestion is long-lasting, consider following it with a dose of **Rhus Tox. Rhus** often follows **Bryonia** in cases of indigestion. Look for the patient to become more restless; he will now want to keep moving to keep his nausea in check. Look at his mouth for indications—his tongue will be dry, and the tip of the tongue will have a red triangular patch on it.

Other remedies that combine indigestion with constipation include **Cocculus, Sepia, Lycopodium, Lachesis,** and **Silicea.**

Cocculus is an excellent remedy for acute indigestion. The keynote of this remedy is that the **Cocculus** patient will complain of a sour taste in his mouth, and of an acid feeling in his stomach. Think of the common symptoms associated with travel sickness: the queasiness and dizziness, with overwhelming nausea, vertigo, and vomiting, and you have a picture of this remedy. The **Cocculus** patient's abdominal muscles feel weak. His head, chest and abdomen feel empty, hollow, and raw. The patient will have a metallic taste in his mouth, and his nausea may be accompanied by palpitations.

The **Sepia** patient, like **Nux** and **Sulphur,** may have a chronic sort of indigestion that is linked to his lifestyle. All three of these remedies may have indigestion that is caused by a lack of exercise, but **Sepia** patient experiences this lack of exercise differently than the other two, who tend to live their lives far more in their minds than in their bodies.

The constitutional **Sepia** type is usually a woman, and she usually feels that she needs to exercise constantly to ward off a sensation of heaviness or gravity that haunts her. (It may be said that **Rhus Tox,** with his restless need to keep moving, along with gravity-overwhelmed **Sepia** fill most of our exercise classes, as the patients needing both remedies are addicted to exercise in their constitutional form.) So when **Sepia** does not exercise and move her body enough, she is given to chronic indigestion.

In such cases, look for headache to alternate with indigestion. Even in the acute sphere, consider this remedy first for cases in which indigestion—belching, with a sour taste in the mouth and a sensation of weight in the abdomen—is alternated by or accompanied by a sick headache.

Lycopodium is a major homeopathic remedy that speaks to indigestion, whether it is acute or chronic. Like **Carbo Veg,** this is a remedy that may be needed on Thanksgiving Day, when all of us overeat. But where the gas escapes from the **Carbo Veg** patient in belches, it becomes intestinal gas for the **Lycopodium.**

It is safe to say that the **Lycopodium** patient has more intestinal gas than any other remedy. Look for him to have to open his belt and pants while he is still at the table. He seems to fill with gas after only a bite or two of food. In chronic cases, the **Lycopodium** patient will come to the table very hungry, but will be filled up with gas after only a bite or two of food.

The **Lycopodium** patient will feel as if his insides were fermenting. There is a constant rolling, rumbling, and swishing of fluids and gas inside his abdomen. This will be particularly true if he eats dairy or foods containing wheat and other grains. He will crave sugar, but will become ill from it.

The **Lycopodium** patient's indigestion will be accompanied by long-term constipation, in which stools are passed only with the greatest difficulty.

In the case of patients who need **Lachesis,** their digestion has become erratic because their diet has become erratic. Acutely, it is often needed during times of deadline stress or vacation travel. The **Lachesis** patient becomes ill from eating his meals at erratic times: sometimes early, sometimes late, and sometimes not at all. He becomes ill from eating too much in one meal, then having a candy bar at the next, and then eating in the car as he drives to a business meeting.

Lachesis's indigestion is also accompanied by constipation, bloating, belching, and a sensation of heaviness and exhaustion. The patient will suddenly need to lie down after eating. He will feel sluggish and a bit confused after eating. Constipation accompanies the indigestion. Patients needing this remedy, along with **Nux,** crave alcohol, and alcohol may play a part in the indigestion. Unlike **Nux,** this patient is talkative and pleasant. He also may flush with heat, while **Nux** is very cold.

Finally, **Silicea** is a remedy for cases in which the patient is so nauseated that he cannot bear to even drink water. He will insist that the taste of it makes him more nauseous. If he does manage to drink it, he will throw up immediately. In other words, think of this remedy for cases of severe indigestion that involve constipation and vomiting.

The **Silicea** patient's nausea will be worse in the morning. He will awaken already nauseated, with a bitter taste in his mouth, and his nausea will grow worse with every meal he eats.

Silicea is, therefore, in important remedy for both chronic and acute indigestion. In a constitutional case, the **Silicea** patient will, like **Calcarea** and **Sulphur** patients, lose the ability to digest even the simplest things almost completely. But where **Calcarea** will vomit undigested foods and **Sulphur** will have diarrhea in the morning, **Silicea** will experience constipation—he will insist that he can only partially expel his stool before it recedes back into his system.

In all cases, the **Silicea** patient will be exhausted, and will seem shriveled by the indigestion. He is tired in his distress, and rather timid.

Consider this remedy for patients who have recovered from another disease that has left them depleted and incapable of digesting their food. (Also consider **China** and **Phosphoric Acid** for this sort of condition.)

Remedies that combine diarrhea with indigestion include **Calcarea, Pulsatilla, Arsenicum, Mercurius,** and **China.** Also to be considered are **Phosphoric Acid** and **Veratrum,** neither of which is listed in our Objective Materia Medica.

Let's start with the remedies **China** and **Phosphoric Acid.** Both may be considered for cases of indigestion brought on by physical or mental depletion. This could mean that the patient has just recovered, or is in the process of recovering from a serious disease. Or it could mean that the patient has worn himself out and has sat up late at night caring for another sick person. Or it could mean that he has been overstudying for midterms. In either case, it often means that the indigestion has developed after the patient has had the loss of vital fluids, whether it is blood after injury or surgery, or water after diarrhea or vomiting. These are also often remedies needed by elderly patients.

In the case of **Phosphoric Acid,** the indigestion will be accompanied by both diarrhea and vomiting. In the case of **China,** the patient will experience a swollen abdomen and he will pass intestinal gas, which will offer no relief. He will also belch a good deal and will taste his food again and again for hours after he has eaten it. Diarrhea will accompany the indigestion. Both these remedy types will want to rest and to lie down. They will be exhausted in their distress. These two remedies are often used to complement each other; the one most called for will be given first, and the other will be given later to complete the case.

Calcarea can look a good bit like **Lycopodium** when you first consider the case. This is another patient who will want to adjust his pants, and loosen the clothing around his waist after eating. The major symptom will be the pressure that the patient feels in his abdomen. But, unlike **Lycopodium,** this is a sweaty patient, and, unlike **Sulphur,** the sweat is cold. The patient's feet will be cold and wet, and the patient's head will be covered with icy sweat.

In cases of **Calcarea** indigestion, the patient will lack the ability to fully digest his food. Look for the patient to vomit partially digested food, or for the patient to have diarrhea that is comprised of partially digested food.

Pulsatilla is another remedy in which you will find indigestion combined with diarrhea. And, it is important to remember that **Pulsatil-**

656

la is one of our best remedies for truly acute cases of indigestion (along with **Nux, Sulphur, Arsenicum, Carbo Veg,** and **Lycopodium).** In the acute case needing **Pulsatilla,** the patient has eaten rich foods to which he is unaccustomed, so this remedy is also often called for during the holidays—times during which we all go to parties and are faced with rich foods not ordinarily part of our diet. This is especially true for fatty foods.

The **Pulsatilla** indigestion will start with a sensation of dizziness and breathlessness. The patient may feel faint when rising up out of a chair, or especially in a warm, closed room. The patient will feel better from cool, fresh air, even if the patient himself feels chilly in his nausea. Further, he will have a raw, scraping sensation in his throat.

This is a remedy for cases of "morning after" nausea, in which the patient will wake up feeling nauseous and dizzy, He may crave indigestible things or odd foods that he usually would not want, much like the cravings of pregnancy. Indeed, **Pulsatilla,** along with **Sepia,** is an important remedy for those cases of indigestion, heartburn, and cravings associated with pregnancy.

Arsenicum is another excellent remedy for cases of acute indigestion, even for cases of food poisoning. This does not diminish the constitutional power of this remedy; it is also important for chronic indigestion, especially in elderly patients. As the major symptom of the remedy is a burning sensation, you should also think of this remedy for cases of heartburn.

Often the symptoms of indigestion will start with a deep chill. The patient will suddenly become very cold, and may actually tremble from coldness.

The **Arsenicum** patient's indigestion tends to be rather violent. The patient will experience both vomiting and diarrhea in addition to tremendous nausea, and will become even more nauseated by eating or even smelling food. He will, however, be very thirsty, and his symptoms will be relieved by warm drinks. Look for the patient to sip his drinks.

The **Mercurius** patient will also tend to have violent nausea, which he will feel in the pit of his stomach. He will feel a weakness there after eating. The nausea will begin in the pit of the stomach and move upward. Indigestion is accompanied by heartburn.

This patient cannot bear to eat solid foods, especially meats. He will not want warm things, but may crave cold foods and drinks (like the **Phosphorus** patient). His nausea will produce a great amount of saliva in the patient's mouth. The patient will also have a salty or metallic taste in his mouth. The **Mercurius** patient is very sensitive to changes in temperature during his indigestion, and will not be able to bear to be too hot or too cold.

When **Mercurius** is the remedy, the indigestion may be a part of a larger picture of illness. It may be one symptom of flu or a systemic infection, so be sure to take the entire case and know the complete picture of the patient's symptoms.

Veratrum Album is not a remedy listed in our Objective Materia Medica. However, it is an important remedy to know about when dealing with cases of indigestion and diarrhea. Here, again, we have a case of violent nausea, accompanied by diarrhea and vomiting. The nausea will start as a cold feeling in the patient's stomach. The patient's face will be very pale or bluish, and will fell cold., He will have a pinched, pained look on his face. Although he is averse to warm foods, the patient will crave cold food and drink even in his distress. Look for the **Veratrum** patient to have a cold sweat on his forehead throughout his nausea,. Further, he may faint from his nausea.

As with **Bryonia** the **Veratrum** patient's diarrhea may develop after the patient has drunk cold liquids on a hot afternoon.

Also think of **Veratrum** for cases of indigestion accompanied by constipation during very cold weather.

A Few More Remedies to Think of for Cases of Indigestion

Ipecac is an excellent remedy to consider for children with indigestion, and for any patient who experiences a sensation of cold in his face and extremities during his nausea. This patient's symptoms combine nausea and vomiting. He will vomit and vomit, and will continue with dry retching after all food and drink has been eliminated. The patient will have a "sinking sensation" in his stomach that will warn him that he will soon vomit.

Chamomilla is another good remedy for acute cases in which the patient experiences nausea, pressure, and bloating high up in the abdomen. The patient will have a bitter taste in his mouth, and a pain in his stomach that extends up under his ribs. This patient will have foul breath, and belches that smell of rotten eggs. He will be worse and will sweat after eating or drinking. He will be nauseated by any food, but is particularly offended by coffee. He will be thirsty for cold things.

This is an irritable patient who cannot be consoled or satisfied.

Graphites may be considered either an acute or constitutional remedy for patients with indigestion. Consider this remedy when the patient feels as if he has a lump trapped in his throat and must either retch or swallow hard in order to clear the blockage.

Indigestion begins within two hours of eating, and starts as a sensation of a constrictive pain in the patient's stomach.

The patient will have a terrible taste in his mouth, like rotten eggs, and his breath will have the same odor.

The **Graphites** patient is unique in that the burning pain in his stomach will actually make him hungry, and he will be improved if he eats. He will especially feel better if he drinks milk (as with **Hydrastis).**

In severe cases needing **Graphites,** look for indigestion to occur from any indiscretion in the patient's diet. Look for diarrhea to accompany indigestion.

Hydrastis is an excellent general remedy to consider for cases of severe indigestion.

The patient will experience a constant, deep pain in his stomach and a burning sensation throughout his system. Even the patient's tongue will feel burnt. The patient's sense of taste will be lacking or warped. Nothing will taste right. Everything tastes burnt, peppery.

The patient will belch up sour fluid. He will vomit anything he eats, with the possible exception of milk, which may soothe his stomach. He may also drink water without vomiting.

Anacardium, which is not contained in our Objective Materia Medica, is an excellent remedy for acute indigestion as well as heartburn. The **Anacardium** patient may be identified by his foul breath, and by the fact that he may have a difficult time speaking during his nausea. His tongue may be swollen and he may have a great deal of saliva in his mouth when he is nauseated.

Indigestion occurs very quickly after the patient eats, and begins as a bad taste in the mouth and the sensation of a plug in the stomach. Although the patient is nauseated, he will actually feel better if he can eat a little food. He will also feel better after passing gas. He will become worse from drinking, however, especially from drinking anything cold.

Think of **Anacardium** as a remedy for cases of indigestion that develop after emotional stress. It is also an important remedy to consider when indigestion occurs just before the patient has to take an important test (as with **Gelsemium).**

Gelsemium is another excellent remedy to consider for cases in which indigestion is accompanied by anxiety and fear. This is especially true for those who fear public speaking or test taking, and for the patient who suddenly develops digestive symptoms when he is called upon to do anything that causes anxiety. The patient will suddenly feel a sensation of weakness or cramps in his stomach. He may also feel a sensation of chill up and down his back. Sudden involuntary diarrhea may accompany indigestion.

Finally, **Arnica** should be considered as an acute remedy for all cases of indigestion caused by mechanical injury, such as a blow to the stomach. Think of this remedy especially for cases in which the patient vomits or has diarrhea after physical trauma.

Heartburn

Like indigestion, the patient with heartburn may experience pressure, gas, belching, and bloating. In cases of heartburn, however, the pressure either begins in or centers in the upper part of the abdomen. From there, it may move up into the patient's chest and throat. Stomach acids and fluids may move up into the throat as well. And nausea may lead to vomiting.

What we call "acid reflux" involves stomach acids rising up into the throat. This can be an unpleasant acute condition, or a damaging chronic condition. Acid reflux has replaced ulcers as the ailment of young urban professionals in today's world. You may, therefore, find good use for the remedies listed here.

I think that perhaps the best and most commonly used general remedy for heartburn is **Phosphorus.** In cases calling for this remedy, nausea and pressure high in the abdomen are accompanied by acid and other, watery fluids rising into the back of the patient's throat. Look for the patient to "gulp up" these fluids. This is also the remedy for those who suddenly experience a regurgitation of sour fluid after eating. The pains in the patient's stomach and throat will be burning in nature. He will feel as if his entire digestive system has become acidic.

The patient needing **Phosphorus** may also experience vomiting and may vomit after every meal. This is especially true for the **Phosphorus** patient who is averse to warm foods and craves only cold thing. The patient may vomit foods and drinks when they warm in his stomach.

Think of **Phosphorus** as the most common general remedy for heartburn.

Another remedy for the patient suffering from heartburn is **Arsenicum.** In this case the patient will feel a burning sensation in the pit of his stomach, either very soon after eating, or hours after eating in the dark of night, usually around midnight. The burning will flow up into the patient's throat, causing him to retch and/or vomit. The patient will feel better from vomiting.

Think of the remedy **Carbo Veg** for the patient who suffers from the sudden flow of sour, acid fluid up into his throat (what used to be known as "water brash"). As is always the case with this remedy type, the patient will feel a sensation of suffocation with the heartburn. It will usually begin as a sensation of burning and acidity in the patient's stomach, followed by a sense of pressure that moves upward and a sudden flow of fluids. The patient will be bloated, belching and sour.

This is a great remedy to think of when heartburn occurs after overindulgence.

If heartburn occurs specifically after the patient has been drinking too much or eating spicy things, think of **Nux.** While the key to understanding **Carbo Veg** has to do with bloating, belching, and a sensation of suffocation, the key to understanding Nux is sensitivity. The Nux feels toxic from his indiscretion, and physically sensitive, especially in the area around his waist. He will also feel sensitive to light, noise and cold.

If the patient says that his dinner is repeating on him, consider the remedy **Pulsatilla.** This is for the patient who will retaste his dinner again and again for hours. He may also experience stomach acids rising in to his throat. In all circumstances, he will also feel acid deep down in his stomach.

In his distress, the **Pulsatilla** will not be able to bear being closed in a warm room. He will have to have open air to feel better. The **Pulsatilla** patient may vomit if he is contained in a too-warm room.

Think of **Pulsatilla** also for the patient who has overdone his eating or celebrating. He will especially become ill from eating rich foods to which he is not accustomed, or from eating fatty meats, especially pork. Nausea may also result from eating pastries, icy cold foods, and fruit. Pain in the stomach generally will begin an hour after eating.

Also think of this remedy for cases of heartburn accompanied by hiccough that begins after the patient smokes tobacco.

For the woman who experiences heartburn during pregnancy, think of **Sepia.** Here, too, the heartburn will begin as a sensation of burning in the patient's stomach and will move upward from there into her chest and throat. The patient may also experience water brash, just like the **Carbo Veg** patient. And look for the patient who needs **Sepia** to experience a churning sensation in his stomach, and a sensation of weight and heaviness in his chest and stomach. The patient may complain of a sensation of something twisting about in his stomach that rises up into his throat. He will be nauseated at the thought and, especially, the smell of food, and also at the thought of sex.

Finally, think of the remedy **China** if heartburn is becoming chronic, and if the patient has burning pains after every meal. In cases needing this remedy, the patient will have a deep hunger and will long for food, but it will lie undigested in his stomach after he has eaten it. The patient's digestion is very slow, possibly because he is still in the process of recovering from a serious illness, or is depleted in some other way. Soon after he eats, he will begin to regurgitate food and bitter, acidic fluid up into his throat. He will also belch, but belching brings no relief. His stomach will be chronically sore. He will have the sensation of weight in the stomach and high into the abdomen after eating even a small amount of food.

The patient may feel dizzy during his nausea, and may actually faint. He will retch, and may vomit partially digested foods.

Constipation

Perhaps our two most important remedies for cases of constipation, whether chronic or acute, are **Nux** and **Bryonia.**

Nux is a remedy of the first order, whether it is for constipation that accompanies a cold or other illness, or for constipation created by lifestyle. It should also be considered when constipation is accompanied by hemorrhoids, and it can also be an excellent remedy for pregnant women who experience constipation.

The patient who needs **Nux** will make frequent attempts to pass a stool, but these attempts will fail. (The stools that the **Nux** manages to pass will be large and hard, and will be passed only with the greatest effort on the part of the patient.) He will likely experience a sensation of fullness in his anus and throughout his body. He will have a headache accompanied by this sensation of fullness in his head.

As always, the **Nux** patient is considered to be an irritable patient, and this is especially true of the constipated **Nux:** he is very irritable indeed. So, if the patient in question follows the remedy picture in all but irritability, this tends to contraindicate the remedy.

The **Nux** patient is a sensitive patient, particularly in the area of his waist. He will not want tight clothing around his waist, and will not want anyone or anything to touch him there. He is also sensitive to his environment. He cannot bear bright lights or loud noises, and cannot bear cold in any form. The **Nux** patient may get colder and colder the longer his constipation remains.

He is also something of a toxic patient. Many of the long-term ailments, including constipation, that plague him are of his own creation. Look for ailments to result from overwork, lack of exercise, and a poor diet that often features alcohol and tobacco.

Bryonia is also a remedy that is equally effective for both chronic and acute cases of constipation. These are often linked to colds and flu. As is keynote of the remedy, look for the patient to not want to move due to the discomfort of constipation. Also look for the patient to complain of a sick headache that accompanies the constipation. The headache may be so bad that the patient will not even want to move his eyes, due to the pain.

The **Bryonia** patient will have dry lips and a dry mouth during his constipation. He will lose his appetite for any sort of food, but he will be very thirsty, and will drink great amounts of water from time to time.

Again, what stools are passed are passed only with the greatest effort. Look for the stools to be small, hard, and very dry. Often they will appear to have been burnt.

Like **Nux,** the **Bryonia** patient can be very irritable. He is often referred to as the "Bryonia Bear." He can be very difficult if he is disturbed or disrupted. He will want to be left alone.

Additional Remedies for Cases of Long-Lasting or Chronic Constipation

Other remedies to consider for cases of constipation that seem to be long-lasting or chronic are **Lycopodium, Calcarea, Carbo Veg,** and **Graphites.**

Acute cases of constipation that are successfully treated by the remedy **Lycopodium** almost always develop as part of another condition, like a cold or flu. But the chronic cases of constipation that **Lycopodium** treats almost always involve a poor diet and a lack of exercise. In this way, **Nux, Lycopodium, Carbo Veg,** and **Sulphur** have a good deal in common. Where the diet itself may differ—with **Nux** wanting alcohol and red meat, Lycopodium wanting dairy foods and wheat, and **Sulphur** wanting fast foods, salt, grease, and sugar—it is the lack of a proper diet that can create long-term havoc for all of them.

Whether it is an acute or chronic condition, look for the **Lycopodium** patient's constipation to be accompanied by a great deal of intestinal gas. The patient will have to undo his pants while he is still at the table because of the pressure from the gas that forms while he eats.

This patient, like the **Carbo Veg** and the **Calcarea** patient, is beset with a weak digestion, and suffers from bloating and gas pains.

The **Lycopodium** patient will experience a chill in the region of the anus and a burning pain in the rectum before feeling the need to pass stool. The stool will be hard and small, difficult to expel, and incomplete. Note that hemorrhoids may accompany constipation for the **Lycopodium** patient. Also note that, in chronic cases, constipation and diarrhea may alternate.

The **Lycopodium** will be soothed by drinking warm drinks. Note that drinking cold things may bring on diarrhea.

The **Calcarea** patient is noteworthy here because he alone, of all the remedy types, will feel better for being constipated. In fact, most will say that they never feel better than when they are constipated.

As with other patients who suffer from chronic constipation, the **Calcarea** patient usually has brought the condition on himself through poor diet and a lack of exercise. In

Calcarea's case, the poor diet is an odd one. **Calcarea** patients, especially young **Calcarea** patients, may crave strange foods that cannot be digested. These are the children who eat paste, dirt, and chalk.

This is a patient who will experience a cold sweat as a part of his constipation, especially when he attempts to pass a stool. The top and back of his head will be covered in a cold sweat, as will his feet, which will be sweaty enough to leave his socks damp and smelly.

The **Calcarea** stool starts out hard and solid, becomes soft, and ends up sticky and pasty. Look for the stool to contain undigested foods.

Note that the mild and pleasant **Calcarea** patient becomes moody and difficult when he has passed a stool.

The **Carbo Veg** patient is another who refuses exercise, but in this case the type of diet is not an issue. What is an issue is the amount of food eaten, as the **Carbo Veg** tends to always overeat. This is a binge eater, a comfort eater, and a person who eats to celebrate, so the constitutional **Carbo Veg** tends to be overweight. He also tends to have difficulty breathing, and fans himself to take in enough air.

Even as an acute remedy, the joint concepts of overeating and suffocation are important.

For all acute cases of constipation that develop as a result of overeating, think of **Carbo Veg.**

Although **Carbo Veg** is more often thought of as a belching remedy than one for intestinal gas, when it comes to indigestion, in cases of constipation the patient may experience the discomforts of gas. In fact, no stool will be passed without gas.

There will be a good deal of ineffectual urging to stool. This may be accompanied by a deep burning sensation, as **Carbo Veg** is another remedy to consider for cases of constipation and hemorrhoids. Stool is passed only with the greatest difficulty, although it will be soft and sticky. The patient will experience pain in the rectum after passing stool.

Graphites is another remedy for chronic cases of constipation in which the patient has, over a long period of time, lost his ability to fully digest his food.

This is another patient who will tend to be overweight. The **Graphites** patient will also tend to have unhealthy looking skin and hair.

Like **Sulphur,** this is a remedy filled with itching, so look for the patient to be itchy during constipation.

The stool will be large and knotty, and the separate parts will usually be linked together by mucus. This is the major remedy for stools that contain large amounts of mucus. Also, the anus will ache when it is wiped.

Additional Remedies for Cases of Acute Constipation

Good remedies to consider for acute cases of constipation include **Apis, Belladonna, Causticum,** and **Ignatia.** And you should also consider two remedies not listed in our Objective Materia Medica: **Alumina** and **Hydrastis.**

Apis is an excellent remedy for acute cases of constipation. Think of this remedy whenever the patient does not even want to try to pass a stool, since he knows it will be very painful. Sometimes the patient may even be convinced that something inside of him has become weakened by the constipation, and will actually break if he strains to pass stool.

The stool itself will be small and dark. It will be preceded by a sensation of an electric shock in the rectum.

Note that a headache will accompany constipation for the **Apis** patient. The headache will be located in the forehead, although the pain may move behind the patient's eyes.

A headache will also accompany constipation in **Belladonna** cases, but this headache throbs throughout the entire head. The patient's face will be flushed red as well. Look for the pain to be greatly increased if the patient moves his head downward.

Constipation is accompanied by burning pains in the rectum, hemorrhoids, and pain in the lower back. Stool is small, green, and lumpy.

The pain associated with cases of constipation that are helped by **Causticum** is centralized in the rectum. This patient may also suffer from hemorrhoids. The pain of these is worst when he walks, so look for the **Causticum** to walk with difficulty and to be unsteady.

The **Causticum** patient may feel cramping pains in the rectum when he tries to pass stool. The stool will be small, hard, tough, and covered with mucus, so that it shines.

Like the **Causticum** patient, the **Ignatia** patient with constipation will feel better from sitting. This will be especially true if he has hemorrhoids, as his hemorrhoids will always bother him less while he is sitting still.

Think of this remedy for constipation that develops from travel, especially from travel that involves long-term sitting in a car. Also consider for constipation brought on as a result of a shock, bad news, or emotional trauma, and for cases of long-term constipation that may be associated with grief. Finally, the patient needing **Ignatia** for his constipation may have the condition as part of an acute ailment, like a cold or flu.

The **Ignatia** patient may experience nausea and cramps in the stomach as part of the symptom picture. This is also a remedy for patients that belch and hiccough after eating. And look for the **Ignatia** patient to experience chills with his pains. The chill may be so great that the patient literally shakes with cold.

The patient will experience itching and tingling in the anus before attempting to pass stool. Stool will pass with difficulty, but painlessly, but the patient will experience a terrible pain in the rectum after passing a scant stool. Note that the stool may be smeared with blood.

Alumina is another excellent homeopathic remedy for those with cases of constipation, whether they are acute or chronic cases.

The **Alumina** patient will typically sit and strain for a long, long time trying to pass stool. He may sit so long that he becomes cold, weak, and trembling.

The stool itself consists of small balls that may contain clots of bright blood. The patient's rectum will be sore, dry, inflamed, and even bleeding after passing stool.

The patient needing **Hydrastis** will, like **Graphites,** pass a stool that is linked together by mucus, but this stool is yellow and lumpy.

It is accompanied by the passing of intestinal gas. The patient will experience a raw pain while he attempts to pass stool, and this pain will linger long after he has completed this task. The patient may feel faint after passing stool.

The **Hydrastis** will experience a weight and fullness in the stomach after eating. Later, he will experience an empty, aching, "gone" feeling in his stomach that is even worse than the fullness.

Remedies for Cases of Alternating Diarrhea and Constipation

Consider **Phosphorus** and **Pulsatilla** for cases in which diarrhea and constipation alternate, and consider **Sulphur** for chronic cases in which the two alternate.

There is no better remedy than **Phosphorus** for acute cases of digestive disorder, in which constipation alternates with diarrhea. This is especially true when the two alternate during a cold or flu. It is also the remedy of first choice when the two alternate, either acutely or constitutionally, in elderly patients.

Commonly, both the constipated and the loose stool will be accompanied by blood, and both will pass with pain and difficulty. Both will be exhausting to the patient. The patient will experience tearing pains in the anus that are better for application of warm water.

Pulsatilla, on the other hand, is helpful for cases of alternating constipation and diarrhea caused by a sudden change in diet, such as holiday overeating or overindulgence in rich foods that throws off the system. This is especially true when the patient eats fatty foods and meals containing pork.

This disordered digestion will begin with belching and a sensation of weight in the patient's stomach. He will retaste his food for hours after it has been eaten. Further, the patient experiences a rumbling in his abdomen, and the rumbling will grow worse at night.

A keynote of the remedy is that, whether the patient is constipated or suffering from diarrhea, no two stools he passes will be alike. His whole digestive system has been thrown out of balance and the ever-changing stool is the result.

As always, the **Pulsatilla** patient will be unable to bear being in a warm, enclosed space. He will need open air to soothe his nausea.

When the digestive system has been chronically thrown out of balance by a poor diet and a lack of exercise, there is no more important remedy to consider than Sulphur. In fact, there is no more potent an ally than the remedy **Sulphur** whether the patient is suffering from acute or chronic troubles, from diarrhea or constipation. And whether the patient is beset with diarrhea or constipation, the formula of the symptoms is the same: the patient will feel hot, sweaty, and itchy. Look for the patient's anus to itch as he attempts to pass stool.

When he is constipated, the **Sulphur** patient will often feel as if he might faint while trying to pass stool. His entire body will be covered in a hot sweat. His rectum will burn. In fact, should he fail to pass stool on his first attempt, the Sulphur may not want to try again, because the pain is just too great.

The stool he does pass will be hard and lumpy, and may contain mucus, or blood and mucus.

Note that this is a remedy for those with hemorrhoids, and that the hemorrhoids may be internal or, especially, external, and will both itch and burn. This is a remedy for those who have hemorrhoids during pregnancy.

And, finally, there is the remedy **Opium,** which is not a part of our Objective Materia Medica. **Opium** is the remedy to consider when the patient has chronically suffered from either diarrhea or constipation or both, and has taken many different allopathic medicines for his condition over the years. His entire system has been so distorted that now it seems impossible for him to have a normal stool. This patient may suffer through days of painful constipation, followed by days of painful diarrhea. His abdomen is distorted and pressurized. There will be a sensation of weight throughout the patient's abdomen.

This is a patient with little enough appetite to begin with, but he will lose his appetite completely while he is constipated. Any stool that passes will be comprised of small, hard, black balls.

Remedies for Constipation in Young Children

For cases of constipation in young children, consider **Veratrum** and **Silicea.**

Veratrum is often called for in acute cases of constipation in young patients. It is especially helpful for cases in which the child's system seems to have come to a complete stop and there is total inactivity of the rectum. In these cases the patient will try, but no stool passes at all. The patient will have a cold sweat on his forehead when he attempts to pass stool, and he will be able to do so only with great straining and forcing.

When they pass, the stools will be large, thin, and flat.

If the young patient has chronic constipation, the remedy of first choice is **Silicea,** especially if he is small for his age and does not seem to be thriving. **Silicea** may also be an acute remedy and a remedy for older patients, but it will be especially effective for the young patient who experiences heartburn and constipation and seems unable to digest his food (like **Calcarea).** The young **Silicea** who has chronic constipation will typically be a small, thin child.

Straining to pass a soft stool is keynote of the remedy, as is the stool that only partially seems to pass, before it recedes again. Stool passes only with the greatest straining, and the patient may retain stools for fear of pain associated with its passing. The patient may experience cramping pains in the rectum after trying to pass stool.

This is also a remedy for those with hemorrhoids. These hemorrhoids will protrude when the patient strains to pass stool.

This is also a remedy to consider for women who experience constipation each month before and during their period.

Diarrhea

Perhaps the best general remedy for the patient with diarrhea, and a remedy that you should always have on hand, is **Podophyllum.**

It is such a good remedy because it lacks a specific keynote, just like **Ferrum Phos** for patients with fever. The **Podophyllum** patient may have morning diarrhea that drives him out of bed (like **Sulphur),** or he may have diarrhea that is preceded by severe cramping in the abdomen.

The **Podophyllum** patient will feel worse each time he eats, and may have a bout of diarrhea following each meal.

The stool will be watery, sputtering, and profuse, and will pass in gushes.

Think of this remedy for cases of young children with diarrhea during teething. It is also an excellent remedy to consider for cases of diarrhea in the summer heat (consider **Bryonia** for this as well). Consider **Podophyllum** for cases, especially in young children, in which stool is passed involuntarily during sleep.

As noted above, **Sulphur** is the other remedy to consider when the patient is driven out of bed in the morning by sudden, painless diarrhea. While the consistency and the amount of the stool may vary, look for the patient to have a hot sweat during diarrhea and to experience itching in the rectum.

The stool in this case will be changeable, like the **Pulsatilla's.** It can be yellow, brown, or green, and may or may not contain undigested food. Sour or bitter vomiting may accompany or alternate with diarrhea.

Sulphur is also an excellent remedy for diarrhea in young children. Again, the diarrhea will be accompanied by hot sweat. The child may awaken suddenly screaming with diarrhea.

An important aspect if the **Sulphur** case has to do with odor. The smell of the **Sulphur** diarrhea will be just terrible, like rotten eggs. That smell will linger on the patient for hours and hours. His breath, too, may be foul.

Consider this remedy for cases of diarrhea in which stool is passed involuntarily when the patient laughs or when he passes gas.

Two remedies to consider for cases of diarrhea that often include vomiting are **Arsenicum** and **Veratrum.** In either case, the acute diarrhea may be a part of a cold or flu.

The **Arsenicum** patient will usually display a picture that involves diarrhea, vomiting, anxiety, burning pain, and chill. The diarrhea can be severe. It will be dark, bloody, and very offensive. The **Arsenicum** patient will feel a burning pain and a sensation of pressure in his rectum. This pain will be soothed by warm applications. Both the pain and the diarrhea will be worse at night.

Consider **Arsenicum** for cases that involve diarrhea associated with alcohol abuse, tainted food—especially meat—or involve the patient becoming cold after drinking cold things.

Remember, the **Arsenicum** is a restless patient, although the **Arsenicum** with severe diarrhea may be so depleted that he takes to his bed. This is also a chilly patient who must wrap up to keep warm, yet he may want cool air on his head and face, especially when his digestive upset is accompanied by headache. He will only want that cool air on his face, however, and will want the room and his body kept warm. He will also want warm liquids, which will help relieve his symptoms.

This will be an anxious, worried patient. His diarrhea may be caused by fear or anxiety about his health.

The **Veratrum** patient may also experience diarrhea and vomiting. Like the **Arsenicum,** this is a chilly patient. Look for his body to be covered in an icy cold sweat during his nausea and diarrhea. Yet this patient will want the windows wide open, and will be thirsty for cold things, which will bring him relief. Like the patient needing **Bryonia,** look for the **Vera-trum** patient's diarrhea to be caused by drinking cold water on a hot afternoon. The stool will be watery, green, and odorless. It will be expelled in large amounts.

Note that, as a remedy that may be helpful both for patients with diarrhea and with constipation, **Veratrum** is very much linked to the weather. Consider this remedy for diarrhea in hot weather and for constipation in cold winter weather.

Patients needing **Bryonia,** which shares **Veratrum's** link with summer weather, will often experience diarrhea after drinking cold things, especially beer, or eating cold fruit on a hot summer day. Consider this remedy as the first-choice when the patient gets diarrhea after becoming overheated. There will be frequent bouts of diarrhea. Look for the diarrhea to be worse in the morning, especially when the patient gets out of bed in the morning.

The stool will be yellow and mushy, with lumps of tough mucus in it.

China also shares this picture of diarrhea that occurs after eating cold things on a hot day. The diarrhea associated with this remedy is painless but debilitating. The stool is very offensive. It may be bloody, and may contain undigested foods.

You should also think of **China** as a remedy of choice for cases of chronic diarrhea in children. Look for the child's pupils to be dilated and his body cold to the touch during and after diarrhea. The child's face, particularly his nose and chin, will be especially cold.

The other remedy to consider for diarrhea in young children is **Chamomilla.** This remedy is especially useful for cases in which diarrhea accompanies teething. The stools will be bright green and will contain undigested food. They will be slimy and mix mucus and blood, and will have a terrible odor, like rotten eggs.

The **Chamomilla** patient will be angry, and will be a difficult patient to treat. He may even strike out at those who attempt to help him.

The **Chamomilla** may experience painful diarrhea that is preceded by colic and cramping pains. Look for the patient's face to have one cheek that is hot, red, and perhaps even sweaty, and the other cheek cold and pale.

Some common remedies that are very handy in treating patients with diarrhea are **Colocynthis, Dulcamara, Aconite, Pulsatilla,** and **Gelsemium. Aloe,** a remedy that is not included in our Objective Materia Medica, should also be considered.

Colocynthis is useful for cases of both chronic and acute diarrhea. Think of this remedy for cases in which diarrhea is preceded by or accompanied by severe cramping pains. These pains will be soothed if the patient bends over forward or applies pressure to the area of the abdomen.

The cramping, as well as the nausea, will occur suddenly and in waves. Pain and diarrhea may both develop after the patient has a bout of anger or indignation. The **Colocynthis** patient will not lose his appetite due to his diarrhea. He will continue to have quite a healthy appetite in spite of it all. His stool will be frothy, watery, or gelatinous, and yellow, and will be accompanied by both pain and intestinal gas. Chronic diarrhea will be watery and worse in the morning. The stool will have a musty odor to it.

Dulcamara is a remedy to consider for cases in which the patient experiences diarrhea after getting cold and wet, or after sleeping on the damp ground. It should also be considered for patients who take on a chill after being overheated. Often, the diarrhea will relate to times of the year—especially spring and fall—during which the days are hot and the nights are cold.

Usually the patient will experience a cutting pain in the area of his navel just before the onset of diarrhea. The patient will also experience a sensation of cold in his abdomen.

The stool will be slimy and may contain blood. Typically, it will be green or yellow. Diarrhea will be worse at night.

Cases of diarrhea that are treated with **Aconite** may also involve the weather. Think of this remedy for cases when diarrhea suddenly occurs after the patient has been in contact with a cold, dry wind. This may be the case with the child who is bundled up and sent out to play, and becomes overheated by his wraps, only to take a chill from the wind. Perhaps more important, think of **Aconite** for cases of diarrhea brought on suddenly by fright, shock, or strong emotion.

The patient may experience stitching and itching pain in his anus. The stool will be frequent in small amounts. It will be green and look as if it had chopped herbs in it.

Pulsatilla is another remedy to consider for cases of diarrhea caused by emotion. Usually the illness begins when the patient is nervous or anxious. It may also be caused by fright. Often, **Pulsatilla** is used to treat timid patients who are chronically given to diarrhea. The diarrhea will be worse at night. It will be accompanied by bloating, heartburn, and flatulence. The patient's abdomen will rumble with water every evening.

Pulsatilla is an excellent remedy for acute cases of diarrhea in which the stool is always changing and no two stools are alike. The diarrhea is often caused by indulgence in too-rich foods, especially fatty foods, like pork. Diarrhea may also be caused by eating onions. Sometimes overindulgence in pastry and baked goods may lead to gastric distress.

Remember, this is a patient who will be worse for being trapped in a warm, closed room. He may need to go for a walk in order to overcome his nausea.

Gelsemium is another remedy whose symptoms derive from emotional causes. In this case, diarrhea will be caused by fear, grief, or hearing bad news. The key that separates **Gelsemium** from other remedies is that the **Gelsemium** patient becomes ill from *anticipation.* He anticipates the worst of future events. Most often, the **Gelsemium** patient will experience diarrhea when he is called upon to speak in public, or when he needs to take an important test. He thinks he will make a fool of himself by speaking or will fail the test, even if he is fully prepared.

The diarrhea will be sudden and without warning, and the patient will have to run to the bathroom. Nausea and diarrhea will be accompanied by a chill that runs up and down the patient's spine.

The stool will be painless and copious. It may be yellow or green.

Cases combining cramping in the abdomen and diarrhea suggest the remedy **Aloe.** Patients needing this remedy will feel a constant bearing-down sensation and a sensation of weight in their rectum. The rectum will bleed, and will feel sore and hot. This pain will be relieved by applications of cold water. Further, the patient will feel a weakness in his sphincter muscle, and will feel as if he has lost control of his bowels. There will be a sense of insecurity in the patient's rectum in that he will not be sure if stool or gas will pass. Diarrhea will pass without effort.

The patient will have a strong urge to pass stool every time he eats or drinks, particularly when he drinks beer. The urge will be sudden, and will send the patient hurrying to the bathroom. The stool is has a good deal of mucus and is jellylike.

Additional Remedies for Cases of Chronic Diarrhea

For cases of chronic diarrhea, consider the remedies **Calcarea, Phosphorus,** and **Phosphoric Acid.**

As noted earlier, the remedy **Calcarea** has the general theme of poor digestion. The **Calcarea** patient will have difficulty taking nutrition from his food, even though he is often overweight. Often he will have a swollen and distended abdomen.

While the patient suffers from chronic diarrhea, he may have difficulty passing urine, which will have a strong odor. Like all of the **Calcarea** patient's discharges, the urine will be sour smelling.

The patient's stool will be chalky, gray, or green, and claylike in texture. Often, the stool will begin hard, become pasty, and finish as a liquid. Usually it will contain undigested food. The diarrhea will be accompanied by a sour smell to the patient's whole body and by a cold sweat on the patient's head and feet.

The **Calcarea** patient has the unusual symptom of always feeling better when constipated. Therefore, expect the **Calcarea** with diarrhea to be most unhappy. This is a depressed or angry patient.

Think of **Phosphorus** as a remedy for those with chronic diarrhea that is worse in the morning. The diarrhea may be accompanied by vomiting. Look for the patient to become weaker and weaker as diarrhea continues. Look for his appetite to lessen, although the patient will remain thirsty for cold liquids. The patient may become nauseated and may vomit as the liquid is warmed in his stomach.

The **Phosphorus** patient will feel as if he has no control over his diarrhea, and that his sphincter will remain open and relaxed and unable to control stool. His stool will be very fetid, and will be passed with intestinal gas. It will be watery, with green mucus and white flakes in it. Blood may also be in the stool.

Note that, as with **Arsenicum,** burning pains run all through the remedy **Phosphorus.** The patient will suffer from burning pains in his stomach, his abdomen, and his rectum.

The remedy **Phosphoric Acid** is related to **Phosphorus,** except that those needing it are even more exhausted and debilitated than those needing **Phosphorus.**

This is a remedy for painless chronic diarrhea. It is especially helpful for very young patients who are weak and sickly in general, and for very old patients who are exhausted and disinterested in their condition. It is keynote that those needing this remedy are apathetic. Patients will tend to be indifferent to everything, even their own health. The patient's face will be pale and sick looking. The skin on the face will be tight and tense, as if egg white had dried on it.

The stool in this case is almost completely involuntary and odorless, although it is accompanied by a great deal of flatulence. And, although the patient is exhausted, the passing of stool is not especially debilitating. The **Phosphoric Acid** patient may experience diarrhea accompanied by heartburn. Ailments may develop after the patient has been worn down by a serious, long-term illness, or from long-term grief and by loss of vital fluids.

Hiccoughs

The remedies for hiccoughs are to be considered as more than Band-Aids, since hiccoughs represent an acute ailment, but I felt they should be grouped with the others dealing with indigestion and related ailments.

Three homeopathic remedies should be considered first when hiccoughs occur after a meal or after eating and drinking. They are **Nux, Pulsatilla,** and **Carbo Veg.** In all three cases, the hiccoughs will represent only one portion of a picture of digestive upset.

Perhaps first among these is the **Pulsatilla** patient, who will get hiccoughs after overindulging, especially in foods that are not part of his regular diet. Therefore, these are holiday hiccoughs brought on by too many trips to the buffet table. The **Pulsatilla** patient will first experience a little nausea in his stomach and a little belching. Then the hiccoughs will begin, usually about an hour after the patient has finished eating. He will be unable to bear being in a warm, closed room, and will seek cold for relief from his hiccoughs. Cold air, either from an open window or a walk outside, and cold water, usually drunk in large quantities, will soothe the hiccoughs.

The **Carbo Veg** hiccoughs will usually begin about a half hour after the patient finishes his meal. It is likely that he will have overeaten. The **Carbo Veg** patient will feel bloated, will belch, and will have a sensation of suffocation in addition to his hiccoughs. **Carbo Veg** hiccoughs can be quite long-lasting, and can interfere with the patient's already weak ability to take in sufficient air. So look for the **Carbo Veg** to be fanning himself and/or seeking moving air to soothe his hiccoughs. His hiccoughs will also be improved when he sits up straight in a chair.

Hiccoughs are often a part of **Nux's** sensation of indigestion. This is perhaps because hiccoughs are caused by a muscle spasm, and muscle spasms and twitches of all sorts are common for the **Nux** patient. His face can be filled with twitches, especially around his eyes. In the same way, he will fall prey to spasmodic hiccoughs. As with the **Carbo Veg** patient, the hiccoughs will tend to develop after the patient has eaten, or overeaten. In **Nux's** case, the meal might easily have contained a good deal of alcohol.

Typically, the hiccoughs will begin two to three hours after the patient has eaten. The hiccoughs, when they arrive, will usually be accompanied by heartburn and a queasy feeling in the pit of the stomach. Unlike the **Carbo Veg** patient, who tends to just let his belches and hiccoughs out, the **Nux** patient will attempt to stifle and control his hiccoughs, but to no avail. Often, he will erupt in a single "hic." Usually he will seek to control his hiccoughs by controlling his breathing. He may, in fact, stop breathing to try to stop the hiccoughs. Just as **Nux's** hiccoughs are slow to develop, they will also be slow to fade, and they can be quite long-lasting.

As always, the **Nux** is an irritable patient. His hiccoughs will both embarrass and anger him.

Magnesium Phosphoricum, or **Mag Phos,** which is not listed among the remedies in our Objective Materia Medica, is another excellent remedy for hiccoughs. We commonly associate it with muscle cramps of all sorts, especially the cramps associated with PMS.

The hiccoughs associated with **Mag Phos** are long-lasting, stubborn, and very unsettling, the kind that seem to take over the patient's body. The hiccoughs will be improved if the patient sips warm liquids.

Another remedy picture in which the hiccoughs are improved if the patient sips warm liquids is **Arsenicum.** These hiccoughs are, in fact, caused by the patient drinking cold water or other liquids. The hiccoughs may also be caused by fever.

If a patient's hiccoughs begin after he suffered a bout of coughing, consider the remedy

Tabacum. This remedy is usually associated with travel sickness, and is not a part of our Objective Materia Medica.

If a patient's hiccoughs start after he has vomited, consider the remedy **Veratrum,** which is not a part of our Objective Materia Medica. The hiccoughs may also be caused by the patient drinking warm liquids.

Finally, there is **Ignatia.** Think of **Ignatia** for hiccoughs that begin after an emotional upset, or if the patient is put in a room with people who are smoking. These will be very loud hiccoughs that inspire laughter from everyone else in the room and cause terrible embarrassment for the patient. They will bounce off the walls and echo down the halls. Look for **Ignatia** hiccoughs to suddenly appear and to end just as suddenly.

Motion Sickness

This is another section in which the remedies are more than Band-Aids and can be curative for the given situation. But if we look deeper to understand why some of us are vulnerable to the nausea associated with vehicular travel and some of us are not, we begin to suspect that we are indeed using something of a Band-Aid if we only treat each episode of travel sickness and do not treat the underlying cause at some point.

There are four major remedies for those who suffer from travel or motion sickness. The three that are listed in our Objective Materia Medica are **Nux, Petroleum,** and **Cocculus.** The one remedy that is not listed is **Tabacum.**

Perhaps the best single remedy is **Cocculus.** Think of this remedy for the patient who first gets lightheaded or giddy when he becomes nauseated in a car, boat, or plane. He finds that his mouth is producing a great deal of saliva, and then becomes nauseated. He is likely to vomit, and is unable to even bear the smell of food after that. He will become worse by eating or drinking anything.

These are exhausted patients who just want to go and lie down, and they will feel better if they can lie down and be quiet. However, they will again become very nauseated if they attempt to rise up from their prone position. You will know the **Cocculus** patients by how unsteady they are on their feet, and how awkwardly they move about.

Like **Cocculus,** the patient who needs Petroleum will tend to have a great deal of saliva in his mouth. Usually the attack of motion sickness will begin with a sensation of emptiness in the patient's stomach. Then the patient will feel lightheaded and nauseated. This is a weak patient who may vomit. He will become very much worse (as with **Nux)** if he has to endure light or noise. Either or both are insufferable to him.

Note that the **Petroleum** patient has an odd keynote symptom: he will feel a terrible pain in the back of his head during his nausea. Further, the muscles in his neck and shoulders will become very tight and rigid.

Finally, and this is also keynote, the **Petroleum** patient will actually feel better if he can eat anything. This is the only remedy type with this symptom.

Some people believe so strongly in **Nux's** ability to help those who suffer with travel sickness that they take a dose or two to act preventatively before they get in any vehicle. And, indeed, **Nux** is one of our great remedies for those with travel sickness. **Nux** motion sickness will usually begin with a sensation of cold in the pit of the stomach. And the **Nux** patient, who is very sensitive to any trouble with his stomach and very, very sensitive to cold in any form, will know immediately that he is in trouble. He will be dizzy. He will have no appetite or desire to drink. Note, however, that even though the **Nux** patient will have terrible nausea, he usually will not actually vomit. Instead, the patient will retch and retch.

Typically, a sick headache will be a main feature of the travel sickness. The patient will feel as if a nail were being driven into his head.

As always, the **Nux** patient who is nauseated will be irritable, and he will become increasingly sensitive to his surroundings, especially to light and noise, as his nausea increases. He will feel that he has to remove himself from other people and from all aspects of life. The people around him will have to sit still and be quiet while the **Nux** suffers alone.

The **Tabacum** patient presents a picture of general nausea that includes a great deal of sweating, which separates this remedy from the others. The other symptom that helps identify the **Tabacum** is that this patient will tremble and may actually faint from his distress. The **Tabacum** will vomit, and, while vomiting, will be covered in an icy sweat. Look for his face to become very pale. Nothing will improve the lot of the **Tabacum** patient; no body position, food, or drink will soothe his ills. But the smell of cigarette smoke can make him very much worse.

Remedies for Air Sickness

Two remedies will be of particular help for the patient who becomes ill while traveling by plane. They are **Borax,** which is not listed in our Objective Materia Medica, and **Rhus Tox.**

The keynote symptom for those needing **Borax** is that they fear and dread downward motion. Therefore, this is an excellent remedy for those who are terrified of airplane travel, especially those who become panicky if the plane hits turbulence or while it is landing.

Remember, in the case of this remedy, it is more the fear of the motion than any physical upset caused by the motion. The patient needing **Borax** will also have trouble with a roller coaster, or a car traveling through mountain terrain.

If airplane travel causes actual physical symptoms such as nausea and vomiting, then **Rhus Tox** may well be the remedy of first choice. The **Rhus Tox** patient will be terribly nauseated. Even the smell of food may cause him to vomit. However, he will be very thirsty and will want to drink a great deal of water. Look for his mouth and tongue to stay very dry in spite of his drinking.

Where downward motion is worst for the **Borax,** upward motion is worst for the **Rhus Tox.** Look for the patient to become worse if the plane rises, or if he himself rises from a prone position.

As always, the **Rhus** patient with travel sickness is a restless patient. He will toss about as he tries, unsuccessfully, to get into a comfortable position.

Remedies for Motion Sickness with Vomiting

If the major feature of the patient's motion sickness is vomiting, and if the patient continues to have dry heaves after he has emptied his stomach, the remedy to consider is **Ipecac.** In fact, no matter what the cause, Ipecac is the remedy to remember for the patient who combines nausea with copious vomiting, especially when vomiting offers the patient no relief.

The **Ipecac** patient will seem to be in a continuous state of nausea from the moment the vehicle begins its motion. He will usually be chilly, but, in his nausea, heat may alternate with chilliness. He will also have a great accumulation of saliva in his mouth. As with **Nux,** look for the patient's face to have ticks and twitches.

The **Ipecac** patient will feel worse in a sitting, or, especially, a stooping position. He will feel worse from eating, or, especially, drinking anything cold. He will also be worse for smelling cigarette smoke.

Toothache

The remedies listed in this section will get you through the night when you find yourself suddenly dealing with a child who has a terrible, throbbing tooth pain. But remember: these really are only Band-Aids. If you have a tooth that is decayed and that decay has exposed a nerve, the only way to truly "cure" that tooth is to get to the dentist and get it filled. These remedies will help make the pain manageable until you can get there, nothing more, unless, of course, the pain is caused by some factor other than decay, like sinus pressure. Then the remedies may have a more permanent impact. Either way, the presence of tooth or teeth pain should be reason enough for you to seek the skilled guidance of a medical professional.

Toothache involves many subjective symptoms that can only be experienced by the patient and that are not visible or tangible to the practitioner, so all cases of toothache will involve a case taking that involves questioning the patient in addition to studying his symptoms. Wherever it is possible, I will list objective symptoms that will help guide you in the selection of an appropriate remedy.

While any of the remedies listed will work for all patients whose symptoms match the remedy's picture, there are some remedies that are especially effective (and possibly more often needed) for children. These remedies include **Aconite, Belladonna, Chamomilla, Coffea,** and **Ignatia.**

The symptom that links all of these remedies is that those who need them will be wound up. They will be restless and unwilling to calm down. They may be angry, and may experience wild mood swings. They may even strike out in their pain, seeking to harm those who would help them.

The **Aconite** toothache will start very quickly, as will **Belladonna's.** Both of these patients will have heads that are red and hot, with dry skin. Both will be feverish with toothache.

The **Aconite** patient will be restless and will wander around the room in pain, unwilling and unable to sit down and rest. His pain will overwhelm him; it will become the only thing in his life.

The **Belladonna** patient will be worked up and perhaps angry, but not nearly as restless. In fact, he may want nothing more than to go lie down in a cool, dark place. He will very much want to sleep, but his pain will not let him rest. The **Belladonna's** pain will start suddenly, and may fade just as quickly.

The **Belladonna** patient's tooth will be aggravated by any contact with cold. This will be especially true once he has gone to lie down and rest.

Belladonna is a thirsty patient. Look in his mouth: his mouth and throat will be very dry, and may also be inflamed and red. Look at his face as well—it may be swollen as well as red and hot.

Finally, the **Belladonna's** pain is throbbing in nature, and along with the toothache he may have a throbbing headache that runs through his entire head.

Where the **Belladonna** patient's whole face is swollen, the **Chamomilla** patient's face will most often be swollen and red hot only on the side with the painful tooth. Look for the other side of the patient's face to be cool and pale. In addition, look for his gums to be red and swollen.

Chamomilla is the first remedy to think of for children with toothache, or with the pains associated with teething. (Another remedy that is commonly called for to soothe children with teething pain is **Mag Phos** —this pain will be soothed by drinking warm liquids or by warm applications.) But remember not to limit this remedy in your thinking, as **Chamomilla** is an excellent remedy to keep in mind for patients of all ages who suffer from toothache.

Chamomilla is the first remedy to think of in cases of toothache that start in the night, and for toothache in which the pain is overwhelming. The patient becomes angry in his pain, and the worse the pain, the more violent he becomes. Sometimes the **Chamomilla** patient may cry because of his pain. But look at the patient's face and you will see that these tears appear to be tears of rage. The pain is made worse from contact with cold air and from drinking warm drinks. Hot coffee especially will cause agony.

To understand the patient who needs **Coffea,** think of how you would feel if you suddenly had a cup of strong coffee with full caffeine after not having had caffeinated coffee for years. Your pulse would race; you would not be able to just sit down and rest. The patient with a **Coffea** toothache acts in just this way. He is restless, frantic, and cannot settle down. Further, the patient will tremble and shake, and will tend to be hyperaware of all his senses. Light and noise especially will make him frantic.

This is a toothache that is worse from heat of any sort, especially from hot food or drink. The pain will be soothed by cold, so the patient will want an icepack on his cheek.

Like the **Chamomilla** patient, the **Ignatia** patient will undergo a complete change of personality during his toothache pain. Where **Belladonna, Aconite,** and **Coffea** patients may become frantic and a bit difficult, both **Chamomilla** and **Ignatia** will become raging beasts. Like the **Belladonna** and **Chamomilla** patients, the **Ignatia** patient's face will be distorted and swollen.

The **Ignatia** patient's pain will involve a sense of pressure. Any simple pressure on the tooth, such as from chewing, will cause great pain. The pain will be so great the patient may feel that his tooth is broken.

This is a toothache that tends to start in the morning, especially first thing in the morning. The pain will become worse if the patient drinks hot coffee or smokes tobacco. The patient may be so sensitive to the smell of tobacco that he may become worse simply by smelling a cigarette burning.

It is keynote of the type that the **Ignatia** patient's pain may cause him to cry. And because this patient is upset and irritable, he may refuse to cry in front of others, but will be heard crying in pain in his bedroom.

Toothaches and Temperature Modalities

I find that perhaps the best way to determine which remedy to use for toothache is to depend on modalities, which is to say that it is helpful to know what makes the pain better, and what makes it worse.

There are four simple rubrics that will help your find your remedy: Sometimes toothache pain is improved by warmth, and sometimes it is aggravated by warmth. And sometimes it is improved by cold, and other times it is aggravated by cold.

For toothache pain that is improved or soothed by warmth, consider the remedies **Arsenicum, Sulphur, Rhus Tox, Nux,** and **Mercurius.**

It should come as no surprise that a remedy as useful as **Arsenicum** would also be of help to those with toothache. And it should come as no surprise that those needing this remedy will be improved by warmth. The **Arsenicum** patient is *always* improved by warmth.

Just as some remedies are more often suggested for children with headache, **Arsenicum, Carbo Veg,** and **Calcarea** will be commonly used in older patients with toothache, and for cases of toothache in which gums are inflamed and swollen and bleed easily. In some cases, the gums will have also receded. You may find that all, or at least more than one, of the patient's teeth will hurt at one time. All these patients may also experience a sensation of their teeth being loose as well as sensitive and painful.

Arsenicum, as well as **Sepia,** is commonly used as a remedy for women who have toothache during pregnancy.

In cases that need **Arsenicum,** look for the patient's pain to extend from the tooth into the jaw, cheek, ears, or temples. Further, the tooth may be more sensitive than painful. It may throb. It may feel as if it has come loose. It may feel as if it is too large for the patient's head. And the sensitivity will be soothed by the patient sipping warm liquids.

The fact that **Sulphur** is listed among those remedies that are improved by warmth may seem odd, in that the **Sulphur** patient is almost always improved by cold. The simple fact is, when it comes to **Sulphur,** temperature is just not that helpful. You will also find it listed among the remedies that are made worse by warmth, and, surprisingly, those made worse by cold. These patients will be especially aggravated by drinking cold water.

So don't hang onto the temperature modalities with this remedy. What is keynote is that the **Sulphur** toothache will be better when the patient is indoors, and will grow a great deal worse whenever he goes outside. (This is often true of **Sulphur,** and is certainly true of the hay fever that **Sulphur** treats.)

Look for the old combination of symptoms to accompany a **Sulphur** toothache—the patient will be hot and sweaty, especially on his head, and his face will be reddened in his pain.

It is also keynote of this remedy that the patient is worse when in bed at night, worse from the heat of his bed. So look for the **Sulphur** patient's toothache to become worse at this time.

It should not be at all odd that the **Rhus Tox** patient is better from warmth, as **Rhus** is *always* improved by warmth. For example, the **Rhus Tox** backache is better if the patient takes a hot shower, and a **Rhus Tox** sore throat is better if the patient drinks warm liquids. So, too, with the toothache; the patient is better from warm applications and from drinking warm things. Not only will the **Rhus Tox** toothache be better from warm things, it will become a great deal worse from cold things. (Again, cold will almost always aggravate a **Rhus Tox** patient's symptoms, whatever they might be.) Weather will greatly affect the action of this remedy. Look for the toothache to be worse in cold, wet weather.

In fact, this toothache may develop every time the weather changes and becomes cold and wet.

Look at the patient's gums for indications. They will be red and swollen. Look at the patient's tongue. It also will be red, and may be swollen. More typically, look for it to have a red triangle on its tip. The patient will complain that his gums itch and/or burn during his toothache.

The remedy **Nux** is well known for the sensation of pain that is like a nail being driven into the patient's head. This is the sensation associated with the **Nux** headache, and it is also the pain sensation associated with the **Nux** toothache. The pain will center in the sore tooth and radiate from there through the patient's whole head.

This is a toothache that starts in the early hours of the morning, or that is worse in the early morning. The pain of the toothache will also become worse if the **Nux** patient thinks about his pain, and the increased pain will anger him as well.

Cold, as always, is the great enemy of the **Nux** patient. Cold in any form, from cold drinks to the slightest draft of cold air, will make the tooth throb. So the **Nux** patient will need to be kept warm, but note that the pain will become worse if he is in a room he finds too warm. Look for the **Nux** patient's teeth to chatter during toothache.

While the **Mercurius** toothache is also made better by warmth, it is important to note that the **Mercurius** patient is easily stressed by any change in temperature at all. He will be sensitive to both cold and warmth if either is carried beyond his fragile ability to adapt to temperature change. In fact, no other remedy is as sensitive to temperature change as **Mercurius.**

The patient needing **Mercurius** may have something worse going on than just a decayed tooth. He may, indeed, have an infected tooth. Look for the patient's mouth to be filled with saliva, and for his tongue to be swollen. Look for the indentations of the patient's teeth on the sides of the tongue. And this patient will have terrible breath, breath that lets you know that something is seriously wrong.

The **Mercurius** is a sweaty patient. Look for a cold, chilling sweat to accompany his pain. This is also a patient who is worse at night. Often, toothache will suddenly develop at night and awaken the patient from his sleep. This is a patient given to night sweats—his whole body will be covered with sweat while he sleeps.

The quality of the **Mercurius** patient's pain is stinging. The patient will complain that his tooth pain extends into his ears, especially when he swallows.

For toothache that is made worse by warmth, consider the remedies **Bryonia** and **Pulsatilla.** Also consider **Chamomilla, Coffea,** and **Sulphur,** which are described above.

Pulsatilla is another major remedy for those with toothache. Again, this is for the patient who is being driven wild by his pain, when the pain is truly unbearable.

Look to the patient's mouth for a clue to this remedy. His mouth will be very dry, and yet the patient has no thirst. The painful tooth will feel better for cold applications, and much worse for warm. Therefore, you will find that this patient, rather oddly, will want to hold cold water in his mouth, although he will not want to drink it.

Now look at the patient. Usually, the **Pulsatilla** will be a chilly patient, even in a warm room. And yet, he will not be able to bear being in a warm, enclosed space. He will need fresh air, or will want to go for a walk in order to get out of that place. And yet, through it all, he is chilly.

Another habit that may give away the need for **Pulsatilla** is rocking. The **Pulsatilla** patient will tend to rock, as if in a rocking chair, when he is in pain. So look for him to rock, whether the condition at hand is a toothache, a headache, or indigestion. Sometimes this clue alone will be enough to make a successful diagnosis.

Often, a headache and an earache on the same side of the head as the painful tooth will accompany the **Pulsatilla** toothache. Sometimes it will be accompanied by a one-sided headache, again on the same side as the painful tooth.

Finally, the patient's demeanor will give you a clue. This is a weepy patient who feels sorry for himself in his distress. He will also be clingy, and will want you to take care of him. He will not want to be alone.

Bryonia, on the other hand, will want to be left alone. And, because this is an irritable patient, you will likely want to leave him alone.

Like the **Pulsatilla,** the **Bryonia** patient's mouth will start out dry. He will put off drinking for as long as possible because of the pain. But soon his thirst will win out over his pain, and he will drink great amounts of cool water.

The pain in his tooth will be worse from warmth, especially from eating or drinking anything warm. This is a toothache that is likely to start at night or become worse at night. It may awaken the patient as he sleeps, but he will try to stay still with his pain, as the pain increases if he moves or speaks.

This is another remedy for cases of tooth decay. It may involve decay that has spread to more than just one tooth.

As with **Nux,** the **Bryonia** toothache may be accompanied by constipation.

For toothache that is made better by cold, consider the two remedies **Bryonia** and **Pulsatilla,** both of which are described above.

For toothache that is made worse by cold, consider the remedy **Staphysagria.** This is also our leading remedy for cases of toothache that involve multiple decayed teeth. (Other remedies, including **Rhus Tox, Belladonna, Nux,** and **Sulphur** will also be worse for cold, and are described above.)

Staphysagria is always called for when the pain of a condition is simply too great for a patient to withstand, as it is here. The pain associated with the toothache will seem so great when you observe the patient that you will doubt that anyone could have such severe pain. You may even question whether the patient is reporting his pain truthfully.

The patient will experience chill along with his pain. Look for a cold sweat to appear on his face and head. Look for his hands to be cold and sweaty as well.

Since this is a remedy for those who have neglected their teeth, you may actually see teeth in the patient's mouth that are blackened by decay. This is highly uncommon in this day and age, at least in most parts of the world, but do consider this remedy when decay seems to have spread from tooth to tooth. You should especially consider this remedy when the patient's gums seem inflamed or ulcerated, when the gums surrounding the tooth are swollen, and when the patient reports that his gums hurt just like his teeth.

This is another remedy in which the tooth will be aggravated by anything cold, from applications to food and drink. Think of this remedy when nothing can soothe the patient or his pain.

Less Common Remedies for Toothaches

For the toothache that is worse for any sort of pressure, consider the remedy **Plantago,** which is not a part of our Objective Materia Medica. (Note that **Ignatia,** which is discussed above, is also worse from any sort of pressure, and **Belladonna** is actually improved from gentle pressure, such as that caused by pressing your teeth together.)

The odd thing about the patient with a toothache that requires **Plantago,** is that it will be better while the patient eats, although the tooth will be very sensitive to pressure and any sort of touch. This seems to defy logic, but something in the gentle pressure of eating will actually soothe the tooth.

Consider this remedy for the patient with a toothache that, like **Mercurius,** extends into the patient's ear. But, in this case, look for the pain in the tooth and the pain in the ear to alternate and shift suddenly with no apparent cause. Also, the pain of the toothache may extend upward into the patient's eyes. Again, the pain may shift without warning. The toothache will become worse from any contact with cold air.

For the toothache that is not usually caused by decay, but, instead is the result of sinus pressure, consider the remedy **Dulcamara.** (Note that the **Rhus Tox** toothache, which has already been discussed, may also be caused by sinus pressure, as well as by weather change.) This is a great remedy to remember for those of us with sensitive teeth that become painful during the spring and autumn. Often these painful teeth will be part of an overall picture of allergy.

Consider this remedy for cases in which the patient has more than one painful tooth. Most commonly, the teeth in question will be the upper molars on each side of the mouth. As these teeth are located near the sinuses, they can become tender when a spring or fall allergy means sinus pressure.

The same may be said for sensitivity of the teeth that occurs during or after a cold. In just the same way, sinus pressure will create sensitive teeth. In either case, look for the teeth to become aggravated during cold and, especially, damp weather. Consider this remedy especially for toothache that recurs seasonally or with changes in the weather. (For information on another remedy that can also, to a lesser degree, be useful for the patient whose tooth pain is caused by sinus pressure and allergies, look for the remedy **Sabadilla** under Hay Fever below.)

For the patient whose toothache has become chronic, or may be the result of mercury fillings, consider the remedy **Hepar Sulph.** This is a toothache that is worse from any pressure, worse if the patient bites down or chews. The patient's toothache will also be worse at night, and worse if the patient is in a warm room (like **Pulsatilla).** Therefore, look for the patient to be awakened from his sleep by the toothache.

Look for the patient's face to be swollen. The patient's gums will also be swollen and will bleed easily. Look for the patient's face to take on a yellowish color.

As is often the case with those needing **Hepar Sulph,** it is possible that an infection is present. The sore tooth may be accompanied by a sore throat, swollen glands, and a general oversensitivity to the environment. Think of this remedy (and **Mercurius)** especially in cases involving an infected tooth. Also think of this remedy for those who have multiple mercury fillings that are still painful.

And, finally, don't forget the remedies **Arnica, Hypericum,** and **Calendula,** all of which are helpful in recovering from dental surgery. Turn to the section of this book dedicated to First Aid for more information on the uses of these remedies.

Hay Fever

When it comes to hay fever, we can speak only of Band-Aids, because the treatment of allergies in all their forms requires the most individualized of all homeopathic treatments. The exact nature of sensitivity and its resulting symptoms differ from person to person, sometimes subtly, sometimes profoundly. Therefore, we have to be in our top form with this case, to bring even temporary relief to the patient with hay fever until he can see a medical professional.

Given the difficulty of the task at hand, we may be tempted to run to the health food store to buy a mixture of remedies that claim to stop hay fever in its tracks. There is only one problem with this—I have yet to find such a mixture that works long term. Many a patient will suddenly find his sinuses opening and his eyes clearing when the first drops hit the tongue. But, within a handful of hours, that same patient will be splashing drop after drop on his tongue to no avail. If he continues to use the drops, he will, within days, find that he is experiencing renewed allergies, complete with new symptoms as he begins to prove some of the many remedies contained in the drops.

No, allergies—even seasonal allergies—demand to be treated with a single remedy, and they often respond better to that well-selected remedy in a potency lower than 30C. I have often found that the 12C potency works very well, as does the 9C, in the treatment of hay fever and other allergies.

In treating the patient with hay fever, I beg you to not try more than one remedy before getting the patient into a medical professional's office. If you give remedy after remedy in your attempt to find the right one, you may confuse the case to the point that your poor patient will simply have to suffer through the entire season without homeopathic help. So consider the remedies carefully, and select the remedy that seems to be the best match. Then, whether you succeed or fail, get that patient to a professional, because clearing away allergies can be a difficult task.

The remedy that, to me, presents the very picture of hay fever is one that is not in our Objective Materia Medica. It is a small remedy that doesn't have a wide range of uses. And yet, in the case of hay fever, it is second to none. The remedy is **Sabadilla.** The most important symptom of this remedy is sneezing. Look for the **Sabadilla** patient to sneeze and sneeze and sneeze. He will have long bouts of sneezing at one time. He may sneeze a dozen times at once, and still will not be able to stop sneezing.

Taking a page out of the remedy **Sulphur's** book, the **Sabadilla** patient will present a picture of heat and sweat. Look for his entire body to be covered in a hot sweat during his bouts of sneezing. But he will lack the third aspect of the **Sulphur** picture—he will not itch. Except for his nose—the inside of the patient's nose will itch terribly.

The patient will feel hot, both internally and to the touch. His throat especially will feel hot. And yet, the patient is chilly.

The patient's nose will flow with clear and thin and watery mucus, or it will stop flowing altogether and be totally stopped up. It is common that the patient's nose will also bleed during and after allergy attacks.

The patient's eyes will be red, inflamed, and will flow with tears. His eyelids will burn. He may experience weakness of sight during allergy attacks. His face will be hot and red. His lips will feel hot to the touch, and the patient will feel as if they had been scalded. The patient's mouth will be dry, and yet he is not thirsty. He will be unable to bear anything hot or cold in his mouth.

Also, to a lesser degree, you should consider **Sabadilla** for cases of toothache caused by sinus pressure and allergies, like **Dulcamara** and **Rhus Tox.** The patient's molars will become tender, with shooting pains, and his gums will be bluish. In cases needing **Sabadilla,** the toothache will be a secondary symptom to the overwhelming allergy.

The symptoms of allergy for the **Sabadilla** will always become worse if the patient smells flowers. The slightest smell of a flower will bring on a long, difficult attack. It is said that the patient will have an allergy attack even if he only thinks of the smell of flowers. Note that the patient will also be unable to bear the smell of garlic or fruit.

Note that a severe headache in the forehead may accompany the patient's hay fever. Also, the patient may have a severe sore throat that will be relieved by warm things, if he can force himself to eat or drink. Finally, the **Sabadilla** patient may have constipation concurrent with his hay fever.

Similar to the **Sabadilla** patient's symptoms and no less important a remedy for those with hay fever is **Sulphur.** And, as always, the **Sulphur** patient's experience of hay fever can be summed up with three words: heat, sweat, and itch.

Itch is often the major symptom. Every part of the patient's body will itch from the allergy, especially his eyes, his nose, and his soft palate. All parts of the patient's body that itch are covered in a hot, thick sweat.

The symptoms that separate **Sulphur** and **Sabadilla,** however, are easy to spot. First, the **Sulphur** patient will be completely and totally thirsty, unlike the **Sabadilla** patient. The **Sulphur** patient will want to drink cold things, from water to beer to soda, but will be willing to drink anything at all if need be. He is thirsty and must quench his thirst. Second, unlike the **Sabadilla** patient, the **Sulphur** patient is always better when indoors. Look for the **Sulphur** patient to not want to go outside at all during allergy season, because he feels so much better when he is inside. He may want the air conditioner on high, he may want fans on all over the house, but he will want to stay inside and seal the house up tight. Third, where the **Sabadilla** patient may experience constipation during hay fever, the **Sulphur** patient will likely experience some diarrhea, which will drive him out of bed in the morning.

Look for burning, heat, and itch to be all over the poor **Sulphur** patient's body. His eyes will burn and itch, and they may feel as if they are filled with sand. His face will tend to be reddened across his cheeks and nose. Look for the patient's lips to be red as well. Look for this patient to typically have a hot head and cold feet. While his head may sweat, he may cover his feet or protect them in shoes. And yet, he cannot bear to have his feet get too hot, either. So watch for the **Sulphur** patient to uncover his feet when they get hot, only to cover them again when they get cold. This will be true during the day and at night; when, in bed, the **Sulphur** sticks his feet out from under the covers. Look for the **Sulphur** to have hot, sweaty hands as well.

Finally, the **Sulphur** patient's allergies will grow much worse if he eats or drinks any dairy products, especially if he drinks milk. Any sort of dairy product will turn his body into a mucus factory.

As with colds, two remedies to keep on hand for the treatment of those with hay fever are **Allium Cepa** and **Euphrasia.** Remember, for the homeopath, the treatment of an ailment involves the uncovering of the totality of the patient's symptoms, and not necessarily the uncovering of the cause of those symptoms. Therefore, if a patient with a cold has the same symptoms as the patient with hay fever, then both will be successfully treated by the same remedy, although one has a condition caused by the presence of a virus while the other was caused by oversensitivity of the immune system.

Therefore, **Allium Cepa** and **Euphrasia,** two remedies most often associated with the treatment of those with colds, are excellent remedies to consider for those with hay fever. Indeed, all the remedies in the section on Colds may be useful for those with hay fever. I suggest that you look at those listings for more complete information, not only on these two remedies, but also on others that may be helpful and that you may want to keep on hand.

Allium Cepa is the homeopathic remedy made from the common onion, so if you think of the symptoms you experience when cutting an onion, you will get the picture of the remedy. The patient with hay fever that can be treated with **Allium Cepa** will have both eyes and nose that are flowing freely. The nasal discharge and the tears flowing from the eyes will be clear, thin, and watery.

However, the tears from the eyes will be bland and will not irritate the eyes, but the nasal discharge will be acrid and will irritate the patient's nose. Therefore the **Allium Cepa** patient is the patient with nostrils and an upper lip that are red, irritated, and crusty.

Euphrasia presents the opposite set of symptoms. Again, both eyes and nose flow with clear, watery discharge, but the **Euphrasia** patient's tears are acrid, and his nasal discharge is bland. Therefore, look for the **Euphrasia** patient to blink or wink his eyes to clear away discharge, and for his eyelids to be swollen. The patient will complain of burning pains in the eyes.

While **Euphrasia** is an excellent remedy for those with hay fever, it is also an excellent remedy for those with conjunctivitis. The flow of tears will be constant. The quality of the flow may, over time, change from clear and watery to thick and yellow.

The discharge from the eyes will be worse when the patient is in open air, also when his is lying down. Look for the eye pain to increase whenever the patient coughs.

Other remedies that you should have on hand in order to treat those with hay fever are **Arsenicum** and **Nux** —two remedies that will mix symptoms of chill with those of allergy—and **Gelsemium,** which will share an overall symptom of exhaustion with both **Arsenicum** and **Nux.**

Like **Allium Cepa, Arsenicum** patients will have an acrid nasal discharge that irritates the nose and the upper lip. And, like **Sabadilla,** the patient needing **Arsenicum** will have bouts of sneezing. The sneezing may be both uncontrollable and long-lasting. Look for the patient to be exhausted by his sneezing. Keynote of the **Arsenicum** case is that the patient will have the sensation of tickling in his nose. It will be located in one specific tiny spot in his nose. The patient will sneeze and sneeze because of the tickling, with no relief.

A sensation of burning will run throughout all of the symptoms. The patient will feel burning pains in his eyes, nose, mouth, and throat. Look for his eyes to be red, inflamed, and swollen. He may feel as if there is sand in his eyes. The rims of the patient's eyes may be scabby or scaly. He will have a profound sensitivity to light.

Finally, look for the **Arsenicum** patient to be greatly exhausted by his ailment. And look for him to feel a sensation of chill during his bouts of hay fever. Look for all of the patient's symptoms to be improved by sipping warm liquids.

The patient needing **Nux** for his hay fever will be even chillier than the **Arsenicum** patient. Even when his face feels hot to the touch, the patient will feel depleted and chilly.

In the case of **Nux,** the patient will have little flow from his nose. His nose will be stopped up, especially at night. In some cases, the patient's nose will flow during the day, only to be stopped up at night. Sometimes, the two nostrils will alternate between flowing and being blocked. The patient's nose will always be blocked up when he is outdoors.

The **Nux** is very sensitive to odors. His hay fever will be triggered by strong odors, especially perfume or by cigarette smoke.

The **Nux** will also be very itchy, and his eyes, nose, and throat will itch constantly. The patient's soft palate may itch as well.

The **Gelsemium,** like the **Nux** and the **Arsenicum,** will seem to be almost overcome by his hay fever, and he will want to lie down. The patient will complain that he feels achy pains all over his body and that he feels exhausted and heavy.

Like the **Arsenicum,** the **Gelsemium** patient's eye discharge will be acrid and will irritate his eyes. Look for his eyes to be red, sore, and swollen. And, as is keynote of the remedy, look for the patient's eyes to be half-open and half-closed. His eyelids will be droopy and heavy. The patient's face will also seem heavy and flushed. He will have a relaxed jaw and will breathe through his mouth. The patient will have a thin, acrid nasal discharge. The discharge will be fluent, as if he has hot water flowing from his nose.

Usually, the irritation of the hay fever symptoms will extend into the patient's throat. The patient will have a hoarse voice or may lose his voice altogether. And the pain will usually travel from the patient's throat into his ear. Swallowing will cause pain in the ear. The pain will become worse from warm food or drink.

These symptoms, then, can help you to select the correct remedy: The **Allium Cepa** has bland eye discharge and acrid nasal discharge. The **Euphrasia** has acrid eye discharge and bland nasal discharge. The **Gelsemium** has acrid eye discharge and acrid nasal discharge. And, like **Arsenicum** and **Nux,** the **Gelsemium** will have a chill, but in this remedy case the chill will only run up and down the patient's back.

Seasonal Allergies

Finally, there are two remedies that are excellent for cases of hay fever that are seasonally linked, one for spring allergies and the other for fall hay fever. These two remedies—neither of which is listed in our Objective Materia Medica—are **Arundo** and **Wyethia.** And there is **Dulcamara,** a remedy that may help in either spring or fall.

Arundo is a small homeopathic remedy that has little use aside from the treatment of those with hay fever. Think of this remedy specifically for those with spring allergies that occur early in the season. The allergies will begin with an itching of the soft palate and the eyes. From there, the itch will spread into the nose. The patient will lose all sense of smell and will begin to itch. This itching may extend to other parts of the body. The patient's head, skin—especially on the chest and arms—and anus will itch as well.

The patient needing **Arundo** will, like the **Arsenicum** patient, also suffers from a tickle in his nose that causes sneezing. Unlike the **Arsenicum** patient, however, the **Arundo** patient will have no flow from his nose. While he has sneezing, sinus pressure, and blockage, he has no flow of mucus.

The **Arundo** patient will also have a sensation of burning in his hands and feet, which will also be hot and sweaty.

The **Wyethia** case will also involve itching. Here the itch will center on the soft palate and will drive the patient crazy. The difference is that **Wyethia** is called for in cases of hay fever that occur in autumn. This patient will have a sore throat with a burning sensation. He will feel as if he must constantly swallow or clear his throat. He may complain that he feels as if the inside of his throat is scalded.

The **Wyethia** patient will tend to lose his voice or become hoarse from talking or singing. His throat will be dry and will feel swollen. The patient will have a hard time swallowing, but he will have a constant need to swallow his saliva. The patient will also have a dry, hacking cough. Look for the cough to be caused by a sensation of tickling in the patient's throat. He may also have dry, mild asthma. As part of his allergy picture, look for the **Wyethia** patient to suffer from a headache centered in his forehead. He will also typically have itching in his right ear and pain in his left ear.

Like **Sulphur,** the **Wyethia** is worse in the late morning, especially around 11:00A.M.. He will be particularly sensitive to his allergies at that time of day, and will feel very thirsty. Along with thirst will come the daily sensation of chill.

Dulcamara is a useful remedy to have on hand for the patient who has spring and/or fall allergies. Think of this remedy for those who are worse during the time of year in which the days are hot and the nights are cold, or for the patient who is worse during changes in the weather, especially at the onset of damp weather. This patient will always be worse outdoors, especially during damp weather.

The **Dulcamara** presents the picture of allergies in which the patient's nose alternates between being stopped up and flowing. When the nose is flowing, look for a constant discharge that can, over time, change from clear and watery to thick and yellow. The slightest contact with cold air will start the nose running. And the **Dulcamara** patient will be very protective of his nose; he will want to keep it warm at all times.

The patient's eyes will also have discharge that is profuse if the patient comes into contact with cold air. Like the nasal discharge, it will begin as clear and watery, but may become thick and yellow over time. The allergies may seem to center in the patient's eyes. Look for the patient's eyelids to twitch when the eyes come into contact with cold air.

Insomnia

From time to time, we all have a night in which it is impossible to sleep. We have received bad news, we are worried about a deadline, or income tax day looms—no matter the cause, the result is that we cannot sleep.

The remedies below will help those who cannot sleep. A 30C potency will be extremely helpful in most cases, although a 200C may be required by the patient who is extremely wound up. Remember that the 30C may be repeated nightly for a handful of nights, while the 200C should be given in single dose. Perhaps the best general remedies for insomnia include **Belladonna, Opium,** and **Arnica.**

It is keynote of the remedy Belladonna that the patient is "sleepy, but cannot sleep." Therefore, this is the first remedy that you should think of for cases in which the patient tosses and turns, thrashes about in bed, but simply cannot go to sleep. Often the patient will be sliding into sleep, but will suddenly jerk awake just at the point of dropping off.

Also remember **Belladonna** for cases of sleeplessness after a nightmare. **Belladonna** is an especially good remedy for young children who are too restless to sleep, and for children who are too terrified to sleep after a nightmare.

Often the **Belladonna** patient will be just exhausted but cannot sleep. He will remove himself to a cool, dark place and lie down. But, just as his eyes close in slumber, they fly open again. The **Belladonna** patient, unlike the **Arsenicum** patient, will not get up and walk the floor in exhaustion, but will just lie there praying for sleep to come.

It should come as no surprise that the remedy **Opium** is a potent homeopathic remedy for those who cannot sleep, since the allopathic drug opium is a powerful soporific. The patient needing **Opium** will lie awake long into the night. The keynote of the remedy is that all of this patient's senses will be increased. He will hear the sounds of the church bell in the town center, and will be sensitive to the smallest sliver of light that comes in under the bedroom door.

This is also the remedy to consider for cases in which the patient feels that his bed is too hot and seeks in vain to find some cool spot so he can rest.

This is also an excellent remedy for those with nightmares that upset the patient's sleep, but usually not waken him. To the patient, these dreams feel overwhelming and imprison-ing—he tries to awaken, but cannot. To the observer, the patient is kicking about, talking or even screaming in his sleep, but does not awaken. The patient's whole body may be covered in a cold sweat during his dream state.

Note that the remedy **Opium** is not includ-ed in our Objective Materia Medica. And it is also important to note that, because of the substance from which the remedy is made, this remedy may not be available for purchase by lay persons in all places. It may be neces-sary to visit a professional homeopath to be treated with the homeopathic remedy **Opium.**

Arnica may be perhaps our most important remedy in combating insomnia. Traditionally, **Arnica** has been the remedy of first choice for those who are unable to sleep because of physical overwork, for example, the laborer whose body aches keep him from sleep. It is especially useful for those who cannot get comfortable in their bed; the bed is too hard and no position of comfort is available. (Think of the fairy tale "The Princess and the Pea," and you will get the idea of the **Arnica** in patient his sleepless distress.)

But **Arnica** is also of great help to those who have overworked their minds. Think of this remedy for the patient who has studied hard for midterms, and now, after the test, cannot relax and sleep. Also think of **Arnica** as an excellent general remedy for those who are sleepless after hearing bad news or after a nightmare. In general, **Arnica** will soothe, heal, and bring needed sleep.

Two other remedies for those who have overworked or overstimulated their minds are **Lycopodium** and **Nux.**

The typical **Lycopodium** sleepless state is one in which the patient has an ongoing conversation with himself. He lies awake to review the work day and criticize his part in it. He will say to himself, "What I should have said to him was..." In this way, **Lycopodium** pa-

734

tient seeks to explain and justify his motivations to himself and bring himself to the place in which he can face another day. Typically, the **Lycopodium** patient will fall asleep just fine in the early part of the evening but will awaken at 4:00A.M. and be unable to sleep again, as the parade of his daily failures works him into a frenzy.

In the case needing **Nux,** the patient has usually kept himself awake and alert, studying or working or driving long distance, with the aid of coffee and other stimulants. Now that he has reached his goal, the **Nux** patient will find that he cannot get to sleep. This is a patient who is talking too fast, rushing about physically, and, underneath it all, just plain exhausted. He may turn to alcohol and drugs to help bring himself down. Note that palpitations and/or constipation may accompany insomnia.

In a more chronic state, consider this remedy first for cases of patients who fall asleep in their chairs after dinner, only to go up to bed and to not be able to sleep. It is also helpful for those who drop off to sleep in their beds nice and early, only to awaken around 3:00A.M. and not be able to go back to sleep. Either way, the **Nux** patient will lie awake, restless and angry, until the first glow of dawn shows against the window. He will then fall into a deep, deep sleep, only to be awakened an hour or so later by his alarm clock. He will then be impossibly irritable until he has had his coffee. He will speak to no one, and it is best not to speak to him until his caffeine jolt awakens him.

The constitutional **Nux** will find himself chronically sleep deprived. With the exception of that brief early morning sleep, his sleep leaves him unrefreshed. Worse, for some **Nux** patients, life becomes a cycle of chemistry, as he uses increasing amounts of alcohol to relax him to sleep in the evening, and increasing amounts of stimulants, like coffee, to get him through his long, exhausting day.

Two remedies will be very helpful to the patient who cannot sleep due to fear and anxiety. One remedy—**Aconite**—is most helpful in the acute sphere. The other— **Arsenicum** —is more often a remedy in cases of chronic insomnia.

Like the symptoms associated with the remedy, the cases of insomnia that **Aconite** treats will start suddenly. The patient has had bad news, or is awake waiting for a child to return home, convinced that something terrible has happened. This is a theme common to the remedy—something bad has happened, something bad is happening, something bad will happen.

No matter the tense of the verb, the **Aconite** patient will be awake and restless, worried and anxious. He may be sleepless because a murderer is on the loose and he is sure that he will come to his door, or he may be sleepless after a physical shock, like a near-miss traffic accident. Whatever the cause, something has temporarily robbed him of his sense of well-being. What is left is a vulnerable, fearful patient.

The **Aconite** patient will be restless; if you can get him to bed, he will toss and turn. But, more likely, he will refuse to stay in bed and will walk the floor in restless anxiety.

The picture that **Arsenicum** presents will be much the same. This is a patient motivated by fear. This is the patient who, night after night, will hear noises in the dark that rob him of peace of mind and sleep.

The **Arsenicum** patient will fear intruders, robbers, and rapists. This patient is sure that he will leave himself and his loved ones in danger if he does not stay vigilant. Some **Arsenicum** patients will move from their beds to the front of the house, and will sit watch by the windows or doors. Nearly all will refuse to stay in bed. They will get up and walk the floors long into the night. Look for midnight and the time thereafter to be the worst for the Arsenicum patient. He will usually totally exhaust himself and find some sleep later in the night. Also look for the Arsenicum to be the patient who, in his sleeplessness, decides to put the time to good efforts. Thus he is writing his novel or doing the dishes while others are asleep.

Early Night Insomnia

For cases of disturbed sleep or for sleeplessness in the early part of the night, consider the remedies **Chamomilla, Pulsatilla,** and **Lachesis.**

Chamomilla is the remedy to consider for cases of insomnia in which sleeplessness in the early stages of the night combines with restlessness. Note that, along with **Nux, Chamomilla** is most often used in treating cases of acute insomnia brought on by drinking coffee. This patient is, like **Nux,** also restless and irritable. He will be worked up by the caffeine, so that he feels palpitations and the blood pumping through his body. He is restless, irritable, and demanding. He walks the floor in his wound-up state.

And note that **Chamomilla** is also the remedy of first choice for cases of insomnia in young children, especially when the child demands that he be the center of attention, or demands to be carried. Think of this remedy first for the child who keeps getting out of bed again and again and who wills himself to stay awake.

The **Pulsatilla** will also find difficulty sleeping in the first part of the night. But this patient will actually tend to fall asleep. He goes to bed on time, lies down with the light out, and fades into a half sleep. In this stage, he grows too hot and kicks off his covers. Soon, the **Pulsatilla** patient will be too cold, and will try to find his covers. In his vague sleep state, he will likely not find them, but will toss and turn and try to awaken enough to pull his covers back on. In this way, the **Pulsatilla** patient works his way through a night of light, unrefreshing sleep.

But the king of unrefreshing sleep is **Lachesis,** and those needing the remedy **Lachesis** fall into two camps. Those in the first camp can actually sleep, but they will find that their sleep is unrefreshing. In fact, they will find that all of their symptoms are actually worse after they have been sleeping than they were before. The other camp of **Lachesis** patients will be unable to sleep. Most commonly, they will be just falling off to sleep when they will suddenly be jarred awake, like **Belladonna.** Most often, the **Lachesis** patient will suddenly awaken with the sensation of suffocation, feeling that they will stop breathing if they fall asleep.

Note that this feeling of suffocation can develop at any time in the night, and that the **Lachesis** patient will awaken at any time from this sensation. Most often, however, look for the sensation to occur in the early evening just as he is drifting off to sleep. (Like the **Carbo Veg** patient, the **Lachesis** patient may be comforted by moving air, and may be able to sleep if he has an electric fan aimed at him.)

The **Lachesis** may also be sleepless after having imbibed in a quantity of alcohol. He may lie in his bed and drift into an alcohol-induced half-sleep, unable to attain a real rest.

And, finally, **Lachesis,** along with **Belladonna,** is to be considered for cases in which the patient awakens in the middle of the night from terrifying nightmares. Note that both the **Belladonna** and the **Lachesis** patient will tend to have truly terrifying dreams, filled with noise, color, and blood. Sometimes the suffocative feelings linked to the **Lachesis** patient's awakened state will be the clue you need in selecting this remedy.

(Note that, the remedy of choice is **Phosphorus** for the young child who has nightmares of monsters, or who feels there are monsters in the closet or under the bed and makes you check these places before he can sleep. This will also be the child who is terrified of the dark. The **Phosphorus** child's reaction to his fear will always be the same—he will want sleep with his parents in their bed.)

"Christmas Eve" Insomnia

Not all sleeplessness is caused by overwork, nightmares, or anxiety. Sometimes, pleasant news and situations can lead to sleeplessness, what I call "Christmas Eve Syndrome." In cases of insomnia due to good news or anticipation of upcoming happy events, like weddings, consider the remedy **Coffea.** While the patient needing **Coffea** may be overstimulated by bad news and anticipation of sorrowful events, more often than not, the stimulation is due to the anticipation of happy things such as Christmas presents and lotto wins.

This is the patient who lies in bed completely awake, his mind flying in a thousand directions all at once. He may feel as if he has drunk a gallon of coffee, but he has had none.

Insomnia and Emotional Upset

From time to time, we all experience a case of "nerves"; a time when our emotional sense of balance is replaced with feeling of anxiety, fear, or shock.

In seeking a homeopathic remedy to help restore balance, it is important to try and understand if the cause of the upset is in the present or past, or if the patient lives in apprehension of future events.

Be aware that some emotional distress may be based in a chronic complaint, or be locked away deep in the patient's heart. In these cases, treatment should only come from a medical professional. The remedies listed here are given only so that the patient may be helped during the brief time it takes for him to get into the professional homeopath's office.

For the patient whose anticipation of future events has thrown off his emotional balance, think of the remedies **Aconite, Coffea,** and **Gelsemium.**

The **Aconite** type patient most commonly anticipates that "something bad is going to happen." He has a free-floating anxiety that all will not be well soon. He may even predict his own death, either through illness or from a sudden, horrifying event.

But he may also be living with the sense of dread that "something bad is happening" right now. This will be especially true of a parent who becomes upset when his child fails to return home on time. He begins to picture all the worst-case scenarios possible.

Finally, the patient **Aconite** may be responding to sudden bad news.

No matter whether the anxiety is based in the past, present, or future, the result is the same: shock. This is a patient in shock over a set of circumstances or fears. He is impatient, restless and thrashing, and cannot be comforted or quieted. He will walk the floor in anxiety and fear.

Usually the **Aconite** patient will make little sense. His fears flow through him, growing larger and larger, and his train of thought and conversation will follow no logical pattern. He will be overly sensitive, and may become hysterical. Oversensitivity to physical pain is common to the **Aconite** patient, who is already in a state of emotional oversensitivity. He will also be overly sensitive to his surroundings. He will not tolerate noise, and music in particular will upset him. He will also not be able to deal with those who try to comfort him by speaking softly and comfortingly.

The **Coffea** patient, on the other hand, will be thrown out of balance by the anticipation of happy events, like a wedding. And yet, the patient will be worse for his excitement—he is too worked up, too excited. Think of this patient as one who, after a lifetime without caffeine, has his first cup of coffee. He has palpitations. He cannot sit still. He cannot sleep. Look for trembling and/or fainting to accompany this emotional excitement.

The patient needing **Gelsemium,** on the other hand, lives in dread of the future. He is anticipating some event that he dreads failing—perhaps a need to speak in public or a need to take a particularly important test. This apprehension may cause the **Gelsemium** patient to have digestive upsets, especially diarrhea.

Also think of this remedy for cases of students who are poor test-takers. They may study and study and be well prepared, and yet they will forget the information when faced with the test itself. Also think of this remedy for chronically depressed patients. **Gelsemium** is especially helpful for patients who are depressed after a long illness, or because they are faced with a chronic illness. Think of this remedy for patients who seem disinclined to work, or to attempt anything, and particularly for patients who take to their bed in depression.

There several remedies for patients with emotional upsets based on their present circumstances. Among these remedies are **Causticum** and **Chamomilla.** Two other remedies, **Argentum Nitricum** and **Kali Phosphoricum,** which are not listed in our Objective Materia Medica, can also be helpful.

For the patient who is "on edge," and jumps at the slightest noise, there is no better remedy than **Causticum.** This is a patient with a free-form anxiety: he does not know what is wrong, but is sure that *something* is wrong.

This is also a patient who can become very upset through a sense of injustice. He may cry or rage over world issues and political injustice, and will be unable to relax or to let these issues go. He will be very critical of those in the news, political leaders, and those who do not share his political opinions. He will get very upset when reading the newspaper or watching the news on TV. **Causticum** may also be needed by patients who grieve (see **Ignatia),** and, especially by those who worry.

Look for the **Causticum** patient to have pain in his neck during his emotional upset. And look for him to lose his voice through overuse from berating others. He will often lose his voice when he is called upon to speak in public. (Note that, unlike the **Gelsemium,** he will not be terrified of speaking in public. He will simply and mysteriously lose his voice when called upon to do so,)

For patients with emotional upsets that need the remedy **Chamomilla,** the upset will always involve rage. While **Nux** may be a remedy needed by a patient who is chronically irritable and critical, **Chamomilla** is the remedy to think of for cases in which the patient's rage is so great that others fear exactly what he will do. Nothing pleases the **Chamomilla** patient, and everything annoys him. He flies into a rage if his dinner is not on time or the food is not to his liking. This is a patient who cannot be comforted or calmed when he is in a rage. He may be very violent, and may strike out physically, hit, or throw things.

Note that, like the **Staphysagria** patient, the **Chamomilla** patient is overly sensitive to his environment and everything in it. He is also, like **Staphysagria,** overly sensitive to pain, and may react with a response far greater than the pain itself. Thus, some **Chamomilla** patients may equate rage with pain, and may become enraged when they have any pain, such as a toothache.

Note that the **Chamomilla** patient is not aware of the fact that he is out of control. He is so involved in his rage—which feels totally justified to him—that he will not understand the implications of his actions while in his rage.

Argentum Nitricum patients, on the other hand, are very aware of the cause of their fear and of the fear itself. If you ask them, they will be able to tell you exactly what they are afraid of, and they can be afraid of any number of things. They fear crowds and parties, and especially fear meeting new people. They fear enclosed places and small spaces. They are afraid of heights—some **Argentum** patients will be so afraid of heights that they can be terrified by standing at the foot of a building and looking *up.* They are afraid of water, especially of deep, dark water when they cannot see the bottom. Many **Argentum** patients will especially fear having to cross bridges. They will feel the impulse to jump off a high bridge.

The response of the **Argentum** patient to his fear is to run or to walk away very quickly. This remedy type will walk faster than any other type. **Argentum** will help those who are riddled with fear and who have impulsive, irrational responses to their fear. It will be of help to those with full-blown panic attacks. It can also be a remedy for those with stage fright and fear of examinations (see **Gelsemium).**

Note that some **Argentum** patients may experience digestive upset, especially diarrhea, as a result of their fear and panic. In this way, the remedy type will resemble **Gelsemium.**

Kali Phosphoricum is an important remedy for those in depression, for those who have come to the conclusion that everything in their life is just too difficult and simply give up after a prolonged period of struggle and stress. This is also a remedy for those who fear meeting people, or simply dread having to deal with people, which makes them feel exhausted and depleted.

Remember, for the remedy **Kali Phos** to be helpful, the patient will need to have a history or struggle or stress—perhaps having had a long-term period of caring for a loved one who has now passed on, or a long period of extreme poverty and struggle for money. Often those needing this remedy will not seem to be in need. Indeed, they will seem to be bland, unconcerned people, but they are people living lives of quiet desperation.

Each little task takes on huge proportions to the **Kali Phos** patient. Everything seems to be too difficult to accomplish. And this patient can be riddled with fears, especially night terrors. He will have deep fear of illness and of death. Look for **Kali Phos** patients to be cruel to those they actually do need and love. They can be very cruel to their spouses or their children.

In the acute sphere, think of **Kali Phos** for those who are aloof, uncaring, and unconcerned, and for those who avoid crowds, and duck responsibility.

For those whose emotional upset is based upon past injustices and abuse, the remedy of first choice is **Staphysagria.** There is no better remedy than **Staphysagria** for those who have been harmed, especially those who have been a victim of a crime. The **Staphysagria** patient has been harmed unfairly, and knows this, but feels powerless to do anything about it. Some **Staphysagria** patients will be angry; others will be entitled to be angry, but do not know how. Either way, this patient has been frozen by the harm he has experienced. He is trapped in the moment of abuse and cannot move beyond it. **Staphysagria** is an excellent remedy for victims of childhood abuse, no matter how many years have passed since it occurred.

The **Staphysagria** patient may be fearful and distrustful of others. He not only is upset by the past, but he also fears the future. In some cases, the **Staphysagria** patient will be so fearful that he will not be able to sleep at night; he will only sleep during the day, and will keep watch at night. And just as the **Staphysagria** will either be very angry or incapable of anger, he will not be able to speak in a normal voice. He will speak either in a very quiet voice or a very loud voice.

Finally, the **Staphysagria,** like the **Chamomilla,** is overly sensitive to his environment and, especially, to pain. He will often experience pain as if he had been knifed, whether it was caused by a cut or a headache. In fact, the idea of being cut is so central to the remedy that it is helpful for those who have actually suffered from a cut, like those recovering from surgery.

For patients whose emotional upset is based in the past, especially if it involves feelings of grief and/or betrayal, the remedy of first choice is **Ignatia. Ignatia** is a well-known homeopathic remedy for those in grief. But be aware—

Ignatia will not be helpful to those undergoing natural grief associated with the loss of a loved one. **Ignatia** will help only those who fail to pass through their normal grief and move on to other things in life. It will help and soothe those patients trapped in their grief. Note that **Ignatia** is also useful for those who equate the death of a loved one with an act of betrayal, as if the loved one had a choice in the matter and they were abandoned.

Ignatia is helpful to those who experience wild mood swings, and are laughing one moment and crying the next. This patient leaves the people around him walking on eggshells, unsure as to just what will upset this moody, emotional person next.

Note that if these feelings of grief and betrayal are not treated and the patient stops his emotional roller coaster and withdraws into himself, and especially his bedroom, instead, the first remedy to consider is **Natrum Mur.** This remedy can be considered a constitutional equivalent of **Ignatia.** In the **Natrum Mur** case the patient is in a deep depression, and values his privacy above all else. This patient will not show his emotions and will feel that his troubles are "nobody's business."

Natrum Mur can follow **Ignatia** naturally in cases in which **Ignatia** fails to complete a cure.

CONCLUSION

Toward an Objective Homeopathy

Man has but one life, and it is the same for all parts. The normal manifestations of this life we call health; the abnormal manifestations of it disease. If we can always think of disease as a method of life, in a living body, we will have gotten rid of an old error, and have made the first step toward a correct diagnosis, and a rational therapeutics.

—JOHN SCUDDER, *SPECIFIC DIAGNOSIS*

It has been the thesis of this book that, homeopathy in the present day has become mired in the art of conversation to the detriment of its being a medical art.

In earlier times, homeopaths were trained to use all their senses in gathering the information concerning their patients—objective information that would lead those practitioners toward appropriate homeopathic treatments. Today, professional homeopaths and lay practitioners alike have come to depend upon their intake forms, their lengthy question-and-answer sessions, and, especially, their computer software in the selection of a remedy, rather than the witness of their own eyes, ears, and hands. It reminds me, sadly, of students raised in the age of the computer who, as a result, have never learned how to add.

In my experience, many homeopaths have all but removed the objective aspect of case taking from their work. Instead, they rely almost solely upon the patient's subjective experience of his illness in gathering information toward the selection of a curative remedy. And while I take nothing away from that first-hand experience, I would remind these practitioners that Hahnemann himself, along many other past practitioners of the healing art—John Scudder among them—would give equal impact to the words of the patient's loved ones and attendants as to those from the patient himself. Surely the patient who lacks the words to express his experience of the disease state and its impact upon his system cannot give sufficient information to lead the practitioner to a curative remedy.

In taking on the role of the physician, the homeopathic practitioner need not study the work of Johnny Carson and Judge Judy to learn how to interview or to grill his patient. Instead, he is called upon to learn to become a witness to the patient. He must learn to sit with him, to listen to him, and to watch him. He must learn to be a witness to all that the patient consciously shares with him as well as all that the patient shares unconsciously.

It is also important that, as much as we may enjoy building a wall of homeopathic reference books, we gather as much working knowledge as possible—both of homeopathic philosophy and of the remedies that make up our homeopathic pharmacy. It is vital that all students of homeopathy be able to understand and recognize the nature of the ailment in front of them in acute cases that call for homeopathic treatment, and especially in cases that call for first aid. It is also vital that that student have the ability to recognize at least the major homeopathic remedies when they see them "on the hoof."

To this end, I have attempted to create a reference book for students of homeopathy that will give them information as to just what they will see when they are looking at the patient who needs Sulphur, as opposed to the patient who needs Kali Phosphoricum. And I have attempted to present the most common ailments in a manner that is sensual in nature—that describes what one will see, smell, and feel when dealing with a specific patient who needs a specific remedy to be brought back to that state of balance we call health.

I gathered this information together so students of homeopathy will not have to guess which remedy may be curative, but will know which remedy is called for by the objective symptoms at hand. The objective symptoms that the practitioner can witness with his own eyes, ears, and hands.

I have also put together the information within the covers of this book so students just beginning their study of homeopathy will have a reference work that covers both the philosophy and the practice of homeopathy.

But it is my hope that students will outgrow this book in short order, and will have to find new resources to increase their understanding of homeopathy. So, whether the reader's goal is being a wise consumer of homeopathy, being able to treat himself and his loved ones in cases of simple household emergencies, or so excelling in his study of homeopathy that he may ultimately (with much work, study, and a medical license) become a medical professional, it is my hope that he will seek to better understand Hahnemann's healing philosophy.

To this end, I have some suggestions:

First, find yourself a study group. If there is no homeopathic study group near you, consider starting one yourself. You do not need to have a great homeopathic education to coordinate a biweekly or monthly study group.

You only need to be willing to put forth the effort.

And while, in all honesty, I must admit that I know some fine homeopaths who were largely self-taught, I must hasten to say that it is so much harder to learn about homeopathy—or any other topic I can think of—if you are working in a vacuum. In the past, those who were self-taught learned by themselves because they had no other option. As recently as a dozen years ago, there were few study groups and fewer homeopathic educational materials. Today, the market is flooded with books, tapes, and educational materials on homeopathy, all of which can help you get started.

If you would like information on a national network of study groups, or would like to see if there is an established group in your area, contact the National Center for Homeopathy, a national educational organization based in Alexandria, Virginia, as a starting point. Information on how to contact this group is located in the Appendices section.

Second, gather as many books on the subject as you can. This may be difficult, as it can get expensive, and worse, it can be very confusing. It seems as if there are as many opinions on what homeopathy is and how it works as there are books on homeopathy.

But once you wrestle with a few of them, I believe you will conclude, as I have, that this is a good thing. Disagreement leads to questions, and questions, ultimately, lead to answers—even if they only lead to answers that tend to change and evolve as the years go by.

This, too, is a good thing. Homeopathy is a living healing art. It is in a constant state of evolution and change. And as it grows and changes, we who study it change and evolve as well. And that is an excellent thing.

As you begin your study, be aware that, unlike the allopathic practitioners, the homeopathic practitioners tend to agree on very little and tend to argue a good deal. It makes for some very interesting gatherings and the chat rooms are seldom dull.

Now, as to the books you'll need: get as many materia medicas as you can afford to buy. Study them. Read what one author has to say about Sulphur, and then see what the others have to say as well. Remember, no one "owns" homeopathy, and no one author understands it in all its aspects. So don't be afraid to question the author's understanding of a remedy or remedies. Don't be afraid to take what you can from each author you read, and to, ultimately, form your own opinion. That is what you are supposed to do.

Also, be aware of what I call the "homeopathic wolves." They lurk all over the place. What I mean by this is to be wary of those presenting themselves as knowing everything about homeopathy. They know the complete history as if they had lived it. They know every remedy, every potency, and all of their uses. In my experience, the more these wolves claim to know, the more ignorant they are of the true precepts of homeopathy—the understanding of which tends to make a person humble. In my experience, the more an author, teacher, or practitioner of homeopathy is willing to admit to not knowing the ultimate answers, and the more willing he is to be questioned by his students or readers, the better. Further, the finest homeopaths I have ever known were those who, in their hearts, still considered themselves to be a student of homeopathy and never its master.

If you don't know how to study the materia medica, here's what I suggest you do. Start either with Arnica (if acute prescribing is of greatest interest to you) or Sulphur (if constitutional work is of greater interest to you) and read that remedy. Learn it. Study it in as many materia medicas that you can lay your hands on. Then, after you have studied that remedy, go to the bottom of the listing and look at the section of the entry that compares it to other remedies; that compares and contrasts the dynamics of Arnica or Sulphur with the dynamics of other remedies. Then study those remedies, how they are like Arnica or Sulphur, how they are different. Study those remedies in as much depth as you can, and then work with the remedies that can be compared with them.

This way, you will form a treelike structure of remedies, all of which have some basis of comparison built in. You can, if you want, actually draw this tree of remedies, adding each one as you study it. This is a good tool to being able to begin to identify families of remedies that can cluster around specific types of patients and specific types of ailment.

Now, as to the repertory: I've said it before in other parts of the book, but I'll say it again. Where you need to have many different materia medicas to get many different insights into the remedies, you will need only one repertory. But finding that one can be difficult.

You will have to look at a lot of repertories to find the one that is set up in the manner closest to the way you would set it up yourself.

You see, a repertory is only an individual homeopath's notes as to what symptoms suggest what remedy. Therefore, they are all organized differently. Some are organized by the symptoms, starting with the spiritual/mental and then moving into the body, from the head down to the feet. Others are alphabetically organized, so that symptoms involving the nose will not be located anywhere near those involving the ear. Both of these methods of organization are great, but you will need to work with the one that is easiest for you. After all, you will be using the repertory to look up the symptoms that you have gathered in your case taking. Time will be of the essence. You will be under some pressure to find not only a remedy, but also a curative remedy. Therefore, you are going to have to be able to find specific symptoms in very short order.

So search through the repertories on the market and find the one you like best. Buy it and study it. Don't, whatever you do, simply put it on the shelf until you need it. Believe me, you won't be able to find a thing at that time, and you will end up rushing through self-help books (like this one), hoping that the answer is included there.

You will have to have done your study in advance to do yourself or anyone else any good when a remedy is needed. There is no way around it, especially with that repertory. I hope that yours will be dog-eared with use long before it is ever actually needed.

From there, get the books that seem to speak to you. Books on philosophy. Books on history. Self-help books. Let your heart lead you and you won't go wrong.

Finally, don't be afraid to move on when you have learned what you came to learn. This means that, even if you were the one who started the study group, don't be afraid to leave it if the time comes when your own study of homeopathy has taken you to a new understanding or a new way of studying, working, or being. I have found that there are many ways of studying, and just as many ways of practicing homeopathy. It is up to you to find your path and your niche.

It's almost thirty years now that I have been studying homeopathy. Sometimes—especially in the early years of my study when there were no study groups to my knowledge, few books on the subject, and no Internet to connect with others out there sharing my interest—I studied alone, trying to piece together information as best I could, and sometimes I studied as a part of a surprisingly large group. I have seen the study of homeopathy thrive, and I have seen interest in it ebb. And I have walked away from the whole thing—exhausted, frustrated, and confused—on more than one occasion.

But there are some things I learned early on that have stayed with me. First, that healing—true healing that does not involve a suppression or temporary lifting of pain only to have it return again worse than ever—is possible. That you can be made well through homeopathy. Truly well, with all that is associated with illness being released once and for all, so that it cannot and will not return. Second, I have learned that this sort of healing involves a catalyst, which is what the remedy truly is.

This always reminds me of the crazed healer Paracelsus, who said that healing is like lighting a fire in a fireplace. When you are about to strike that match, you don't have to stop and ask yourself just how much energy you are going to have to apply to that wood in order to bring about a fire as a response. No, you only have to strike the match, place that spark of energy to the wood, and trust that the natural process of combustion will begin.

In the same way, healing is a natural process, that takes the same catalyst, the same spark. And that is what the remedy is. It is that burst of energy that can catch fire in our whole beings, body, mind, and spirit. We have only to trust the natural process and allow the natural process to be well.

And so, your study of homeopathy is a study of natural, universal principles. The process of the "healing combustion" is as natural and universal as the principle of "for every action, there is an equal and opposite reaction," which is the very heart of homeopathy.

Therefore, your study of homeopathy will involve as much unlearning as it will learning. You will have to unlearn much of what you thought was true, and a good bit of what you may have wanted to be true.

It seems, therefore, that it is not very likely that you can truly study homeopathy and not have it, in some very fundamental way, change you.

Which leads me to the last tiny bit of advice I have for you as you begin your study of homeopathy: Let it change you.

Appendices

Taking a man in entirely, we find a distinct expression when he walks, stands, sits or lies. Every part of the man talks to us, his hands, his arms, his legs, his feet, even his 'calves may wink,' as described by Dickens in one of his Christmas stories.

—JOHN SCUDDER, *SPECIFIC DIAGNOSIS*

APPENDIX ONE

A Bibliography of Books Related to This Volume

The following are books that have been helpful to me, not only in my understanding of homeopathy, but also in the creation of the book you hold in your hands. To make this list more useful, I have divided it into the specific areas of interest contained in this volume, from the history of homeopathy to its practice, and to the philosophy and practice of traditional Chinese medicine. I recommend all the books listed here.

If you want more information on the history and development of homeopathy thought and practice, consider these books:

Coulter, Harris. *Divided Legacy: A History of the Schism in Medical Thought* (4 volumes). Berkeley, CA: North Atlantic Books, 1975–1994.

Handley, Rima. *A Homeopathic Love Story: The Story of Samuel and Melanie Hahnemann.* Berkeley, CA: North Atlantic Books, 1990.

Winston, Julian. *The Faces of Homeopathy: An Illustrated History of the First 200 Years.* Tawa, New Zealand: Great Auk Publishing, 1999.

Wood, Matthew. *The Magical Staff: The Vitalist Tradition in Western Medicine.* Berkeley, CA: North Atlantic Books, 1992.

If you want to learn more about homeopathic philosophy and practice, consider these books:

Bailey, Philip. *Homeopathic Psychology: Personality Profiles of the Major Constitutional Remedies.* Berkeley, CA: North Atlantic Books, 1995.

Close, Stuart. *The Genius of Homeopathy: Lectures and Essays on Homeopathic Philosophy.* New Delhi, India: B. Jain Publishers Ltd., 1993 (reprint).

Cook, Trevor M. *Homeopathic Medicine Today: A Modern Course of Study.* New Canaan, CT: Keats, 1989.

Eizayaga, Francisco Xavier. *Treatise on Homeopathic Medicine.* Buenos Aires, Argentina: Ediciones Marecel, 1991.

Hardy, Mary and Dotty Nonman. *The Alchemist's Handbook to Homeopathy.* Allegan, MI: Delta K Trust, 1994.

Kent, James Tyler. *Lectures on Homeopathic Philosophy.* Berkeley, CA: North Atlantic Books, 1979.

McCabe, Vinton. *Homeopathy, Healing and You.* New York, NY: St. Martin's, 1997.

Roberts, H.A. *The Principles and Art of Cure by Homeopathy.* New Delhi, India: B. Jain Publishers Ltd., (reprint).

Vithoulkas, George. *The Science of Homeopathy.* New York, NY: Grove, 1980.

Vithoulkas, George. *A New Model for Health and Disease.* Berkeley, CA: North Atlantic Books, 1991.

Whitmont, Edward C. *Psyche and Substance: Essays on Homeopathy in the Light of Jungian Psychology.* Berkeley, CA: North Atlantic Books, 1991.

Whitmont, Edward C. *The Alchemy of Healing: Psyche and Soma.* Berkeley, CA: North Atlantic Books, 1993.

If you want more books on self-treatment, consider these:

Castro, Miranda. *The Complete Homeopathy Handbook.* New York, NY: St Martin's, 1990.

Castro, Miranda. *Homeopathy for Pregnancy, Birth and Your Baby's First Year.* New York, NY: St. Martin's, 1993.

Curtis, Susan and Romy Fraser, *Natural Healing for Women.* London, England: Pandora, 1991.

De Schepper, Luc. *Musculoskeletal Diseases and Homeopathy.* Santa Fe, NM: Full of Life Publishing, 1994.

Lessell, Colin B. *The World Traveler's Manuel of Homeopathy.* Saffron Walden, England: C.W. Daniel, 1993.

Lockie, Andrew. *The Family Guide to Homeopathy: Symptoms and Natural Solutions.* New York, NY: Simon and Schuster Fireside, 1993.

Lockie, Andrew and Nicola Geddes, *The Women's Guide to Homeopathy.* New York, NY: St. Martin's, 1994.

McCabe, Vinton. *Practical Homeopathy.* New York, NY: St. Martins, 2000.

Moskowitz, Richard. *Homeopathic Medicine for Pregnancy and Childbirth.* Berkeley, CA: North Atlantic Books, 1992.

Nauman, Eileen. *Poisons that Heal.* Sedona: Light Technology Publishing, 1995.

Panos, Maesimund B. and Jane Heimlich, *Homeopathic Medicine at Home: Natural Remedies for Everyday Ailments and Minor Injuries.* Los Angeles, CA: Tarcher, 1976.

Ullman, Dana. *The Consumer's Guide to Homeopathy.* New York, NY: Tarcher Putnam, 1995.

Ullman, Dana with Stephen Cummings, *Everybody's Guide to Homeopathic Medicines.* New York, NY: Tarcher Putnam, 1984.

768

Zand, Janet, Rachel Walton, and Bob Roundtree, *Smart Medicine for a Healthier Child.* New York, NY: Avery, 1994.

Editions of The Organon of Medicine:

There are many, many different editions of the *Organon* on the market. The best, in my opinion, combine the 5th and 6th editions into one work.

You will note that there are only three editions listed here. I list them because I consider them to be the best. And, among the three, the best by far is *The Organon of the Medical Art,* a new translation by Steven Decker that has been masterfully annotated by Wenda Brewster O'Reilly, Ph.D. I've marked it with a star.

Hahnemann, Samuel. *The Organon of Medicine.* New Delhi, India: B. Jain Publishers Ltd. (reprint).

Hahnemann, Samuel. *Organon of Medicine.* Blaine, WA: Cooper Publishing, 1982.

*Hahnemann, Samuel. *The Organon of the Medical Art.* Redmond, WA: Birdcage Books, 1997.

Materia Medicas:

There are many *Materia Medicas* on the market. Those listed here are all part of my own shelf of homeopathic reference works. Note that I have decided to list some that are long out of print, because, thanks to the Internet and, especially, to Bibliofind (a division of Am azon.com) and eBay, it is now possible to find and purchase these works. And, happily, the Indian publisher B. Jain has reprinted many works of classical homeopathy that previously were almost impossible to find.

Note also that I have placed a star next to the *Materia Medicas* I consider especially fine and that were of help to me in creating my Objective Materia Medica.

*Allen, Timothy Field. *A Handbook of Materia Medica and Homeopathic Therapeutics.* Philadelphia, PA: Hahnemann Publishing House, 1889.

Boericke, William. *Pocket Manual of Materia Medica with Repertory.* New Delhi, India: B. Jain Publishers Ltd. (reprint).

Boger, C.M. *A Synoptic Key to the Materia Medica: A Treatise for Homeopathic Students.* New Delhi, India: B. Jain Publishers Ltd. (reprint).

Coulter, Catherine. *Portraits of Homeopathic Medicines* (2 volumes). Berkeley, CA: North Atlantic Books, 1986, 1988.

*Hahnemann, Samuel. *Materia Medica Pura* (two volumes). New Delhi, India: B. Jain Publishers Ltd. (reprint).

*Hering, Constantine. *The Guiding Symptoms of our Materia Medica* (10 volumes). New Delhi, India: B. Jain Publishers Ltd., 1997 (reprint).

Jouanny, Jacques. *The Essentials of Homeopathic Materia Medica.* Boiron S A, France: Boiron, 1984.

Kent, James Tyler. *Lectures on Homeopathic Materia Medica.* New Delhi, India: B. Jain Publishers Ltd. (reprint). (Note: this is not truly a materia medica; Kent did not leave us a materia medica of his work. However, this collection of the lectures that Kent gave his students on specific homeopathic remedies belongs on the reference shelf of every student of homeopathy.)

*Mathur, K.N. *Systematic Materia Medica of Homeopathic Remedies with Totality of Characteristic Symptoms and Various Indications of Each Remedy.* New Delhi, India: B. Jain Publishers Ltd., 1988.

*Morrison, Roger. *Desktop Guide to Keynotes and Confirmatory Symptoms.* Berkeley, CA: Hahnemann, 1993.

*Murphy, Robin. *Lotus Materia Medica.* Pagosa Springs, CO: HANA, 1995.

Narasimhamurti, *Handbook of Materia Medica and Therapeutics of Homeopathy.* New Delhi, India: B. Jain Publishers Ltd. (reprint).

Nash, E.B. *Leaders in Homeopathic Therapies.* New Delhi, India: B. Jain Publishers Ltd. (reprint).

Phatak, S.R. *Materia Medica of Homeopathic Medicines.* New Delhi, India: Indian Books and Periodicals Syndicate, 1977.

*Tyler, Margaret. *Drug Pictures.* Saffron Walden, England: C.W. Daniel, 1952.

Vermuelen, Frans. *Concordance Matieria Medica.* Haarlem, the Netherlands: Merlijn Publishers, 1994.

Vithoulkas, George. *Materia Medica Viva, Volume One.* Mill Valley, CA: Health and Habitat, 1992.

Zaren, Ananda. *Core Elements of the Materia Medica of the Mind* (2 volumes). Gottingen, Germany: Burgdorf, 1993, 1994.

Repertories:

While I always recommend to my students that they get as many materia medicas as possible, I also recommend that they get only one or two repertories—and that the repertory they choose be structured as close to the way they would structure it as is possible. In other words, it is important that you and the author of the selected repertory think alike. Therefore, you will have to look through a great many repertories before you find the one that works best for you. Then it is important that you become as familiar with this work you can.

I own several repertories, but I find myself reaching for Kent's or Murphy's most often.

Kent, James Tyler. *Repertory of the Homeopathic Materia Medica.* New Delhi, India: B. Jain Publishers Ltd. (reprint).

Murphy, Robin. *Homeopathic Medical Repertory.* Pagosa Springs, CO: HANA, 1993.

Phatak, S.R. *A Concise Repertory of Homeopathic Medicines.* New Delhi, India: B. Jain Publishers Ltd. (reprint).

Schroyens, F. *Synthesis Repertorium.* London, England: Homeopathic Book Publishers, 1993.

Van Zandvoort, Roger. *The Complete Repertory* (3 volumes). Leidschendam, the Netherlands: IRHIS, 1994.

If you would like more information on traditional Chinese medicine, consider these books:

Lee, Jacques K. *The Tongue: Mirror of the Immune System.* Kent, England: Helios Books,

1999. (Note that this book contains information on both homeopathy and TCM.)

Maciocia, Giovanni. *Tongue Diagnosis in Chinese Medicine.* Seattle, WA: Eastland Press, 1995.

Manning, Clark A. and Louis J. Vanrenen, *Bioenergetic Medicines East and West: Acupuncture and Homeopathy.* Berkeley, CA: North Atlantic Books, 1988. (Note that this book contains information on both homeopathy and TCM.)

Qin, B.W. *Elementary Traditional Chinese Medicine.* Hong Kong: Taiping Book Publishers, 1971.

Wang, S.H. *Classic of the Pulse.* Hong Kong: Taiping Book Publishers, 1961.

Zhen, Li Shi. *Pulse Diagnosis.* Brookline, MA: Paradigm Publications, 1981.

APPENDIX TWO

A Source Guide to Homeopathic Remedies, Organizations, Websites, and Materials

This is a listing of the names, addresses, phone numbers, and, where possible, websites and e-mail addresses for our nation's leading homeopathic educational groups, professional societies, pharmacies, and providers of homeopathic educational materials and books.

In addition to this list, I add one more web address, which I consider to be the finest homeopathic site on the Internet. For just about everything to do with homeopathy, including free book downloads, chat groups and links to every other site, set your web browser to the Homeopathy Home Page at www.homeopathyhome.com.

I also suggest that readers interested in gathering books on homeopathy, especially rare and out-of-print books, not forget Bibliofind (a division of Amazon.com) and eBay. Both of these sites will provide you with more books than you can possibly read.

Homeopathic Educational Organizations

All of these organizations offer education in homeopathy. Some of it is available for lay persons, while some is only for medical professionals. Note, however, that to my knowledge none of these organizations offers a degree or certificate that would allow anyone to practice homeopathy in the United States without another medical license.

National Center for Homeopathy

801 N. Fairfax, Suite #306
Alexandria, VA 22314
(703) 548-7790
(703) 548-7792 (FAX)
info@homeopathic.org
www.homeopathic.org

Desert Institute School of Classical Homeopathy

2001 W. Camelback Road, #150
Phoenix, AZ 85015
(602) 347-7950
(602) 864-2949 (FAX)
disch@igc.org

www.chiaz.com/disch

This is the leading homeopathic organization in the United States. Membership is open to both lay persons and medical professionals, as are the center's classes. This is one of the most useful of the homeopathic web sites.

Homeopathic Educational Services

2124 Kittredge Street
Berkeley, CA 94704
(800) 359-9051
(510) 649-0294
(510) 649-1955 (FAX)
mail@homeopathic.com
www.homeopathic.com

Homeopathic training with clinical experience and long-distance learning programs are available through this organization.

Luminos School of Homeopathy, Los Angeles

1640 Bryn Mawr Avenue
Santa Monica, CA 90405
(310) 772-8235

(310) 581-9610 (FAX)
avgh1@homeopathycourses.com/laschool
www.homeopathycourses.com/laschool

This school offers learn-at-home classes for lay persons. Books, tapes, and remedies are also available.

New England School of Homeopathy

356 Middle Street
Amherst, MA 01002
(413) 256-5949
(413) 256-6223 (FAX)
nesh@nesh.com
www.nesh.com

This school is for very serious students only, and offers a four-year diploma program.

New York Luminos School of Homeopathy

158 Franklin Street
New York, NY 10013
(212) 925-4623
faculty@nyhomeopathy.com
www.nyhomeopathy.com

Classes and seminars for beginners are available.

Pacific Academy of Homeopathic Medicine

1199 Sanchez Street
San Francisco, CA 94114
(415) 695-2710
(415) 695-8220 (FAX)
health@homeopathy-academy.org
www.homeopathy-academy.org

This organization is a merger between the old New York School of Homeopathy and Luminos. It offers a four-year diploma program.

The School of Homeopathy, Devon

82 Pearl Street
New Haven, CT 06513
(203) 624-8783
betsy@homeopathyschool.com
www.homeopathyschool.com

A three-year certification course is offered.

The School of Homeopathy, New York

964 Third Avenue, 8th Floor
New York, NY 10015
(212) 570-2576
(212) 737-2489 (FAX)
kathy@homeopathyschool.com
www.schoolofhomeopathynewyork.com

This school offers a correspondence course in homeopathic philosophy and practice.

Teleosis Foundation

P.O. Box 7046
Berkeley, CA 94707
(510) 558-7285
(510) 528-1998 (FAX)
teleosis@igc.org
www.teleosis.com

The foundation provides courses and clinical study.

Teleosis School of Homeopathy

5A Lancaster Street
Cambridge, MA 02140
(617) 547-8500
info@teleosis.org

www.teleosis.com

Weekend classes and clinical experience are available.

Professional Homeopathic Organizations

To the best of my knowledge all of the organizations listed here are open only to those medical professionals whose license and practice apply.

Academy of Veterinary Homeopathy

P.O. Box 9280
Wilmington, DE 19809
(866) 652-1590
(866) 652-1590 (FAX)
office@theavh.org
www.theavh.org

American Association of Homeopathic Pharmacists

33 Fairfax Street
Berkeley Springs, WV 25422
(800) 478-0421

info@homeopathyresource.org
www.homeopathyresource.org

American Institute of Homeopathy

801 N. Fairfax Street, Suite #306
Alexandria, VA 22314
(888) 445-9988
www.homeopathyusa.org

Council for Homeopathic Certification

1199 Sanchez Street
San Francisco, CA 94114
(866) 242-3399
(415) 869-2867 (FAX)
chcinfo@homeopathicdirectory.com
www.homeopathicdirectory.com

Homeopathic Nurses Association

4 Kellcourt Drive
Attleboro, MA 02703
(505) 586-1166

(508) 223-5301
(508) 223-1801 (FAX)
wellnessnurse@5pillars.com
www.homeopathicnurses.org

Homeopathic Pharmacopoeia Convention of the United States

P.O. Box 2221
Southeastern, PA 19399
(610) 783-0987
(610) 783-5180 (FAX)
hpus@aol.com
www.HPCUS.com

Homeopaths without Borders (North America)

P.O. Box 1550
Basalt, CO 81621
(970) 927-9550 (FAX)
hwb@igc.org

North American Society of Homeopaths

1122 E. Pike Street, Suite #1122

Seattle, WA 98122
(206) 720-7000
(208) 248-1942 (FAX)
nashinfo@aol.com
www.homeopathy.org

Homeopathic Pharmacies

The businesses listed below sell homeopathic remedies, some by kit, some by single remedies, most by both. Many supply other homeopathic products as well, from books to tapes to software.

1-800-HOMEOPATHY

P.O. Box 8080
Richford, VT 05476
(800) HOMEOPATHY
(877) 999-0090 (FAX)
info@1800homeopathy.com
www.1800homeopathy.com

Apthorp Pharmacy

2201 Broadway
New York, NY 10024
(212) 877-3480
(212) 769-9095 (FAX)

Arrowroot Standard Direct

83 E. Lancaster Avenue
Paoli, PA 19301
(800) 234-8879
(800) 296-8998 (FAX)
customerservice@arrowroot.com
www.arrowroot.com

Boiron

6 Campus Boulevard, Building A
Newtown Square, PA 19073
(800) BOIRON-1 (Information line)
(800) BLU-TUBE (Orders only)
(610) 325-7480 (FAX)
info@boiron.com
www.boiron.com

Dolisos

3014 Rigel Road
Las Vegas, NV 89102
(702) 871-7153

Hahnemann Laboratories, Inc.

1940 Fourth Street
San Rafael, CA 94901

(888) 427-6422
(415) 451-6981 (FAX)
info@hahnemannlabs.com
www.hahnemannlabs.com

Homeopathic Educational Services

2124 Kittredge Street
Berkeley, CA 94704
(800) 359-9051 (Orders only)
(510) 649-0294
(510) 649-1955 (FAX)
mail@homeopathic.com
www.homeopathic.com

Homeopathy Works

33 Fairfax Street
Berkeley Springs, WV 25411
(800) 336-1695 (Orders only)
(304) 258-2541
(877) 286-0601 (FAX)
Info@homeopathyworks.com
www.homeopathyworks.com

Kent Homeopathic Associates, Inc.

710 Mission Avenue
San Rafael, CA 94901
(877) YES-KENT
(415) 457-0678
(415) 457-0688 (FAX)
kha@igc.org
www.kenthomeopathic.com

Luyties Pharmacal

4200 Laclede Avenue
St. Louis, MO 63108
(314) 533-9600

Note: this company develops and sells computer software only

Minimum Price Homeopathic Books

250 H Street
PMB 2187
Blaine, WA 98230
(800) 663-8272 (Orders only)
(604) 597-4757
(604) 597-8304 (FAX)

orders@minimum.com
www.minimum.com

Santa Monica Homeopathic Pharmacy

629 Broadway
Santa Monica, CA 90401
(310) 395-1131
(310) 395-7861 (FAX)
info@smhomeopathic.com
www.smhomeopathic.com

Similasan Corporation

1321-D South Central Avenue
Kent, WA 98032
(800) 426-1644

Standard Homeopathic Company

210 West 131st Street
P.O. Box 61067
Los Angeles, CA 90061
(800) 624-9659 (Orders only)
(310) 768-0700
(310) 516-8579 (FAX)
shcinfo@hylands.com

www.hylands.com

Washington Homeopathic Products

4914 Del Ray Avenue
Bethesda, MD 20814
(800) 336-1695

Weleda Inc.

175 North Route 9W
Congers, NY 10920
(800) 289-1969, ext. 212
(800) 280-4899 (FAX)
rx@weleda.com
www.weleda.com

APPENDIX THREE

The Wisdom of John Scudder

The following information is taken from the 1874 book I include these detailed passages because Scudder's work is long out of print and very difficult to find.

Scudder on "Facial Expression"

"The fact has already been noticed that mental states find easiest expression in the usual channels of innervation, and through those muscles in common use. This is not only true of mental activity, but is also true of disease. There is not disease without a wrong of the nervous system, and I think I may add with truth, that there is no wrong of life that is not represented upon the surface through the nervous system. We may not be able to read it, because our senses have not been trained to observation, and we have not sufficient experience, but the fact that disease is thus expressed should stimulate to study.

"The face will show clearly the *right* life that we call health; and the *wrong* life we call disease. If one will closely study the expression of the face in health, and compare it with the expression seen in sickness, this fact will be clearly seen. It not only tells us of impaired life, but also of the kind of impairments, and of the remedies that will remove the wrong, and restore health. It will be well to make this study with reference to—1st: The condition of the brain; 2nd: With reference to the condition of the sympathetic nervous system, and associated spinal cord; 3rd: With reference to the condition of the circulation and the blood; 4th: With reference to local disease; 5th: With reference to pain; 6th: Resistance of disease...

"Pain and suffering are distinctly expressed in the features, yet not always in the same way. Firm contraction of muscles is the most common expression. Thus every reader will recollect the contracted brow as evidencing pain, especially pain with irritation of the nerve centers. We involuntarily associate contraction of the structures about the eyes, and the wrinkled skin, with pain or with suffering. But we have the evidence of pain in their region without muscular contraction; indeed, there is the reverse, drooping of the tissues, the expression is sad, of the exhaustion that follows excessive grief, and we are assured that there is enfeebled circulation in the brain, and the pain is the expression of atony.

"It is very important to make these distinctions in order to select remedies. Pain is the result of two very opposite conditions—an excited circulation and an enfeebled circulation...

"Pain in the abdomen, pelvis, or lower extremities, finds expression in the mouth. Acute pain almost always finds expression in contraction of the mouth; when very severe lips are firmly drawn in, the angles of the mouth retracted, and somewhat depressed. In some cases, the angles of the mouth are drawn in, and there is that action of the muscles of the upper lip that gives it and the cheeks a full expression.

"I hardly need call attention to the fact, that some patients *resist* disease by an influence of the will, and that sometimes this effort is very important. Others yield to it from the first, and thus favor its progress. Every one has made these observations, and will recognize the importance of knowing whether a patient resists or yields, as it may determine whether he will recover or die."

Scudder on "Expression in Motion"

"We not only find disease expressed in position and in persistent muscular contraction, as heretofore named, but it is also shown in motion. We see a man standing or sitting and observe that his soft tissues seem to sit on him like a badly fitting suit of clothes, and we think at once of impaired nutrition and degeneration of tissue. But it may be only a want of innervation, from habitual torpor of the nervous system. Set him in motion, and we will soon see whether this is so or not, for there are none so sluggish in this respect, but what they may be aroused.

"We notice the movements of the person that we may confirm the diagnosis of expression, especially as regards the important point of undue irritation and circulation, or impaired innervation and circulation. The quick, restless movement is characteristic of the first. The desire to lie still, and the slow movements, of the second. Possibly there is no evidence of disease more definite that this, and it should be allowed it full weight in diagnosis.

"In some cases the rapid movement is but a means of removing excessive excitement of the brain and spinal cord, as in great grief or joy, or in cases of severe, but temporary pain. In such cases it may be looked upon as a means of relief, for if the excessive emotions, or pain were pent up, the person might suffer severely from it.

"But in other cases, whilst it tells of nervous irritability, the bodily movements give no relief, but even intensify the wrong, besides causing exhaustion. In these cases we endeavor to get bodily rest from the first, as a means of allaying the nervous excitation. Every one will have noticed the influence of the physician, nurse, or friend who with kindness but firmness, insists on keeping still. The hand placed upon the body of the sufferer to give support, seems to strengthen the will power, and frequently with an effort on the part of the patient comes rest and relief.

"There is a case of restlessness from an enfeebled and atonic condition of the nerve centers that requires notice. The unsteady movement, or the evidence of exhaustion following it, with the anxious, depressed countenance, tells the story. In the other case we will find almost continued tension of the muscular system...

"Increased movement is not associated with structural, or even with severe local functional disease, so that unless it points to a wrong of the cerebro-spinal centers we do not regard it as an unpleasant symptom. In ordinary colic the patient is restless, and seems to get relief from motion, but in the severer forms of colic, called 'bilious' ... he remains very still."

Scudder on the "Color of the Surface"

"As has already been named, the education of the eyes to distinguish colors is of much importance in diagnosis; and the reasons will be obvious to the reader. There is no property of living bodies so sensitive as color. It is usually thought of as evanescent, changeable, fleeting, and the expression of poetry in this regard, but represents the results of close observation.

"The florist is guided by it to a very considerable extent. When he visits he greenhouses in the morning, his eye closely scans the plants with reference to their health. Change of color, even so slight that it would not be noticed by an ordinary observer, is to him evidence of disease. He recognizes in change of color, the escape of gases from his flues, want of ventilation, a wrong in the temperature, the want of, or a wrong plant food, the presence of parasites, etc. He not only makes his 'diagnosis' from change of color, but gives the prognosis as well.

"The farmer, without any special training, or knowing why, recognizes the wrong color in his plants, and speaks of their sickly appearance. If he has been a close observer, there is something about their expression, and usually in their color that tells him of the character of the wrong—from drought, from wet, from too much heat, from cold, from atmospheric changes, from want of plant food, from excess of certain foods, or from a wrong kind. He recognizes the coming of blight, rust, mildew, and the various parasitic diseases, by these changes, before the diseases are fully developed.

"These are familiar examples, and should prompt to diligent study on our part. For, if in the vegetable world, disease may be recognized in changes of color, should it not be a means of diagnosis in animals and man? And if so definite in determining the kind of disease in vegetable life, will it not be equally definite in determining the kind of disease in vegetable life, will it not be equally definite in determining disease in man? It will be noticed further that color has reference to the *life;* to the life of the blood, to the nutrition of tissue, to the oxygenation and decarbonization of the blood, and to the waste and excretion.

"Even here the popular expression should have stimulated professional inquiry—he has a healthy color—what is the color of health? He has a sickly appearance, what is a sickly color? If the popular mind recognizes health in color, is it not well that we should make a careful study of it?

"Color in man has two sources—from the blood; from pigment—and it is well to distinguish these. In the first case the changes of color are referred to wrong of the blood; in the second they are referred to changes in the quality of character of the pigmentary matter of the body...

"In making examinations with reference to the blood, we select parts where the circulation is free and the epidermis or epithelium is thin—where the skin is thin, and the mucous membranes delicate. We examine the nails, the lips, the cheeks, the hands, sometimes the feet, the tongue, and mucous membranes of the mouth.

"What is the color of health as shown from the blood? It is rosy, a light shade of carmine and lake, and is clear, transparent, and offers no darkness, or admixture with blue, purple or brown. As the finger is pressed upon the surface, or pressed over it, toward the heart, the rosy color is removed, leaving the structures clear and transparent, and the color comes back quickly when the pressure ceases. If is difficult to describe color in words, but if the reader will now make his examination of health he may readily learn to distinguish the color of health.

"The shade of rose color in mucous membranes differs somewhat from the skin, because it is modified to some extent by the pigment of the rete-mucosum. It is well to get a clear idea of it by examinations of the lips, the tongue, the mucous membranes of the mouth, and fauces. The color of mucous membranes is quite changeable to a slight degree, even in health, having shades of blue, violet, white, probably from the secretions in the mouth, and the food and drink; and we never regard these slight variation as diagnostic.

"The pigment color of health varies in different races and in different individuals. But if we say it is somewhat transparent and clean, we may express its character for all races...

"In studying color, especially that given by the presence of blood, it is well to note that it may be changed in quality (so to speak), and in kind. Change in quantity has reference in increased circulation, and an increased amount of blood in the capillaries; change in kind, to the condition of the blood.

"Simple *excess* may be noticed from any cause increasing the circulation to the surface, or to a part. We observe this excess of color in slight acute disease, where the activity of the heart is increased, and there is general vascular excitement...

"If a part of the surface shows this excess, we at once think of its relations to internal organs and functions. If of the upper portion of the face and eyes, we refer to wrong to the brain. If of the cheeks, one or both, we refer to the respiratory organs or apparatus of circulation. If of the mouth and lower part of the face, we refer to the abdominal viscera...

"We not only find an excess, as above named, but in other cases a defect in color, showing poor blood ... or an impaired circulation to the surface. The pallor of anemia is shown in all parts of the body, and is associated with evidence of impaired nutrition ... In deficient circulation to the surface, we have want of color, but no evidence of want of blood in totality, or impaired nutrition."

Scudder on the "Examination of the Tongue"

"'Let me see your tongue,' says the doctor at every visit, what he expects to learn from 'seeing the tongue' he would be puzzled to tell you, unless it was that the patient was 'bilious.' Of course habitually seeing the tongue in disease will, unconsciously, many times, grown some knowledge of it diagnostic value, and if the physician is a close observer, it will give him valuable aid in determining the character of disease. But many men are so little in the habit of using their eyes, and thinking for themselves, that they learn but very *little.*

"If we think for a moment, we will see that the tongue may tell us of—a) the condition of the digestive apparatus; b) the condition of the blood; c) the condition of the nervous system; and d) of the functions of nutrition and excretion. As these are important inquiries, indeed just the things we want to know, we will make the tongue talk as plainly as possible.

"We find the expression of disease in—a) its form; b) its condition of dryness or moisture; c) its coating; d) its color; and e) its motion. It is well to think of the subject in this methodical way, even though we are not able to follow it wholly in this study.

"The common idea of physicians is, that the tongue expresses the condition of the stomach and intestinal tract, and it should be examined with reference to this; few think that it may give further information. Being a part of the digestive tract, supplied by the same nerves, and invested the same mucous membrane, we would naturally expect it to show something of the condition of parts below.

"If we say that its condition may be taken as the type of condition of the parts below, we will not be far out of the way. True, there are many exceptions, but the rule is a very good one, and will hardly lead to serious error. The mind at once recognizes the changes of form, movement, condition, color and secretions, as expressions of local disease. It will not be far wrong, if it recognizes them as expressions of disease of the entire digestive apparatus.

"*Change of form* is quite expressive, and rarely leads us into error. The *elongated* and *pointed* tongue expresses the condition of irritation and determination of blood to stomach and intestinal canal very distinctly, and it is safe practice to give it full weight and be very careful in the administration of remedies. As it is associated with excitation of the nerve centers, this is to be taken into consideration, when we value the evidence with reference to the stomach and bowels...

"The *full* tongue, broad and thick, is the evidence of atony of the digestive tract, especially of the mucous membranes...

"The *pinched, shrunken* tongue expresses a want of functional activity in the digestive tract. It is the tongue of an advanced acute disease, and is usually associated with dryness. 'Want of functional activity' hardly expresses the condition, for the life of the digestive apparatus has suffered to such and extent that there can be but little function...

"The *fissured* tongue in chronic disease points us to lesion of the kidneys inflammatory in character. In some cases, the fissures are transverse only, but in severe cases they are somewhat irregular, and by pressing the tongue down it is seen to separate in irregular patches of prominent villi. The symptom is so definite, that one can be assured of inflammation when this tongue presents.

"The conditions of *dryness* and *moisture* are important evidences of the condition of the intestinal tract. If the tongue is dry, we are sure the stomach and intestinal canal can do but little digestive work, and give it as much rest as possible ... If the tongue is dry we are confident that there is want of secretion from the intestinal canal and associate glands, and indeed that there is a condition present which will prevent the action of direct remedies to favor secretion ... Moisture, on the contrary, expresses a condition favorable to functional activity. True, there may be impairment of function, as when the tongue is full, showing atony, or heavily coated, showing increased mucous secretion, or dirty, showing depravation of the blood and secretions.

"If in acute diseases with dryness of the tongue, we observe it becoming moist, we are confident of improvement, of the establishment of secretion, and indeed of all vegetative processes. Having this meaning, it is nearly always regarded as a favorable symptom.

802

"The coating of the tongue are observed with care, as they are thought to be especially symptomatic of the condition of the digestive tract and the liver...

"The vivid *whiteness* of the tongue, evidently a change in the epithelium, evidences simple functional wrong, and is associated with the febrile state. If observed at other times, it may be taken as an indication that the stomach and digestive tract want rest.

"The *fur* which has consistence is evidently upon the tongue and can be scraped off—evidences impairment of function and the wrong is generally in proportion to its thickness. If uniformly distributed it may be regarded as having reference to the entire intestinal tract; if restricted principally to the base, we think of greater wrong of the stomach. The heavily loaded tongue would call our attention to accumulations in the bowels, and would prompt the means (mild) to secure their evacuation...

"*Yellowness* of coating is thought to arise from wrong in the hepatic function, and to point to the use of 'liver remedies...'

"The *bright redness* of the *tip* and *edges*, especially of the papillae, is evidence of irritation with determination of blood. It always suggests care in the use of remedies, rest to the stomach, and the special agents named to remove irritation...

"The *broad, pallid* tongue—marked want of color in the tongue itself—evidences the want of the alkaline elements of the body...

"The *deep red* tongue, (usually contracted and dry), evidences the want of an acid...

"From what has been said, the reader will draw the conclusion that impairment of nutrition and secretion will be indicated by a marked dryness and contraction on the one hand; or increased moisture and relaxation on the other. In the first case there is undue excitation, and if we select remedies to increase secretion or excretion, they will be of a sedative character. In the other case, there is a want of innervation, and the remedies will be those which will give stimulus and tone."

Scudder on "The Pulse"

"Among the most important of the functions of life is a normal circulation of blood, indeed it seems to serve as a basis for the performance of all other functions. Healthy life is dependent upon a regular and uniform circulation of blood, and disease must follow any considerable or continued variation in this function.

"Whilst the heart is the center and principal source of power of the circulation, every vessel does its part in aid of the movement of the blood. We have, therefore, to determine by the pulse the condition of the heart, the condition of the arteries, the condition of the capillaries, and to some extent the condition of the veins. As these movements are stimulated and co-ordinated by the sympathetic nervous system, it should also tell us of wrongs of innervation. As the movement of the blood depends, to a certain extent, upon its organization and condition, it may also determine for us something of the wrongs of this fluid.

"We will probably study the pulse to better advantage if we analyze it, and think of its elements separately. Put your finger on the radial artery and carefully observe the movement. It first divides itself into: a) a dilation of the artery and b) a succeeding contraction. The wave of blood forced forward by contraction of the ventricles, gives us the arterial dilation, whilst the contraction of the artery may represent the subsequent filling of the ventricles from the arteries.

"With regard to *frequency of pulse* we are in the habit of saying—as is the frequency so is the impairment of all vegetative functions—of the appetite, digestion, blood-making, nutrition, excretions from skin, kidneys and bowels—wrongs of the blood, the activity of zymotic poisons, etc. There may be exceptions to this general rule, but it is so constant that we find it important to act upon it in every case of disease. Given, frequency of pulse, the questions at once suggested are—What is the cause? What is the remedy?

"Frequency of pulse is associated with frequent respiration. The proportion is usually five beats of the pulse to one respiration. Thus an adult man in the sitting position will make thirteen to fifteen respirations each minute, and the proportionate pulse will be sixty-five to seventy-five beats per minute. The relations of the frequent respiration to various wrongs of function will be known to the reader, and evidently a slower respiration is something to be desired in all cases of disease, and something that must be obtained in some cases if the patient recovers health...

"But frequency is only one of the wrongs of the circulation, and but a part of the information we should obtain from the pulse. Frequency has reference to the rapidity of the blood-waves—the number that passes under our finger in one minute. In addition to this we have to notice that there are peculiarities in the blood-wave, and in the cufrent after this wave has passed. The pulse has volume—referring to the size of the artery. It has varying impulses in the wave of the blood, and also in the interval between the waves.

"Volume, or increased size of the artery may have reference to the amount of blood, it its increased circulation, or to some obstruction to its free movement. We will have a large pulse in the plethoric, we may expect a small one in the anemic, and these conditions will be determined by other evidences. If the artery is large, and the person is not plethoric, we ask the question—is it dependent upon a more rapid movement of the mass of the blood, especially to the surface, or is it dependent upon an obstruction to the surface, or is it dependent upon an obstruction to its movement through the capillaries? Freedom in the pulse-wave indicates the one, and a want of freedom—oppression—indicates the other condition.

"The *sharp* impulse of the wave of blood, as it strikes the finger, may be referred to lesions of the nerve centers, especially the sympathetic. The wrong is of irritation, and calls for remedies that relieve it. If the impulse is sharp, the wave short, and the inter-current vibratile, the irritation is extreme...

"The *oppressed* pulse is marked by a want of power in the stroke, and more especially by a feeling as if the current in advance of the wave broke its force. Evidently the blood-wave does not measure the amount of blood passing through the artery. It refers us to obstruction in the capillary vessels or possibly an impairment of the large vessels as well, or a wrong in the blood unfitting it for circulation.

"If the finger is carefully trained it will notice a variation in the surface of the wave, as well as in its length. Many times it is distinctly felt as two waves—a first sudden and short, and a second full, even and prolonged. The first may be called the *shock-wave,* and the second the *systolic-wave* which represents the movement of the blood from the heart.

"The shock-wave *sharp* and *pronounced* may always be referred to undue excitation of the nerves distributed upon the vessels and an undue contraction or tension of their walls.

"The *full, strong* systolic-wave may be referred to excitation of the heart and strength of its movements.

"The *short* systolic-wave evidences a want of cardiac power, and especially of impaired innervation from the spinal cord and the sympathetic.

"The inter-wave current sometimes gives valuable information, and it is well for the reader to observe it carefully in health and learn its normal condition. We find in disease that it has more or less volume, has more or less strength, and has more or less of the vibratile quality.

"When we speak of a *full* pulse, we have reference to the inter-wave current as well as to the wave, and the condition of sthenia will be determined by this. It is strong life in a state of excitation.

"If now we add *hardness,* we have added an especially lesion of innervation, of excitation steadily maintained.

"If we speak of a *small* pulse *hard,* we refer it to impairment of life from activity, still maintained.

"If we speak of a *small* pulse *soft* and easily compressed, we refer it to deficient innervation.

"If we have a *small* pulse *vibratile,* we say it is the expression of impaired life, with great excitation of the nerve centers.

"If we have an empty pulse, the inter-wave current hardly perceptible, it is the evidence of impaired life with enfeebled innervation from the sympathetic.

"There are other changes of the pulse which might be noticed, but they are difficult to describe and learn. I do not think that we can tell every lesion by it, as Chinese doctors believe, but to the educated touch it gives most valuable information with regard to the most important functions of life. I doubt not many physicians can locate lesions with very great certainty from it alone; that they can distinguish lesions of the brain, lungs, digestive apparatus, urinary apparatus, etc., and determine, to some extent, their character.

"But in the practice of medicine, there is something of more importance than locating a disease, or even determining the character of the lesion. The important object is to associate the evidence of disease with remedies for their cure, and to make the expressions of the disease point to the medicine:

"The *full* pulse with *strength* means medicine—Veraturm. Whether full and hard, full and bounding, the special sedative named is at once suggested...

"The *full* pulse *doughy* (lacks the marked vibration) means Lobelia; or if marked and associated with fullness of mucous membranes and purplish discoloration, Batisia...

"The *full* pulse *open,* is kindly influenced by Podophyllum...

"The *full* pulse *vibratile* calls for Gelsemium, usually associated with Veratrum.

"The *full* pulse *oppressed* calls for Belladonna, alternated with Veratrum...

"The *small* pulse usually means Aconite.

"The *small* pulse *vibratile* Aconite and Gelsemium.

"The *small* pulse *oppressed* Belladonna and Aconite.

"The *small, soft,* easily compressed pulse, Aconite...

"The *small* pulse, *frequent,* easily compressed, the wave of blood giving the sense of squareness as it passes under the finger, Opium.

"Want of power in the impulse suggests Digitalis, Capsicum.

"The *sharp stroke* of the pulse with tremulous wave between strokes means Rhus."

Scudder on "Temperature"

"Among the evidences of disease, none are more definite and important than changes in temperature. Heat is not only force in the animal body, but it is also a condition of life; a man has activity through it, and he has life by it. The theory of Samuel Thomson—'Heat is life, cold is death,' was very simple, and had much of truth in it—it was just one-third of the truth. Cold is death, but so is too high a temperature, and an unequal distribution of heat.

"The human body maintains its healthy functions at a temperature varying from 98° to 98.5°. This is a condition absolute for health. If the temperature varies from this above or below, disease must result. We may state the proposition in a different form—no disease can exist without changing the temperature of the body, either raising it, depressing it, or rendering it unequal. Thus, change of temperature becomes an absolute evidence of disease, though it may not point out the character or location of the lesion."

Scudder on "Diagnosis by the Ear"

"The ear may not be as important in diagnosis as the eye or touch, yet we purpose employing it to its fullest capacity. To the routine physician who asks questions and depends for his knowledge of disease upon what the patient tells him, it is the organ of greatest importance. But we have already seen that we do best when we study disease with our senses, and depend but little upon what the patient says.

If the reader will refer back to our study of facial expression, he will notice the statement that wrongs of life find expression through the usual channels of expression; where the nerve currents have been most in the habit of flowing in health, they incline to flow in disease. Mankind use the facial muscles to express their feelings or sensations, and hence disease is expressed in the face. For the same reason we should expect to find wrongs of life expressed in the voice, in all animals using the voice, and especially in man who finds it a principal instrument of expression.

812

"As we come into the sick room we give attention to the voice of the sick persons, quite as much as we do to what he is saying. We find that it expresses strength and weakness, is free or difficult from local disease, and shadows forth the condition of the brain in its tone, which varies from the listlessness of atony to the querulousness of excited feebleness, and the excitation of over-activity.

"In studying the voice as the expression of disease, we recognize its three-fold bearing as it refers us to a general impairment of life, a lesion of the brain, and to lesions of the respiratory apparatus. If we did not keep these sources of wrong in view we might make serious mistakes. IF, for instance, we have feebleness of voice, it may be due to general impairment of the brain, to deficient innervation from the spinal cord, or to a lesion of the respiratory apparatus.

"Whilst strength of voice is usually regarded as evidence of good vital power, and a good respiratory apparatus, it will not do to place too much dependence upon it in these regards. It certainly evidences good innervation from the brain to the spinal cord. But if these nerve centers are sound, active and well supplied with blood, we may have a strong voice, even though the body at large is nearly exhausted. Usually it is a favorable symptom.

"Feebleness, on the contrary, evidences a lesion of atony, either of the body at large, of the brain or mind, of the spinal cord, or of the respiratory apparatus...

"It is difficult to give a name to the peculiar expression of voice associated with nervous irritation and vascular excitement, yet the reader will learn to recognize it readily, and may frequently be able to determine these characters of disease by simply hearing the patient speak. There is a sharpness, and want of smoothness, representing pretty accurately in degree the amount of disease...

"The oppressed voice, hollow and unsteady, evidences a general impairment of life...

"Sharpness of voice suggests nervous excitation and will sometimes point to the remedy, as in the peculiar sharp accentuation of the Rhus voice...

"The voice is the function of the larynx, and its changes will point us to disease of this organ. The croupous cry and voice is quite as distinctive as the croupous cough. If it evidences moisture, we have mucous croup; if it is dry and metallic, pseudo-membraneous croup; if variable in tone and character, spasmodic croup.

"In chronic disease of the larynx, roughness of the voice is one of the first symptoms. As the disease progresses, we have various changes in the voice and difficult use of it, as characteristic symptoms.

"In chronic bronchitis we also find change, but not similar in kind. It may give the voice shrillness, as in irritative bronchitis, or dullness, hollowness or reverberation, as in asthenic bronchitis."

Scudder on "Diagnosis by the Sense of Smell"

"The sense of smell has less development in the majority of men than any other of the senses—as some writer has remarked—'it is yet in the savage state.' It may not be of much use in diagnosis, and yet the little it may tell us we want to know. It requires education, as do the others, and we must learn to distinguish pleasant odors from stinks, and thus be able to analyze stinks, and determine their influence on the human body. It is possible that some persons will never be able to recognize the genus 'stink,' much less be able to assort them for our present purpose.

"It is well for the physician to commence educating his nose at home, and to start with a realization of the fact that all unpleasant smells are noxious to the human body. It requires very little exercise of reason to reach this conclusion, for if the thing was not unpleasant or noxious to the economy, the nose would not give the warning of unpleasantness. What is the evidence of disease to the person suffering? Unpleasantness; the very expression used, 'person suffering' tells the story of disease. Is disease ever pleasant? No. Are causes of disease ever pleasant? No. Do causes of disease ever pleasantly impress the senses? You might answer yes, but I say no again."

Scudder on "Information from Patient and Nurse" (Case Taking Questions and Answers)

"We neglect no source of information with reference to the origin, condition, or progress of disease, and whilst careful not to be guided by information from nurse, friends and patient, we wish to give it its true value. Attention has already been called to many sources of error. To a want of knowledge and care in observation on the part of nurse and friends, as well as their prejudices and tendency to distortion. To the want of knowledge on the part of the patient, want of language for description, and the impairment of his powers of sensation and reason from disease.

"The elements of uncertainty are thus very great, and we have to pursue our inquiries with much care. Questions should never be suggestive, but should be so put as to let nurse or patient tell you what they know, or to require but the simple and direct answer, yes or no. Careful attention to these points and continued guard upon the tongue, will soon form a habit of examination that will lessen the danger of erroneous information.

"We prefer to get information from attendants with regard to the general condition of the sick, and the performance of the essential functions of life. From the patient we desire to know his sensations, as these are changed by disease.

"A first examination may take the following course: How long sick? What are the seeming causes of the sickness? How did it commmence? What has been noticed with reference to the progress of disease up to the present time? How does the patient rest in the daytime? At night? What food and drink does he take? How often does he have a motion of the bowels? How does he pass urine? These questions may seem suggestive, and once in a while they may take a simpler form as—Does he sleep? Does he eat? Does he drink?

"It is most absurd for the attendant to attempt a description of the sensations of the sick, and yet they almost always volunteer to do it. Many times they will be continuously making suggestions to the patient, and lead him into erroneous statements. They will probably have formed some theory of the disease, will bend everything to the support of their theory. Physicians are very frequently guilty of this, and should try to get rid of the bad habit which they condemn in nurses.

"The question—How do you feel? Elicits a loose, wandering description of the patient's sensations, and is only important in that it suggests special questions and examinations. The question—Where do you feel it? Is pertinent, and will elicit valuable information of local disease. It does not do to take if for granted that the patient's anatomical or physiological knowledge is perfect, and that his reference to heart, lungs, stomach, liver. The directions at once follows—put your hand on the place. It is a little singular to find after a patient has located a disease in his own mind, the hand meanders about with uncertainty, trying to find its location. If the unpleasantness is marked, and means local disease, the patient has no difficulty in placing his hand upon the exact spot.

If there is anything uncertain in the patient's manner or method, and especially if uneducated, we wish him to describe his sensations, with the hand upon the affected part. In many cases we will find that the description commences to wander as soon as the hand is removed. There is a reason for this; with hand upon the part, the mind is directed to it and concentrated, extraneous ideas are rejected, and the description is of actual sensations."

About the Author

Vinton McCabe is an author and educator. In his more than fifteen years as president of the Connecticut Homeopathic Association, he taught the philosophy and practice of homeopathic medicine to thousands of laypersons and medical professionals alike. He also developed educational materials into a number of published books, including *Practical Homeopathy* and *Homeopathy, Healing, and You.*

Back Cover Material

Household Homeopathy

A Safe and Effective Approach to Wellness for the Whole Family

Homeopathy is an alternative medical practice that treats a health condition by administering minute doses of a remedy that would produce symptoms of that condition in a healthy person. Homeopathy is the full expression of holistic medicine, one that sees all people as whole beings in body, mind, and spirit, in whom all symptoms must then be both interconnected and interrelated. As a specific form of medical treatment, homeopathy dates back just over 200 years, but the underlying principles of homeopathy go back to the time of Hippocrates.

Those who wish to gain a practical understanding of homeopathy know that study and dedication are required. This book makes the subject of homeopathy as down to earth and as practical as it can be and provides food for thought. It discusses the most common homeopathic remedies—such as Arnica, Hypericum, Calendula, Aconite, and many others—and how they can be used most safely and effectively. *Household Homeopathy* teaches you how to promote healing in yourself and your loved ones in your own home. It covers the importance of how to handle the remedies, how to select them, and how to use them wisely.

From short-term solutions to long-term fixes, virtually every common health condition—from headaches and sore throats to digestive ailments and motion sickness—can benefit from the homeopathic approach to wellness. There will be no need to turn to unnecessary and potentially harmful medications to relieve everyday health complaints. This will also mean fewer trips to the doctor's office and reduced medical expenses. Armed with the information in this book and the will to fully understand homeopathic treatments, anyone can take control of their well-being and that of their loved ones safely and effectively.

ABOUT THE AUTHOR

Vinton McCabe is both an author and an educator. In his more than fifteen years as president of the Connecticut Homeopathic Association, he taught the philosophy and practice of homeopathic medicine to thousands of laypersons and medical professionals alike. He also developed educational materials into a number of published books, including *Practical Homeopathy* and *Homeopathy, Healing,* and *You.*

Nosebleeds,
Nux Vomica,

5131
O'Reilly, Wenda
Brewster,
Onions,
Opium,
Organon of Medicine,
Overeating,

5132
Pain,
Palpitations,
Panic attacks,
Parasites,
Patient, Not the Cure, The,
Patients,
　answers,
　improvement of,
　physical traits,
Pattern discrimination,
Petroleum,
Phosphoric Acid,
Phosphorus,
Phytolacca,
Pien, Cueh,
Plantago,
Podophyllum,
Poison ivy,

Polypharmacy,
Potency,
Predisposition,
Pregnancy,
Premenstrual syndrome (PMS),
Psora,
Psoric,
Pulsatilla,
Pulse,
　diagnostic tool in homeopathy,
　diagnostic tool in TCM,
　fast,
　hard,
　intermittent,
　irregular,
　slow,
　soft,

5134
Radiation,
Rage,
　See Anger,
Reactions,
Reflexology,
Remedies,
　care of,
　creation of,
　giving and taking,

Sprains,
Stage fright,
Staphysagria,
Stings,
Stitches,
Strains,
Stramonium,
Strokes,
Styes,
Sulphur,
Sunburns,
Surgery,
Sweating,
Symphytum,
Symptom modifiers,
    duration and onset,
    location,
    modalities,
    sensation,
Symptoms,
    alternating,
    chief complaint,
    common,
    concomitant,
    determining,
    disappearance of,
    equal and opposite,
    functional,
    general,
    improvement of,
    in case taking,

keynote,
lack of improvement
of,
mental,
modifying,
objective,
specific,
subjective,
totality of,
types,
unchanged,
worsening,

5136
Tabacum,
Taste,
TCM,
    case taking,
    diagnostic tools in,
    face color as
    diagnostic tool in,
    generalization,
    pulse as diagnostic
    tool in,
    tongue as diagnostic
    tool in,
    twelve pulses,
Teething,
Temperature,
Tendons,
Three laws of cure,

infected,
lacerated,
Wry neck,
  See Torticollis,
Wyethia,

5140
X-scale of potency,

5141
Yellow Emperor,
Yin and yang,

5142
Zinc,

Books For ALL Kinds of Readers

At ReadHowYouWant we understand that one size does not fit all types of readers. Our innovative, patent pending technology allows us to design new formats to make reading easier and more enjoyable for you. This helps improve your speed of reading and your comprehension. Our EasyRead printed books have been optimized to improve word recognition, ease eye tracking by adjusting word and line spacing as well as minimizing hyphenation. Our EasyRead SuperLarge editions have been developed to make reading easier and more accessible for vision-impaired readers. We offer Braille and DAISY formats of our books and all popular E-Book formats.

We are continually introducing new formats based upon research and reader preferences. Visit our web-site to see all of our formats and learn how you can Personalize our books for yourself or as gifts. Sign up to Become A (RHYW) Registered Reader.

www.readhowyouwant.com

4/15 (4) 11/14